Teen Health Series

Eating Disorders Information
For Teens, Third Edition

Eating Disorders Information For Teens, Third Edition

Health Tips About Anorexia, Bulimia, Binge Eating, And Body Image Disorders

Including Information About Risk Factors, Prevention, Diagnosis, Treatment, Health Consequences, And Other Related Issues

Edited by Elizabeth Bellenir

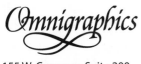

Omnigraphics

155 W. Congress, Suite 200
Detroit, MI 48226

Bibliographic Note

Because this page cannot legibly accommodate all the copyright notices, the Bibliographic Note portion of the Preface constitutes an extension of the copyright notice.

Edited by Elizabeth Bellenir

Teen Health Series

Karen Bellenir, *Managing Editor*
David A. Cooke, M.D., *Medical Consultant*
Elizabeth Collins, *Research and Permissions Coordinator*
Cherry Edwards, *Permissions Assistant*
EdIndex, *Services for Publishers, Indexers*

* * *

Omnigraphics, Inc.
Matthew P. Barbour, *Senior Vice President*
Kevin M. Hayes, *Operations Manager*

* * *

Peter E. Ruffner, *Publisher*
Copyright © 2013 Omnigraphics, Inc.
ISBN 978-0-7808-1269-7
E-ISBN 978-0-7808-1270-3

Library of Congress Cataloging-in-Publication Data

Eating disorders information for teens : health tips about anorexia, bulimia, binge eating, and body image disorders, including information about risk factors, prevention, diagnosis, treatment, health consequences, and other related issues / edited by Elizabeth Bellenir. -- Third edition.
     pages cm. -- (Teen health series)
 Audience: Grade 9 to 12.
 Includes bibliographical references and index.
 Summary: "Provides basic consumer health information for teens about causes, prevention, and treatment of eating disorders, along with healthy eating tips. Includes index, resource information and recommendations for further reading" --Provided by publisher.
 ISBN 978-0-7808-1269-7 (hardcover : alk. paper) 1. Eating disorders--Juvenile literature. 2. Eating disorders in adolescence--Juvenile literature. I. Bellenir, Elizabeth.
 RC552.E18E2836 2013
 616.85'2600835--dc23
                                                                                    2012036612

Table of Contents

Preface

Part One: Eating Disorders And Their Risk Factors

Chapter 1—Facts About Eating Disorders...3

Chapter 2—Identifying Healthy Eating Patterns.............................9

Chapter 3—Causes And Risk Factors For Eating Disorders 17

Chapter 4—Eating Disorders—Not Just A Women's Issue 25

Chapter 5—Eating Disorders In Female Athletes 29

Chapter 6—Negative Body Image May Contribute
To Eating Disorders... 37

Chapter 7—Genetics And The Impact Of Culture
On Eating Disorders 41

Chapter 8—Media And Eating Disorders.. 47

Chapter 9—Eating Disorder Statistics... 59

**Part Two: Understanding Eating Disorders And Body Image
Disorders**

Chapter 10—Anorexia Nervosa... 65

Chapter 11—Bulimia Nervosa.. 71

Chapter 12—Binge Eating Disorder.. 77

Chapter 13—Emotional Eating... 83

Chapter 14—Night Eating And Sleep Eating Syndromes 89

Chapter 15—Orthorexia... 93

Chapter 16—Eating Disorders Not Otherwise
Specified (EDNOS)... 97

Chapter 17—Pica 101

Chapter 18—Substances Abused In Eating Disorders 105

Chapter 19—Compulsive Exercise 109

Chapter 20—Female Athlete Triad 113

Chapter 21—Body Dysmorphic Disorder And Bigorexia 119

Part Three: Medical Consequences And Co-Occurring Concerns

Chapter 22—Complications Of Eating Disorders.............................. 127

Chapter 23—Obesity And Its Consequences 135

Chapter 24—Oral Health Consequences Of Eating Disorders 151

Chapter 25—The Link Between Osteoporosis And Anorexia 155

Chapter 26—Eating Disorders Impact Fertility
And Pregnancy.. 159

Chapter 27—The Impact Of Other Conditions On Eating
Disorder Symptoms And Treatment............................ 163

Chapter 28—Diabetes And Eating Disorders 167

Chapter 29—Depression, Anxiety, And Eating Disorders 171

Chapter 30—Self-Injury Linked To Eating Disorders........................ 183

Chapter 31—Unresolved Trauma And Eating Disorders 187

Part Four: Diagnosing And Treating Eating Disorders

Chapter 32—Signs And Symptoms Of Eating Disorders................ 193

Chapter 33—Eating Disorders Self-Assessment Test 197

Chapter 34—When You Suspect Someone You Know
Has An Eating Disorder 205

Chapter 35—Diagnosing Eating Disorders 209

Chapter 36—Treating Eating Disorders 213

Chapter 37—Medications And Therapies For
Eating Disorders 219

Chapter 38—Improving Your Body Image And
Self-Esteem... 229

Chapter 39—Re-Establishing Normal Eating....................................237

Chapter 40—Eating Disorders Relapse And Relapse
      Prevention 241

Part Five: Maintaining Healthy Eating And Fitness Habits

Chapter 41—Identifying The Right Weight For Your Height.........247

Chapter 42—What Should You Really Eat?....................................253

Chapter 43—Eat The Right Amount Of Calories For You...............265

Chapter 44—Use Food Labels To Help You Make
      Healthier Choices 279

Chapter 45—Healthy Eating For Vegetarians...............................283

Chapter 46—Healthy Eating For Athletes.....................................287

Chapter 47—Healthy Eating And Weight Management 295

Chapter 48—How To Choose A Safe Weight-Loss Program.........317

Chapter 49—Physical Fitness For Teens..321

Chapter 50—Fitness Safety Tips 329

Chapter 51—Mental Fitness 333

Chapter 52—Developing Resilience..341

Part Six: If You Need More Information

Chapter 53—For More Information About Eating Disorders........349

Chapter 54—For More Information About Nutrition And
      Weight Management..353

Chapter 55—For More Information About Physical And
      Mental Fitness 357

Index...365

Preface

About This Book

For many people, watching what they eat and exercising are important components of healthy lifestyles. For others, however, these concerns become extreme. Some people develop serious disruptions in eating patterns, become fixated on food worries, and experience severe distress about body weight and shape. These obsessions are characteristic of eating disorders.

According to the National Institute on Mental Health, eating disorders—including anorexia, bulimia, and binge eating—frequently first appear during adolescence or young adulthood, although they can also appear earlier in childhood or sometimes not until much later in life. Girls are more than two and a half times as likely as boys to develop an eating disorder, but the issue is not strictly a female concern and many boys are affected. Current statistics suggest that 2.7% of 12–18 year olds may have an eating disorder. Sadly, most of them do not receive treatment.

Eating Disorders Information For Teens, Third Edition discusses the differences between healthy eating patterns and anorexia nervosa, bulimia nervosa, binge eating syndrome, emotional eating, night eating syndrome, orthorexia, pica, and other eating disorders. It explains how to recognize eating disorders, how they are diagnosed, the types of treatment available, and guidelines for relapse prevention. Facts about medical consequences, co-occurring conditions, and other diseases that may be complicated by an eating disorder are also included. A special section reports on healthy weight management and exercise plans. The book concludes with directories of resources for additional information about eating disorders, nutrition, and fitness.

How To Use This Book

This book is divided into parts and chapters. Parts focus on broad areas of interest; chapters are devoted to single topics within a part.

Part One: Eating Disorders And Their Risk Factors explains differences between healthy eating patterns and eating disorders and the types of influences that can lead to disruptions in normal eating patterns. It also offers a statistical look at the prevalence of eating disorders in various segments of the population.

Part Two: Understanding Eating And Body Image Disorders provides facts about the three most common types of eating disorders: anorexia nervosa, bulimia nervosa, and binge eating disorder. It also offers information about sleep eating syndrome, pica, and other lesser-known types of eating disorders, and it discusses other related concerns, including compulsive exercise and body dysmorphic disorder.

Part Three: Medical Consequences And Co-Occurring Concerns summarizes some of the most commonly experienced physical and mental problems associated with eating disorders, including the effects of inadequate nutrition and the risks associated with obesity. It also discusses other conditions that can impact the progression and outcomes of eating disorders.

Part Four: Diagnosing And Treating Eating Disorders identifies frequently seen signs and symptoms of eating disorders, and it provides a self-assessment questionnaire readers can use to better understand whether they need to be evaluated by a healthcare professional for the potential presence of an eating disorder. Information is also included about dietary and mental health treatments, medications, and relapse prevention.

Part Five: Maintaining Healthy Eating And Fitness Habits offers tips for achieving good dietary habits, mental wellness, and physical fitness. It provides suggestions for identifying an appropriate target weight, a sufficient number of daily calories, and an adequate intake of important nutrients.

Part Six: If You Need More Information offers directories of resources for more information about eating disorders, nutrition, weight management, and physical and mental fitness.

Bibliographic Note

This volume contains documents and excerpts from publications issued by the following government agencies: Centers for Disease Control and Prevention (CDC); National Heart Lung and Blood Institute; National Institute of Arthritis and Musculoskeletal and Skin Diseases; National Institute of Diabetes and Digestive and Kidney Diseases; National Institute of Environmental Health Sciences; National Institute of Mental Health; National Library of Medicine; Office on Women's Health; President's Council on Fitness, Sports, and Nutrition; U.S. Department of Agriculture (USDA); U.S. Department of Health and Human Services; and the U.S. Food and Drug Administration (FDA).

In addition, this volume contains copyrighted documents and articles produced by the following individuals and organizations: A.D.A.M., Inc.; Academy for Eating Disorders; Alliance for Eating Disorders Awareness; American Pregnancy Association; American

Psychological Association; Binge Eating Disorder Association; Canadian Mental Health Association; Centre for Clinical Interventions; Children's Hospital of Colorado; Colorado Department of Public Health and Environment; Cornell Research Program on Self-Injurious Behavior in Adolescents and Young Adults; Families Empowered and Supporting Treatment of Eating Disorders; David M. Garner, Ph.D.; LifeMed Media, Inc.; Mirror Mirror; National Association of Anorexia Nervosa and Associated Disorders; National Centre for Eating Disorders; National Eating Disorder Information Centre; National Eating Disorders Association; Nemours Foundation; Northwestern University; PsychCentral; Rector and Visitors of the University of Virginia; Remuda Ranch; River Centre Clinic; SportsMD Media, Inc.; and the Stanford School of Medicine.

The photograph on the front cover is © Image Source Photography/Veer.

Full citation information is provided on the first page of each chapter. Every effort has been made to secure all necessary rights to reprint the copyrighted material. If any omissions have been made, please contact Omnigraphics to make corrections for future editions.

Acknowledgements

In addition to the organizations listed above, special thanks are due to Liz Collins, research and permissions coordinator; Karen Bellenir, managing editor; Lisa Bakewell, verification assistant; and WhimsyInk, prepress services provider.

About The *Teen Health Series*

At the request of librarians serving today's young adults, the *Teen Health Series* was developed as a specially focused set of volumes within Omnigraphics' *Health Reference Series*. Each volume deals comprehensively with a topic selected according to the needs and interests of people in middle school and high school.

Teens seeking preventive guidance, information about disease warning signs, medical statistics, and risk factors for health problems will find answers to their questions in the *Teen Health Series*. The *Series*, however, is not intended to serve as a tool for diagnosing illness, in prescribing treatments, or as a substitute for the physician/patient relationship. All people concerned about medical symptoms or the possibility of disease are encouraged to seek professional care from an appropriate health care provider.

If there is a topic you would like to see addressed in a future volume of the *Teen Health Series*, please write to:

Editor

Teen Health Series

Omnigraphics, Inc.

155 W. Congress, Suite 200

Detroit, MI 48226

A Note About Spelling And Style

Teen Health Series editors use *Stedman's Medical Dictionary* as an authority for questions related to the spelling of medical terms and the *Chicago Manual of Style* for questions related to grammatical structures, punctuation, and other editorial concerns. Consistent adherence is not always possible, however, because the individual volumes within the *Series* include many documents from a wide variety of different producers and copyright holders, and the editor's primary goal is to present material from each source as accurately as is possible following the terms specified by each document's producer. This sometimes means that information in different chapters or sections may follow other guidelines and alternate spelling authorities. For example, occasionally a copyright holder may require that eponymous terms be shown in possessive forms (Crohn's disease *vs.* Crohn disease) or that British spelling norms be retained (leukaemia *vs.* leukemia).

Locating Information Within The *Teen Health Series*

The *Teen Health Series* contains a wealth of information about a wide variety of medical topics. As the *Series* continues to grow in size and scope, locating the precise information needed by a specific student may become more challenging. To address this concern, information about books within the *Teen Health Series* is included in *A Contents Guide to the Health Reference Series*. The *Contents Guide* presents an extensive list of more than 16,000 diseases, treatments, and other topics of general interest compiled from the Tables of Contents and major index headings from the books of the *Teen Health Series* and *Health Reference Series*. To access *A Contents Guide to the Health Reference Series*, visit www.healthreferenceseries.com.

Our Advisory Board

We would like to thank the following advisory board members for providing guidance to the development of this *Series*:

Dr. Lynda Baker, Associate Professor of Library and Information Science, Wayne State University, Detroit, MI

Nancy Bulgarelli, William Beaumont Hospital Library, Royal Oak, MI

Karen Imarisio, Bloomfield Township Public Library, Bloomfield Township, MI

Karen Morgan, Mardigian Library, University of Michigan-Dearborn, Dearborn, MI

Rosemary Orlando, St. Clair Shores Public Library, St. Clair Shores, MI

Medical Consultant

Medical consultation services are provided to the *Teen Health Series* editors by David A. Cooke, M.D. Dr. Cooke is a graduate of Brandeis University, and he received his M.D. degree from the University of Michigan. He completed residency training at the University of Wisconsin Hospital and Clinics. He is board-certified in internal medicine. Dr. Cooke currently works as part of the University of Michigan Health System and practices in Ann Arbor, MI. In his free time, he enjoys writing, science fiction, and spending time with his family.

Part One
Eating Disorders
And Their Risk Factors

Chapter 1

Facts About Eating Disorders

What is an eating disorder?

Eating disorders take several forms: anorexia nervosa, bulimia nervosa, and an atypical eating disorder "not otherwise specified." An eating disorder arises when a person develops a distorted relationship with food and weight, but it involves much more than simple dieting, exercise, or feeling too full.

Both anorexia and bulimia are about eight times more common in females than in males. Young people often work hard to keep their struggles with food secret, so it's hard to know just how many people suffer from eating disorders. Between 1–13% of American high school and college-age women are estimated to be anorexic or bulimic.

Eating disorders often begin with dissatisfaction in appearance and efforts to "eat healthier" or exercise more. But for some people, these behaviors can lead to changes in thought patterns and behaviors that develop into an eating disorder. The thoughts and behaviors become difficult to resist, and emotional and physical health begin to deteriorate.

Sometimes the problem begins with a weight-loss diet, but then something goes wrong. Once five pounds have been lost, the weight goal is lowered another five or ten pounds. Or perhaps the original goal is never quite reached, and instead the teenager's weight goes up and down in a seesaw pattern. Sometimes no actual diet is involved; the teen simply believes that they are much too fat and experiences a relentless drive to be thinner. Eventually, the pursuit of thinness becomes an obsession that assumes more importance than anything else in the person's life.

About This Chapter: "Facts about Eating Disorders, including Anorexia and Bulimia," © 2012 Children's Hospital Colorado (www.childrenscolorado.org). All rights reserved. Reprinted with permission. For more information about Children's Hospital Colorado, Eating Disorder Program, call 720-777-6452.

About Anorexia Nervosa: The symptoms of anorexia nervosa include severe weight loss as part of a drive to be thin, fear of weight gain, loss of menstruation in females, and body image distortion (not perceiving appearance accurately, such as the belief that one is fat, despite being very thin).

About Bulimia Nervosa: People with bulimia nervosa have episodes of binge eating at least several times a week, followed by purging through self-induced vomiting, exercise, laxatives, or fasting. This often leads to weight fluctuations—sometimes large, sometimes small.

What causes eating disorders?

Despite more than 50 years of research, the cause of eating disorders remains largely unknown. We do know that living in a culture that values thinness and promotes dieting increases the risk of kids developing an eating disorder like anorexia or bulimia. In fact, research shows that by the age of seven, many children have already decided that it isn't okay to be fat.

Genetic factors, family history, and certain personality traits, such as perfectionism, also contribute to the likelihood of an eating disorder. The pressure to be slender is especially intense for girls and young women in their teens. Two-thirds of girls between the ages of 10 and 15 have tried dieting. Cultural messages about thinness are directed almost entirely toward women, and puberty is a time when young people are confronted with a rapidly changing body.

An understanding of issues that may have contributed to the onset of dieting and exercise leading to the eating disorder is important, but normalizing eating behavior and weight remains the most important intervention. It is often difficult for the person with an eating disorder to admit that they need help. That's why it may be up to friends, family members, coaches, or teachers to guide the young person to the help they need.

How can I recognize an eating disorder in a child or teen?

Young people go to great lengths to deny and conceal their painful struggles with food. Here are some signs that may help you recognize an eating disorder in someone you know:

- Excessive weight loss. Anorexia is diagnosed when someone is 15% below expected weight (whether because of loss of weight or failure to gain with growth).

- Weight fluctuations. Although people with bulimia usually maintain near-normal body weight, their roller coaster dieting may show up in erratic weight gains and losses.

- Unusual eating habits, such as taking tiny bites to stretch out eating time or compulsively arranging food on the plate.

Binge-Eating Disorder

With binge-eating disorder a person loses control over his or her eating. Unlike bulimia nervosa, periods of binge-eating are not followed by purging, excessive exercise, or fasting. As a result, people with binge-eating disorder often are overweight or obese. People with binge-eating disorder who are obese are at higher risk for developing cardiovascular disease and high blood pressure. They also experience guilt, shame, and distress about their binge-eating, which can lead to more binge-eating.

Treatment options for binge-eating disorder are similar to those used to treat bulimia nervosa. Psychotherapy, especially cognitive behavior therapy (CBT) that is tailored to the individual, has been shown to be effective. Again, this type of therapy can be offered in an individual or group environment.

Fluoxetine and other antidepressants may reduce binge-eating episodes and help lessen depression in some patients.

Source: Excerpted from "Eating Disorders," National Institute of Mental Health (www.nimh.nih.gov), January 10, 2012.

- The person stops eating meals with the family; they might make excuses that they are too busy or eating elsewhere.
- Secretive behavior, especially with respect to eating and bathroom use. A teenager who habitually runs water, plays the radio, or flushes the toilet repeatedly while using the bathroom may be masking the sounds of vomiting.
- Use of laxatives or diet pills.
- Food disappearing on a regular basis.
- Excessive and often obsessive exercise.
- Dull hair and hair loss, splitting or softening nails.
- An absence of menstrual periods related to loss of body fat.
- Dental cavities and gum disease, caused by malnutrition and vomiting.
- Extreme sensitivity to cold, caused by loss of fat and muscle.
- Fine body hair on arms and legs. This is the body's attempt to keep warm.
- Low self-esteem.
- Distorted body image. No matter how thin they get, people with anorexia still believe they are too fat.
- Irritability, depression, or talk of suicide.

- Drug or alcohol abuse. Sometimes, teenagers with eating disorders will turn to substance abuse to relieve feelings of fear, shame, and depression.

What happens if an eating disorder isn't treated?

Without intervention, the consequences of an eating disorder can be tragic. Prolonged dieting, bingeing and purging, and weight loss can all cause severe malnutrition. Almost every organ system is affected by malnutrition, including the brain, heart, liver, kidneys, bone marrow, skin, and reproduction.

For example, the heart rate slows, increasing the risk for potentially fatal heart attacks. Brain tissue is lost, some of it permanently. Girls stop having periods, and the lack of estrogen can lead to osteoporosis (weak bones), which happens in 50% of patients with anorexia. The act of purging causes electrolytes, especially potassium, to get dangerously low, leading to potentially fatal irregular heart rhythms. And vomiting can irritate and even tear the esophagus.

The emotional complications of an eating disorder can be just as devastating as the physical problems. Relationships with family and friends often suffer as the person begins to avoid eating with others or resists efforts by others to help them. The child or teen often feels isolated and depressed. This can get to a point where the person considers suicide, which is the leading cause of death in people who suffer from eating disorders.

Eating Disorders

Eating disorders are serious behavior problems. They include anorexia nervosa, bulimia nervosa, and binge-eating:

- Anorexia nervosa, in which you become too thin, but you don't eat enough because you think you are fat
- Bulimia nervosa, involving periods of overeating followed by purging, sometimes through self-induced vomiting or using laxatives
- Binge-eating, which is out-of-control eating

Women are more likely than men to have eating disorders. They usually start in the teenage years and often occur along with depression, anxiety disorders and substance abuse.

Eating disorders can cause heart and kidney problems and even death. Getting help early is important. Treatment involves monitoring, mental health therapy, nutritional counseling, and sometimes medicines.

Source: "Eating Disorders," National Library of Medicine (www.nlm.nih.gov/medlineplus), January 4, 2012.

What can I do?

As A Friend: Don't comment on your friend's eating behavior or size. If your friend has had anorexia nervosa and gains weight, don't praise him or her for it. What your friend will hear is, "You're fat again."

Remember that you can't solve the problem. You aren't responsible for saving your friend—you can be supportive and concerned, but encourage your friend to talk to a parent, teacher, or counselor. If they don't, tell an adult close to your friend about your concerns.

What help is available?

The important thing to remember is that the person with an eating disorder needs professional help. The person is caught in a cycle of destructive behavior that they cannot break alone, even with all the willpower in the world.

If you think someone in your family may be struggling with an eating disorder, speak with his or her physician or call an eating disorders program that specializes in the treatment of children, young adults, and teenagers. Children, teens and young adults have different problems and pressures than adults, and treatment approaches should address these special concerns.

Chapter 2

Identifying Healthy Eating Patterns

Definition Of A Healthy Body Weight

Dieting Is Not Healthy Eating

Close to a third of the population is overweight, and in addition, eating disorders are on the rise especially among young women. The preoccupation of body image and the pursuit to be thin has professionals looking at weight as they affect the physical and mental health of those involved. The concept of a healthy weight emerged from the recognition that we needed to shift our attention away from only body weight and focus on healthy living in general. Healthy living involves eating well, being active, and feeling good about oneself.

A healthy body weight is a weight range appropriate for a particular height and body build. It should not be confused with a thin weight. A healthy weight is the point at which you feel: fit and flexible, healthy and energetic, and are at a lower risk for weight-related health problems. The healthiness of your weight can be measured using the Body Mass Index (BMI) calculator (available online at http://www.cdc.gov/healthyweight/assessing/bmi/index.html). The calculator uses a person's body weight in relation to their height to define normal, overweight, and obesity.

To achieve a healthy body weight, regular physical activity in combination with healthy eating promises the best hope. The type of physical activity one chooses can range from walking, riding a bike, dancing, gardening, running with your dog… but joining an expensive gym or sport club is not the only option or an excuse.

About This Chapter: "Eating Disorders Not Otherwise Specified (EDNOS)," © 2012 Binge Eating Disorder Association (www.bedaonline.com). All rights reserved. Reprinted with permission. For information about the Eating Attitudes Test (EAT-26), see Chapter 33—Eating Disorders Self-Assessment Test.

Healthy Eating Guidelines

Many people eat for emotional reasons. It is typically triggered by stress, and anxiety, too, often leads to overeating and/or making poor food choices. A study done by the *International Journal of Eating Disorders* compares the daily journals kept by a group of normal-weight women, half of whom were binge-eaters. The key influence on emotional eating, however, is not just negative or stressful events, but rather it's people's response to them. People who are less thrown off by stress tend to focus on how they want to constructively deal with a negative situation, or they simply put it aside and move on. These who tend to experience more disruption due to negative situations are more inclined to stay focused on the problem, mentally replaying a distressing situation over and over again.

Those whose healthy-eating goals are often disrupted by emotions can benefit from finding new strategies to help them respond more effectively to stressful situations. A study found that people gave in to eating temptations every time they didn't have a strategy to deal with stressful situations. Individuals who respond to a negative situation with both positive and negative thoughts and constructive action are able to avoid emotion-based eating. Action responses might include attempts to fix a problem by asking a friend, family member, or associate for their advice, or through calming and soothing yourself by taking a walk, listening to music, or deep breathing. Examples of positive thinking include reminding yourself that the problem is not really as big as it seems or brainstorming different approaches to the problem to find the most effective solution.

It has been observed that many people use food as a means to distract themselves from emotions ranging from simple boredom to frustration to elevated anxiety. Differentiating between biological hunger and other urges to eat and trying to identify the feelings and needs behind non-hunger urges is the baseline for understanding what is behind the hunger. When a rest or distraction or refreshing relief from routine is needed, simply learning to acknowledge it is appropriate to take a break can be freeing. If you're not hungry, use breaks to read, nap, or take a walk.

It is shown that emotional eating can be a significant source of excess of calories. This can result in overweight or obesity, which can increase problems. The American Institute for Cancer Research emphasizes the need to choose portions appropriate to individual needs and to avoid popular super-sized foods. Emotional eating is controlled with healthier foods or smaller portions and by getting whatever help and support you need to learn how to handle non-hunger urges without actually turning to food for temporary solace.

For more information on food and nutrition guidelines visit the Academy of Nutrition and Dietetics (formerly the American Dietetic Association) at http://www.eatright.org.

Nutritional Requirements

Men are from Mars and women are from Venus, but other than origin the genders also see differences in their nutritional requirements. What does everyone need to be concerned about and what health concerns do men and women specifically need to be aware about?

1. Calcium

Women: Calcium is important in lowering a woman's risk of osteoporosis. A diet high in calcium and vitamin D has been proven to lower the risk of bone fractures and regulate blood pressure. For women under 50 years of age, the recommended amount of daily calcium is 1,000 milligrams and 1,200 mg for women over 50 years.

Men: Calcium is important in lowering the risk of osteoporosis in men, but can be harmful in large doses. Studies have shown that men who consumed high levels of calcium saw an increased risk in prostate cancer. For all ages the recommended amount is 800 mg or three servings of dairy per day.

2. Iron

Women: Women require more iron then men because of their monthly menstrual cycles. Signs of iron-deficiency anemia include fatigue, inability to concentrate, and difficulty breathing. If these symptoms appear, speak to a doctor. The recommended amounts of daily iron are 18 mg and eight milligrams for postmenopausal women. The difference is one of the reasons why it's important to choose an age-appropriate formula if you are taking multivitamin supplements.

Men: The recommended amount is eight milligrams for men of all ages. Studies have shown that men with high iron stores were associated with increased risk of heart attacks. It is important to choose an age-appropriate as well as gender-appropriate formula if taking a multivitamin supplement.

3. Omega 3 Fatty Acids

Women: Omega 3 fatty acids are a type of polyunsaturated fatty acids, which have been shown to help lower triglycerides and increase the good HDL cholesterol. They may also act as an anticoagulant to prevent blood from clotting. Omega 3 fatty acids can be found in almost all fish, but they are particularly high in fatty fish such as mackerel, salmon, sardines, and herring. They can also be found in nuts and seeds as well as vegetable cooking oils. There is no official recommendation on how much omega 3 fatty acids women should eat, but the American Heart Association recommends eating fish at least two times a week.

Men: Omega 3 fatty acids benefit men, but only the marine kind from fish oil. Vegetable omega 3, also known as alpha-linolenic acid (ALA) may not be good for men. Still controversial, a high intake of ALA has been linked to higher risk of prostate cancer. Until more is known, men should avoid taking concentrated ALA supplements such as flaxseed oil pills.

4. Protein

Women: Protein provides energy, and it is also important in growth and repair. As a result of the high-protein diet hype, many people eat more protein than required. Excess protein accelerates calcium loss in urine, therefore, women with a high risk of osteoporosis should be careful not to eat too much protein. The average requirement is based on 0.8 grams of protein per kilogram of body weight. For example, a 130 pound woman would need 47 grams of protein daily.

Men: Men weigh more and therefore need more protein. Excess protein accelerates calcium loss in urine, even in men. Thus, men with a high risk of kidney stones should watch their intake. The same calculation is applied to men when determining an individual's average requirement of daily protein. Based on 0.8 grams of protein per kg of body weight a 165 pound man would need 60 grams of protein daily.

In general healthy men and women will do fine with a daily 60 grams (8 oz.) of protein. If you are an athlete, however, your needs and requirements will increase.

5. Fiber

Women: Fiber prevents constipation, hemorrhoids, and diverticulosis and can help reduce the risk for some chronic diseases such as colon and breast cancer. In addition, it may help lower bad LDL cholesterol and total cholesterol, reducing the risk of heart disease. Fiber can also help lower the blood sugar to help manage diabetes. Women under 50 require 25 grams of fiber, while those over 50 require 21 grams. This is equivalent to at least two cups of vegetables and 1.5 cups of fruit.

Men: In a brief statement, men require more fiber than women. Men in general need more calories and in turn they need more fiber. Fiber requirements are calculated to provide the greatest protection against heart disease and are based on energy intake. Men under 50 require 38 grams of fiber, while those over 50 require 30 grams of fiber. This is equivalent to at least three cups of vegetables and two cups of fruit.

Understanding Food Labels And Nutrition Facts

Food labels have become synonymous with cryptic ingredients, hidden macronutrients, and undecipherable content amounts. Grocery shopping for some can be a real headache and stressful experience, but it doesn't have to be. Determining whether or not a product fits into your healthy lifestyle has become easier with the addition of listing the amounts of macronutrients and vitamin and mineral contents. The food label provides good information to help a consumer determine if a particular food product meets his or her nutritional needs.

In 1990, the Nutrition Labeling and Education Act went into effect with the intention that food labels are designed to help consumers make healthy food choices. The U.S. Department of Agriculture (USDA) and the U.S. Food and Drug Administration (FDA) developed these guidelines so that consumers would have access to useful nutritional information. According to this act all packaged food must contain the following information:

- Common name of the product

- Name and address of the product's manufacturer

- Net contents in terms of weight, measure or count, and

- Ingredient list and Nutrition Facts

The most frustrating and yet most sought after component is the Nutrition Facts panel. Required fields include components of common nutrients, such as total fat, cholesterol, and sodium. Each package must identify the quantities of specified nutrients and food constituents per serving. Note the following measurements:

- 1 gram of fat = 9 kcal

- 1 gram of protein = 4 kcal

- 1 gram of carbohydrate = 4 kcal

- 1 gram of alcohol = 7 kcal

Nutrients Listed, Serving Size, Calories (kcal)

Total fat, saturated fats, cholesterol, total carbohydrate, protein, vitamins A and C, calcium and iron, are required on the label. Other nutrients are optional and may be listed at the discretion of the manufacturer. The percent daily values provide an estimate of the percentage of a nutrient from one serving in a typical 2000 kcal diet. Also included is the daily reference values footnote. This reminds consumers of the daily intake of different foods depending on their own nutritional needs. In addition, a few other nutrients relevant to heart health are important to pay attention to when reading a label. At the beginning of January 2006 all labels also included trans fatty acids.

Serving sizes are standardized to make for easier comparison among similar products. They are expressed in common household and metric measures. It is always important to pay attention to a serving size. For example, if you eat four pieces and the serving size is two then you need to double the amount of nutrition content listed on the label.

It is important to find out the total amount of calories. Calories provide a measure of how much energy you obtain after eating a portion of food. Many consumers are surprised to find out that fat-free is not synonymous with low calorie, just as sugar-free is not always low in calories or fat.

The Bottom Line: Regarding Food Labels

Food labels and Nutrition Facts enable consumers to compare products based on key ingredients. When comparing foods, focus on the ingredients that are most important to you. Tips to consider when comparing food labels:

- If you are concerned about your weight, compare products based on both their calories and fat.

- If you have heart disease or high blood pressure, focus on the amount of total fat, saturated fat, trans fat, cholesterol, and sodium. Then choose products that contain less than 20 percent Daily Values for fat, cholesterol, and sodium.

- If you have diabetes, focus on the amount of carbohydrate and sugar added as well as fiber.

Nutrition Myths

Good fats, bad fats, low-fat, fat-free, low-calorie. These are just some of the many terms that get thrown at us as consumers daily by food manufacturers. They are enticing and intriguing especially with Americans' preoccupation with body image. The fact is that we need fats, and reduced fat items have more sugar added to them to enhance the flavor. What you may think is a conscious effort to be healthy may result in unintended outcomes and sabotage. Fats get a bad reputation and are one of the first nutrients monitored when people begin their quest for health. It is true that all fats are not equal and some promote health while others increase the risk of heart disease, it is also true that fats help nutrient absorption, nerve transmission, and maintaining cell membrane integrity. The key is to replace the bad fats with good fats in our diet.

Good fats include monounsaturated fats (MUFAs) and polyunsaturated fats. They lower total cholesterol and LDL cholesterol (bad cholesterol). MUFAs aid in increasing HDL cholesterol and have been found to help weight loss, especially in body fat. Food stuffs that supply MUFAs include nuts, such as peanuts, walnuts, almonds, and pistachios, avocado, and canola and olive oil. Polyunsaturated fats include the well-known group omega 3 fatty acids. Seafood, such as salmon and fish oil, and corn, soy, safflower, and sunflower oils are high of this type of fat.

Bad fats include saturated fats and the highly talked about trans fats. Saturated fats raise total blood cholesterol and LDL cholesterol. They are mainly found in animal products such as meat, dairy, eggs, and seafood. Some plant foods such as coconut oil, palm oil, and palm kernel oil are also high in saturated fats. Trans fats are not found in nature but were invented as scientists began to "hydrogenate" liquid oils so that they can withstand better in food production process and provide a better shelf life. Trans fatty acids are found in many commercially packaged foods, commercially fried food, other packaged snacks as well as in vegetable shortening and hard stick margarine.

To reduce your intake of bad fats consider these simple changes. Avoid using cooking oils that are high in saturated fats and/or trans fats such as coconut oil, palm oil, or vegetable shortening. Instead, use oils that are low in saturated fats and high in monounsaturated and polyunsaturated fats such as canola oil, olive oil, and flax seed oil. Minimize using commercially packaged foods which are high in trans fats, and read labels to look for trans-fat free alternatives. Use lower-fat dairy products such as 1% or skim milk instead of whole milk and trim visible fats and skins from meat products to reduce saturated fats.

The truth about fats and calories is not the only myth surrounding nutrition. Other common myths seen in the dieting and the nutrition world are brown eggs are more nutritious than white, avoid carbohydrates to lose weight, avoid nuts because they are fattening, eating for two is necessary during pregnancy, and red meat is bad for health. All of these "truths" can easily be debunked with the knowledge of dietitians and their work.

1. Brown Eggs Are More Nutritious Than White Eggs

This widely believed myth that the color of the eggshell has an affect on the eggs overall nutritional value has no scientific support. The color has nothing to do with the nutritional value, quality, flavor, cooking characteristics, or shell thickness. It only tells you what breed of hen produced the egg. The white shelled eggs are produced by hens with white feathers and white earlobes whereas the brown shelled eggs are produced by hens with red feathers and red earlobes.

2. Avoid Carbohydrates To Lose Weight

Many low-carb diets convey the message that carbohydrates promote insulin production, which in turn results in weight gain. The problem is many low-carb diets do not provide sufficient carbohydrates to your body for daily maintenance. This means the body will begin to burn stored carbohydrates (glycogen) for energy, and when your body starts burning glycogen, water is released. This water release is the reason for the initial weight loss of a low-carb diet. These diets are often calorie-restricted allowing an average of 1000–1400 calories, compared to

1800–2200 calories needed for most people. Carbohydrates are not the pinnacle of successful weight loss. You can lose weight by healthfully reducing your caloric intake by 500 calories per day in respect to your normal diet.

3. Avoid Nuts Because They Are Fattening

Nuts are caloric and it is easy to overeat them, but when properly portioned, nuts can be part of a healthy diet. Nuts are high in good fats, monounsaturated and polyunsaturated fats, as well as plant sterols, which have all been shown to lower bad LDL cholesterol. Instead of simply adding nuts to your diet, the best approach is to eat them in replacement of foods high in saturated fats.

Diet

Almost every eating disorder starts with a diet. In a person with a genetic predisposition, a diet can set an eating disorder's downward spiral into motion. Seemingly innocent statements of intention may include: "I want to eat healthier;" "I just want to cut back on snacking and sweets;" "I want to get in shape;" or "I want to be vegetarian." These diets often start with dietary changes and oftentimes include increases in activity. The safety and efficacy of dieting is currently controversial, even for those not predisposed to an eating disorder. For those with this predisposition (there is no test for this) a diet can lead very quickly to anorexia nervosa or other eating disorders.

Source: Excerpted from "Eating Disorders Glossary," © 2012 Families Empowered and Supporting Treatment of Eating Disorders (www.feast-ed.org).

---

4. Eating For Two Is Necessary During Pregnancy

The idea that pregnancy allows for women to eat double and ice cream in a free-for-all is a nutrition myth. Generally it is recommended that pregnant women increase their daily intake by 100 kcal in the first trimester and 300 kcal in the second and third trimesters. A daily prenatal multivitamin supplement is recommended and an extra snack before bedtime such as a piece of fruit, a serving of milk or yogurt, and a few biscuits is enough.

5. Red Meat Is Bad For Health

Some studies have linked red meat with increased risk of heart disease due to the saturated fat content, but even chicken can contain as much saturated fat as a cut of lean pork or beef. Poultry is naturally lower in saturated fats but only if you do not eat the skin. Red meat altogether is not bad for your health. Instead of excluding red meat altogether, choose leaner cuts. For beef, choose eye of round, top round roast, top sirloin and flank; for pork, choose tenderloin and loin chops.

Chapter 3

Causes And Risk Factors For Eating Disorders

Causes

There is no single cause for eating disorders. Although concerns about weight and body shape play a role in all eating disorders, the actual cause of these disorders appears to involve many factors, including those that are genetic and neurobiologic, cultural and social, and behavioral and psychologic.

Although much has been written about the roles of families and parenting as causes of eating disorders, there is no solid evidence supporting this claim.

Genetic Factors

Anorexia is eight times more common in people who have relatives with the disorder. Studies of twins show they have a tendency to share specific eating disorders (anorexia nervosa, bulimia nervosa, and obesity). Researchers have identified specific chromosomes that may be associated with bulimia and anorexia.

Biologic Factors

The body's hypothalamic-pituitary-adrenal axis (HPA) may be important in eating disorders. This complex system originates in the following regions in the brain:

- **Hypothalamus:** The hypothalamus is a small structure that plays a role in controlling our behavior, such as eating, sexual behavior, and sleeping, and regulates body temperature, hunger and thirst, and secretion of hormones.

About This Chapter: Excerpted from "Eating Disorders: In-Depth Report," © 2012 A.D.A.M., Inc. Reprinted with permission.

- **Pituitary Gland:** The pituitary gland is involved in controlling thyroid functions, the adrenal glands, growth, and sexual maturation.

- **Amygdala:** This small almond-shaped structure lies deep in the brain and is associated with regulation and control of major emotional activities, including anxiety, depression, aggression, and affection.

Biology, Not Just Society, May Increase Risk Of Binge Eating During Puberty

Biological changes associated with puberty may influence the development of binge eating and related eating disorders, according to a recent study on female rats conducted by researchers funded by the National Institute of Mental Health (NIMH). After puberty, the rats showed binge eating patterns that resemble those in humans, supporting the role of biological factors, since rats do not experience pressures to be thin or other psychosocial risk factors commonly associated with human eating disorders. The study was published online ahead of print on May 16, 2011, in the *Journal of Abnormal Psychology*.

Background

Among girls, symptoms of binge eating or bulimia nervosa often arise around puberty. Past research has largely focused on psychosocial roots for this association, but biological changes that occur during and after puberty are likely to have an effect as well.

Kelly Klump, Ph.D., of Michigan State University, and colleagues tested this theory in an animal model since animals do not experience psychological risk factors during puberty. They used a rat model that can distinguish between rats that are resistant to binge eating (BER) from those prone to binge eating (BEP), based on their individual eating habits.

For this study, the researchers studied binge eating risk from pre-puberty to adulthood in 66 female rats. In addition to their standard food, the rats were provided intermittent access to cake frosting, a highly enjoyable but nutritionally empty and high-fat food.

Results

Over the course of development, all rats ate more frosting as they matured. However, a difference in frosting intake between BER and BEP rats emerged during puberty—no differences in frosting intake were observed in pre-puberty, but large differences were observed in puberty and adulthood.

The researchers noted that rats in the BER and BEP groups ate similar amounts of the standard food and were similar in body weight. This suggests that the BEP rats were not overeaters generally, but were instead, prone to binge eat on high-fat foods only.

The HPA system releases certain neurotransmitters (chemical messengers in the brain) that regulate stress, mood, and appetite. Abnormalities in the activities of three of them, serotonin, norepinephrine, and dopamine, may play a particularly important role in eating disorders. Serotonin is involved with well-being, anxiety, and appetite (among other traits), and norepinephrine is a stress hormone. Dopamine is involved in reward-seeking behavior.

Significance

The findings reveal dramatic increases in binge eating proneness during puberty, suggesting that increases in binge eating and similar eating disorders during and after puberty in girls may be partially due to biological factors.

Similar to binge eating in humans, BEP rats ate much more of the high-fat food but did not increase their consumption of the standard food. Also, all rats preferred the high-fat food, regardless of developmental stage, which is similar to behaviors seen in girls; for example, girls tend to prefer candy over healthier treats at all ages. In both rats and humans, this behavior begins to diverge during puberty, with some consuming much more of the high-fat food than others.

Unlike humans, however, the percentage of binge eating rats (30 percent) was much higher than estimates in humans (3.5–19 percent). According to the researchers, this difference may indicate that binge eating in rats is a "pure" form of binge eating that is unmodified by psychosocial factors—such as social disapproval or guilt—that tends to decrease binge eating rates in humans.

What's Next

More research is needed to develop and validate animal models of the cognitive and behavioral symptoms of eating disorders. Studies exploring the mechanisms underlying developmental changes that occur during puberty, for example the action of ovarian hormones, may also inform research on eating disorders.

Reference

Klump KL, Suisman JL, Culbert KM, Kashy DA, Sisk CL. Binge eating proneness emerges during puberty in female rats: A longitudinal study. *J Abnorm Psychol*. 2011 May 16. [Epub ahead of print] PubMed PMID: 21574664.

Source: "Biology, Not Just Society, May Increase Risk of Binge Eating During Puberty," *Science Update*, National Institute of Mental Health, August 22, 2011.

Imbalances with serotonin and dopamine may explain in part why people with anorexia do not experience a sense of pleasure from food and other typical comforts.

Cultural Pressures

The media plays a role in promoting unrealistic expectations for body image and a distorted cultural drive for thinness. At the same time, cheap and high-caloric foods are aggressively marketed. Such messages are contradictory and confusing.

Risk Factors

In the United States, about seven million females and one million males suffer from eating disorders.

Age

Eating disorders occur most often in adolescents and young adults. However, they are becoming increasingly prevalent among young children. Eating disorders are more difficult to identify in young children because they are less commonly suspected.

Gender

Eating disorders occur predominantly among girls and women. About 90–95% of patients with anorexia nervosa, and about 80% of patients with bulimia nervosa, are female.

Race And Ethnicity

Most studies of individuals with eating disorders have focused on Caucasian middle-class females. However, eating disorders can affect people of all races and socioeconomic levels.

Personality Disorders

People with eating disorders tend to share similar personality and behavioral traits, including low self-esteem, dependency, and problems with self-direction. Specific psychiatric personality disorders may put people at higher risk for eating disorders.

Avoidant Personality Disorder: Some studies indicate that many patients with anorexia nervosa have avoidant personalities. This personality disorder is characterized by:

- Being a perfectionist

- Being emotionally and sexually inhibited

- Wanting to be perceived as always being "good," not being rebellious

- Being terrified of being ridiculed or criticized or of feeling humiliated

People with anorexia nervosa are often extremely sensitive to failure, and any criticism, no matter how slight, reinforces their own belief that they are "no good."

Obsessive-Compulsive Personality Disorder: Obsessive-compulsive personality disorder defines certain character traits (being a perfectionist, morally rigid, or preoccupied with rules and order). This personality disorder is strongly associated with a higher risk for anorexia. These traits should not be confused with the anxiety disorder called obsessive-compulsive disorder (OCD), although they may increase the risk for this disorder.

Borderline Personality Disorder: Borderline personality disorder (BPD) is associated with self-destructive and impulsive behaviors. People with BPD tend to have other co-existing mental health problems, including eating disorders.

Narcissistic Personality Disorder: People with narcissistic personalities tend to:

- Have an inability to soothe oneself

- Have an inability to empathize with others

- Have a need for admiration

- Be hypersensitive to criticism or defeat

Accompanying Mental Health Disorders

Many patients with eating disorders experience depression and anxiety disorders. It is not clear if these disorders, particularly obsessive-compulsive disorder (OCD), cause the eating disorders, increase susceptibility to them, or share common biologic causes.

Obsessive-Compulsive Disorder (OCD): Obsessive-compulsive disorder is an anxiety disorder that may occur in up to two thirds of patients with anorexia and up to a third of patients with bulimia. Some doctors believe that eating disorders are variants of OCD. Obsessions are recurrent or persistent mental images, thoughts, or ideas, which may result in compulsive behaviors (repetitive, rigid, and self-prescribed routines) that are intended to prevent the manifestation of the obsession. Women with anorexia and OCD may become obsessed with exercise, dieting, and food. They often develop compulsive rituals (weighing every bit of food, cutting it into tiny pieces, or putting it into tiny containers.

Obsessive-compulsive disorder is an anxiety disorder characterized by an inability to resist or stop continuous, abnormal thoughts or fears combined with ritualistic, repetitive, and involuntary defense behavior.

Other Anxiety Disorders: Other anxiety disorders associated with both bulimia and anorexia include:

- **Phobias:** Phobias often precede the onset of the eating disorder. Social phobias, in which a person is fearful about being humiliated in public, are common in both types of eating disorders.

- **Panic Disorder:** Panic disorder often follows the onset of an eating disorder. It is characterized by periodic attacks of anxiety or terror (panic attacks).

- **Post-Traumatic Stress Disorder:** Some patients with serious eating disorders report a past traumatic event (such as sexual, physical, or emotional abuse), and exhibit symptoms of post-traumatic stress disorder (PTSD)—an anxiety disorder that occurs in response to life-threatening circumstances.

Depression: Depression is common in anorexia and bulimia. Major depression is unlikely to be a cause of eating disorders, however, because treating and relieving depression rarely cures an eating disorder. In addition, depression often improves after anorexic patients begin to gain weight.

Being Overweight

Extreme eating disorder behaviors, including use of diet pills, laxatives, diuretics, and vomiting, are reported more often in overweight than normal weight teenagers.

Body Image Disorders

Body Dysmorphic Disorder: Body dysmorphic disorder (BDD) involves a distorted view of one's body that is caused by social, psychologic, or possibly biologic factors. It is often associated with anorexia or bulimia, but it can also occur without any eating disorder. People with this disorder commonly suffer from emotional disorders, including obsessive-compulsive disorder and depression. As part of obsessive thinking, some people with BDD may obsess about a perceived deformity in one area of their body, and may repeatedly seek cosmetic surgery to "correct" it. People with BDD are also at higher risk for suicidal thinking and attempts.

Muscle Dysmorphia: Muscle dysmorphia is a form of body dysmorphic disorder in which the obsession involves musculature and muscle mass. It tends to occur in men who perceive themselves as being underdeveloped or "puny," which results in excessive body building, preoccupation with diet, and social problems. Such individuals are prone to eating disorders and other unhealthy behaviors, including the use of anabolic steroids.

Girls With ADHD Are At Increased Risk For Eating Disorders

Girls with attention deficit hyperactivity disorder stand a substantially greater risk of developing eating disorders in adolescence than girls without ADHD, a new study has found.

"Adolescent girls with ADHD frequently develop body-image dissatisfaction and may go through repeating cycles of binge eating and purging behaviors that are common in bulimia nervosa," said University of Virginia psychologist Amori Yee Mikami, who led the study.

"Girls with ADHD may be more at risk of developing eating problems as adolescents because they already have impulsive behaviors that can set them apart from their peers," Mikami said. "As they get older, their impulsivity may make it difficult for them to maintain healthy eating and a healthy weight, resulting in self-consciousness about their body image and the binging and purging symptoms."

The study was conducted with an ethnically diverse sample of 228 girls in the San Francisco Bay area; 140 who had been diagnosed with ADHD and 88 matched comparison girls without ADHD. They were first assessed between the ages of 6 and 12 and again five years later.

Girls with the "combined type" of ADHD (those with both inattention and hyperactivity/impulsivity) were most likely to have adolescent bulimia nervosa symptoms, relative to girls with the "inattentive type" of ADHD (those with inattention only) and girls without ADHD. Girls with both types of ADHD were more likely to be overweight, to have experienced harsh/critical parenting in childhood, and to have been peer-rejected than girls without ADHD. Mikami said she believes these factors could contribute to the bulimia nervosa symptoms.

"An additional concern is that stimulant medications used to treat ADHD have a side effect of appetite suppression, creating a risk that overweight girls could abuse these medicines to encourage weight loss, though we have not yet investigated that possibility," Mikami said.

She warned parents and teachers to be aware that adolescent girls with ADHD may develop an array of female-relevant symptoms beyond the standard ADHD symptoms, to include eating disorders, depression and anxiety.

Source: Excerpted from "Adolescent Girls with ADHD Are at Increased Risk for Eating Disorders, Study Shows" *UVa Today*, March 13, 2008. © 2008 by the Rector and Visitors of the University of Virginia. All rights reserved. Reprinted with permission. The complete text of this article is available at http://www.virginia.edu/uvatoday/newsRelease.php?id=4502.

Excessive Physical Activity

Highly competitive athletes are often perfectionists, a trait common among people with eating disorders.

Female Athletes: Excessive exercise is associated with many cases of anorexia (and, to a lesser degree, bulimia). In young female athletes, exercise and low body weight postpone puberty, allowing them to retain a muscular boyish shape without the normal accumulation of fatty tissues in breasts and hips that may blunt their competitive edge. Coaches and teachers may compound the problem by overemphasizing calorie counting and loss of body fat.

In response, people who are vulnerable to such criticism may feel compelled to strictly diet and lose weight. The term *female athlete triad* is a common and serious disorder that affects young female athletes and dancers. It includes:

- Eating disorders, including anorexia

- Amenorrhea (absent or irregular menstruation)

- Osteoporosis (bone calcium loss, which is related to low weight)

Male Athletes: Male wrestlers and lightweight rowers are also at risk for excessive dieting. Many high school wrestlers use a method called weight-cutting for rapid weight loss. This process involves food restriction and fluid depletion by using steam rooms, saunas, laxatives, and diuretics. Although male athletes are more apt to resume normal eating patterns once competition ends, studies show that the body fat levels of many wrestlers are still well below their peers during off-season and are often as low as 3% during wrestling season.

Diabetes Or Other Chronic Diseases

Eating disorders may be more common in teenagers with chronic illness, such as diabetes or asthma. They are particularly serious problems for people with either type 1 or type 2 diabetes:

- Binge eating (without purging) is more common in type 2 diabetes and, in fact, the obesity it causes may even trigger this diabetes in some people.

- Both bulimia and anorexia are common among young people with type 1 diabetes. The combination of diabetes and an eating disorder can have serious health consequences. Some women with diabetes omit or underuse insulin in order to control weight. If such patients develop anorexia, their extremely low weight may appear to control the diabetes for a while. Eventually, however, if they fail to take insulin and continue to lose weight, these patients develop life-threatening complications.

Early Puberty

There appears to be a greater risk for eating disorders and other emotional problems for girls who undergo early menarche and puberty, when the pressures experienced by all adolescents are intensified by experiencing these early physical changes, including normal increased body fat.

Chapter 4

Eating Disorders— Not Just A Women's Issue

Clinical reports say one out of every ten patients with an eating disorder is a man. Many researchers speculate the true number is much higher. There is a social ideal for men to be lean with defined muscles—as well as great athletes. Certified athletic trainer Tina Bonci said a nutrition plan and realistic weight expectations can prevent some men from developing eating disorders.

Eating Disorder Signs And Symptoms

The symptoms of eating disorders are similar in males and females (except males do not experience irregular menstruation). Here are the most common symptoms for anorexia and bulimia from the National Institute of Mental Health.

- **Anorexia:** Brittle hair and nails, dry and yellowish skin, growth of fine hair over body, mild anemia, muscle weakness, muscle loss, severe constipation, low blood pressure, slowed breathing and pulse, lethargy

- **Bulimia:** Chronically inflamed and sore throat, swollen glands in the neck and below the jaw, sores on the hand, worn tooth enamel, increasingly sensitive and decaying teeth, severe dehydration from purging of fluids, and severe acid reflux.

Dr. Angela Doyle, a clinical psychologist at the University of Chicago, said a young man transitions from having competitive, dedicated habits to an eating disorder when:

- There are problems with school, work, friends

About This Chapter: "Male Eating Disorders May Be More Common than We Think," by Kimberly Weisensee, February 4, 2009, Medill News Service, Northwestern University (http://news.medill.northwestern.edu/chicago). © 2009 Northwestern University. All rights reserved. Reprinted with permission.

- He is unhappy and seems depressed

- He becomes very irritable when he is offered more food

- He does extra work-outs

- He refuses to go out to eat or to be in a situation where he cannot control the food

Resource Suggestions

- National Association of Anorexia Nervosa and Associated Eating Disorders (http://www.anad.org): Founded in 1976, the Highland Park-based association has an online database to find a therapist anywhere in the U.S.

- National Eating Disorders Association (http://www.nationaleatingdisorders.org): The organization's website has extensive information and research—including a section dedicated to men and boys with eating disorders.

- *Help Your Teenager Beat an Eating Disorder*: A book co-authored by University of Chicago psychiatrist Daniel Le Grange to inform and empower parents to take action and help their teens.

(Source for the above information: Angela Doyle, clinical psychologist at the University of Chicago)

Men's Body Image And Eating Disorders

Did you know that men, like women, can struggle with body image issues or an eating disorder? Men may feel a lot of pressure to have a "perfect," muscular body and may focus too much on exercise and dieting. This focus can wind up hurting a man's body, job, and relationships. But medicines and counseling can help men with eating and body image disorders lead healthy lives.

Muscle Mistakes

Some men try to pump up their muscles by taking anabolic steroids. But using steroids in this way can harm your physical and mental health — and it's illegal. Also, injecting steroids raises your risk of getting HIV and hepatitis.

Sometimes, men try natural supplements like creatine to build muscle. Keep in mind that "natural" doesn't necessarily mean safe. Make sure to discuss any supplements with your doctor before taking them.

Source: Excerpted from "Men's Health: Body Image and Eating Disorders," Office on Women's Health (www.womens health.gov), January 10, 2011.

Male Eating Disorders

Contrary to the misconception that eating disorders affect only women, clinical reports show one out of ten patients with eating disorders is a man. And a large but unreported number of these men are athletes.

"There is a high possibility we are under-identifying men with eating disorders because they are less likely to come in," said Angela Celio Doyle, a clinical psychologist in the University of Chicago's Eating Disorders Program. She said the lower rate of male eating disorders makes it hard to get accurate statistics for men. Because eating disorder assessments were developed for women, doctors may be missing nuances specific to men, she added.

Common eating disorders include anorexia, which involves maintaining extremely low body weight, and bulimia, which involves binge eating followed by induced vomiting, laxatives, or diuretics to prevent weight gain.

Male athletes are prone to disordered eating because of pressures in their sport and culture. There is no research on what sports drive specific eating disorders, but Doyle speculates an athlete with an eating disorder will do whatever is necessary to reach a target weight or body image. This may account for why the a high percentage of male athletes with eating disorders are classified with an unspecified eating disorder called EDNOS (eating disorder not otherwise specified).

There is also disordered eating, a subclinical classification that covers a spectrum of eating problems that precede the onset of an eating disorder.

"These are early signs you can catch early and run interference with," said Tina Bonci, a certified athletic trainer. "Disordered eating runs the whole gamut of other behavior that may not meet the clinical criteria [for an eating disorder]." Bonci is the co-director of the athletic training division and sports medicine at the University of Texas. She also is the lead author of the National Athletic Trainers' Association's position statement on disordered eating in athletes.

The trainers' association presented recommendations for preventing, detecting, and managing disordered eating in athletes. Bonci said more education is needed for people who supervise athletes, especially in high schools where she said not enough information is collected in the pre-participation stage to identify athletes with potential or existing disorders.

"We do have cases of disordered eating at our institutions with no protocol in place to manage disordered eating or even diagnose athletes," Bonci said, calling management of athletes with disordered eating a "complex art."

There isn't any research on the differences between men with eating disorders versus women or athletes versus non-athletes. However, Doyle had some clinical observations from more than 10 years of research. Young men tend to gain more weight before they become concerned, whereas women become troubled with their weight before much is gained. She's also seen a subset of young men come to the clinic who are overweight before they develop anorexia or bulimia. A lot of young men initially call their habits healthy living—cutting out trans fats and high fructose corn syrup—and gradually the habits get distorted. While males and females both feel a need for weight management, young men insist they need lean muscles.

"They have this idea to reach an ideal body shape that is very similar to an Abercrombie & Fitch model," Doyle said.

Vigilance and early detection are key, said Bonci and Doyle. Both agree the disorders are fully treatable and beatable, and the process is much easier if the problem is caught early. Bonci said men tend not to self-identify because of shame or embarrassment and go much longer without treatment.

Chapter 5

Eating Disorders In Female Athletes

Eating disorders and disordered eating are seen in both males and females in the general population. However, females are ten times more likely than males to have an eating disorder. Of females with either eating disorders or disordered eating, a certain percentage gravitates towards athletics for several reasons.

First, the personality traits of individuals with eating disorders and of athletes are similar. Second, individuals may move towards athletics because certain behaviors of athletes can disguise behaviors of someone with an eating disorder (i.e., excessive exercise, focus on body shape and size, diet restrictions). Last, although sports do not cause eating disorders or disordered eating, there are a number of risk factors involved in sports which may lead someone who may be at risk for eating disorders towards disordered eating behaviors.

Understanding the risk factors that may trigger eating disorders in female athletes is an important component in preventing disordered eating in young women. Once the risk factors are understood, coaches and those working with young women can take proactive steps in preventing eating disorders in their athletes.

What Places Female Athletes At Risk For Eating Disorders?

There are a number of risk factors both in society in general and in sports that may place an athlete more at risk for an eating disorder. Some risk factors can be changed. Others cannot. Knowing the difference can help those who work with female athletes become aware of how to alter their own behavior, policies, and language to not increase existing risks.

Sociocultural Pressure

Unfortunately, in western society, there is sociocultural pressure for women to be thin in order to be accepted (Beals, K., 2004). Girls are exposed at a very young age to the pressures of being thin via pictures and advertising in the media as well as through television shows and movies. Happy, well-adjusted, and popular characters are portrayed as thin and fit.

Extremely lean female models are still used in the fashion industry and on the runways to market fashion trends. This message alone is a dangerous one as it sets the precedent that clothes can only look good on really thin body frames.

Added to the pressure that western society already places on girls and women to be thin is the additional pressure in "thin-build" sports. These are sports in which the athletes are either judged by their appearance or whose performance is enhanced with leaner bodies. These sports include dance (specifically ballet), gymnastics, distance running, triathlon, diving, figure skating, and cheerleading (Beals, K., 2004).

Individuals who coach these sports need to recognize the inherent risks of these athletes towards eating disorders just by the nature of the sport itself. More than other sports, these coaches need to be cognizant of comments and/or procedures that they follow that may add additional pressure to already at-risk athletes.

Finally, it is important for coaches to recognize that it is the female athlete's perception of her body that is the important factor to focus on rather than the athlete's actual body weight, size, or shape. Many females (athletes or not) have misperceptions about their body size or shape.

If an athlete perceives that her body size and shape is not good enough for her sport (regardless of whether it is or not), it is this perception that may cause disordered eating in the athlete.

Psychosocial Factors

The ability for an individual to be coping effectively with life's stressors is an important psychosocial development that healthy young people develop. Knowing how to deal with adversity and cope effectively with problems may be one key to preventing the development of an eating disorder.

According to Beals (2004), individuals with eating disorders are often those who are raised in dysfunctional families in which there may be overbearing or over controlling parents or physical or sexual abuse. It is the loss of control that the individual feels and the loss of self-esteem that she is trying to gain control of through managing her food intake. Food is the one substance that the individual can completely control.

Second, effective coping mechanisms teach an individual how to handle stressful situations by facing them directly, thinking through possible options, and then acting on the option that best fits the scenario. Healthy coping mechanisms tend to include the ability to talk openly and freely about emotions and fears with family or close friends. A network of close family and friends are one of the most important coping mechanisms that an athlete can have.

Individuals who face adversity on a regular basis without an emotional outlet may learn unhealthy coping mechanisms including shutting down, withdrawing, and hiding their emotions. Although this may be a defense mechanism that a young girl may learn and need to survive while growing up in a dysfunctional family, it can lead to a myriad of problems coping as an adult.

While some people learn to overcome these factors, others may be at risk for eating disorders. While emotional experiences play a role in the background of predisposing an individual towards being at risk for an eating disorder, other personal characteristic are involved. Personality characteristics commonly seen in athletes with eating disorders include the following (Beals, K., 2004):

- Perfectionist
- Achievement-oriented
- Independent
- Persistent
- Tolerant of pain and discomfort
- High self-expectations
- Low self-esteem

An individual who possesses these personality characteristics and who has a history of being raised in a dysfunctional family has a higher risk for eating disorders. What is really interesting is that the personality characteristics listed above are also many of the same ones found in good athletes. It is not a surprise that sports may draw in females who are at risk for eating disorders.

Because certain personality traits are well documented to place athletes at risk for eating disorders, coaches can help identify at-risk athletes by getting to know their athletes on a personal level. Once communication is established between the coach and the athlete, the athlete may be able to open up about difficulties at home.

Becoming a safe mentor for a young female athlete may be one way to identify at-risk athletes, provide an outlet for expressions of emotions in a safe environment, and provide further guidance or referral to a medical professional if necessary.

Age

It is well known in those working with people with eating disorders that most eating disorders are developed in early adolescence during the teenage years.

Teenage years are difficult enough as hormones and bodies change. These alone can create tumultuous times for young people.

However, for those that do not have good coping skills and who already may have low self-esteem, the pressure of trying to fit in and be accepted can be the trigger towards experimenting with disordered eating behaviors.

Understanding how self-esteem can be impacted by changing body shapes and sizes in young females is a really important factor in helping to prevent disordered eating behaviors in young women.

It starts with teaching young girls that everybody has a unique body shape and size. Young girls need to be taught to accept their bodies and to focus on the good rather than the imperfections. Teaching a healthy body image needs to start in the elementary school age children and then be reinforced as these young girls move through puberty.

With the goal of improving self-esteem in young girls is a campaign launched in 2004 by DOVE to help girls and women accept their bodies regardless of their size and shape. DOVE launched the campaign called "Campaign for Real Beauty." The goal is for girls and women to "Imagine a world where beauty is a source of confidence, not anxiety" (www.dove.us).

It is a three phase campaign to reach women of all ages for the purpose of breaking down stereotypical perceptions of beauty by helping girls and women to each find and accept their unique beauty. Part of the campaign is a DOVE Self-Esteem Fund with part of the funds going towards a new program Uniquely ME! developed specifically for the Girl Scouts of America for the purpose of improving the self-esteem of young girls ages 8–17.

This type of program is a necessity for this age group because this is the age group in which disordered eating and eating disorders begin—adolescent females. Because low self-esteem is one of the character traits of an individual at risk for an eating disorder, programs like these are needed and are a valuable resource to programs working with young girls.

Coaches working with this age group need to be especially careful in their comments made to the girls about weight, size, and shape. Understanding that this age group is where disordered eating behaviors take root is critical to helping prevent disordered eating in this population.

Biological Factors

Serotonin is a naturally found neurotransmitter in the brain that has a number of important functions including regulating sleep, body temperature, and mood. Low serotonin levels may create a number of side effects that would only compound problems seen in someone with an eating disorder.

There is some research that has shown that serotonin (a neurotransmitter) levels decreased in women who were on severely restricted diets (1,000 kcal/day). What is interesting to note is that this neurotransmitter was shown to only decrease in women during three weeks of calorie restriction and not in men (Kaye, W.H. and Weltzin, T.E., 1991). This may be one explanation as to why women are more susceptible to eating disorders than men.

Sports Specific Risk Factors

While a number of societal factors may predispose an individual towards eating disorders, a number of sports-related factors may compound the problem. Awareness of these risk factors can help coaches adjust their approaches to sports (especially thin-build sports) to reduce the risk of eating disorders in their athletes.

Exercise-Induced Anorexia

In the early to mid-eighties, a group of researchers (Epling, Pierce, and Stefan, 1983) theorized that extreme exercise might lead to anorexic behavior. Their theory proposed that extreme exercise decreased an athlete's appetite thus the athlete ate less and began to lose weight. As the athlete's weight dropped, the athlete's performance increased which lead to an increase in motivation to exercise. The researchers hypothesized that this cycle led to exercise-induced anorexia.

Although this was a plausible scenario for some athletes, it did not explain the many individuals who already suffered from eating disorders and then pursued sports as an excuse for extreme exercise. While it appears that exercise does play a role in eating disorders, it does not appear that research supports the hypothesis that exercise can cause an eating disorder.

Pressures To Lose Weight

For athletes who incur eating disorders during sports participation, a primary risk factor appears to be the pressure to lose weight. Because dieting is the primary precursor to the development of an eating disorder (Thompson, R.A. and Trattner Sherman, R., 1993), the perception that an athlete needs to lose weight is all that may be needed to trigger disordered eating.

Whether real or perceived, the issue at the center of the problem is the perception of the athlete's own body image. For athletes who may already have a poor self-image, a comment towards an athlete about her needing to lose weight is all that it needs to take to start and athlete towards disordered eating.

Adding to the above pressures of self and the coach, the athlete is at an even higher risk if she is involved in a "thin-build" sport in which the focus during competition is on the athlete's body. Combine all three of these issues and it is not surprising that athletes develop disordered eating behaviors.

While good intentioned, some coaches make the mistake of setting weight limitations for their female athletes. Athletes are weighed at the end of a season and then are required to come back in to the sport for the following season at a specific weight. If the weight requirements are not feasible or guided by sports medical professionals, athletes may turn to pathological eating behaviors to drop weight.

Pressure to make a certain weight for a female athlete may be all the pressure that is needed for an athlete to start dieting, restricting calories, over exercising, or turning to other purging techniques to drop weight. With all that is known about the risk factors for disordered eating in female athletes, there is no place for mandatory weigh-ins or weight restrictions in female sports.

For more information on the pressure of body weight and performance, read "Ideal Body Weight and Athletic Performance" (online at http://www.sportsmd.com/SportsMD_Articles/id/407/n/ideal_body_weight_and_athletic_performance.aspx).

Stress And Trauma

According to Katherine Beals (2004), author of *Disordered Eating among Athletes*, stress and/or trauma can lead to disordered eating in susceptible athletes. Types of stress might include injury, illness, change or loss of a coach, moving away from family or friends, academic challenges, and athletic performance changes.

The trait that all of these stressors are able to evoke is the feeling of being in or losing control over something that was important to the athlete. If the athlete feels out of control in some areas of her life, she may try to regain control through strict control of the food that she eats along with her energy expenditure.

Long term injuries can add a slightly different risk in that the athlete may not be able to exercise or compete with her team for long periods of time. If this is the case, she may try to control her weight through strict calorie restriction since she may be unable to burn up calories through her normal practices and competitions.

This is another factor that coaches and sports medicine professionals need to be cognizant of. Athletes who are identified as those with injuries, illness, or who are experiencing stressful situations need to be carefully monitored to ensure that they have the emotional support they need.

One important role of a good coach is to mentor their young athletes and to help them develop into responsible adults. As much fun as winning is, coaches can impact players for a lifetime if they can offer the emotional support and stability for their athletes during difficult times.

Daily personal contact is one way to provide much needed support for a struggling athlete. The challenge for the coach is to choose to take the time to invest in the athlete off of the field of play and not just on the field. Sending the message that the athlete is more than just a "performer" is a powerful message to athletes who may only perceive themselves as valuable because their athletic ability.

Understanding the risks that may place female athletes at risk for disordered eating/eating disorders is the first step to helping prevent these disorders. While some risk factors cannot be altered, others can be addressed by coaches and others working with female athletes to help minimize the impact and help prevent disordered eating.

If you have any concerns or questions about your nutritional needs, seek the consultation of a local sports nutritionist for appropriate care. To locate a top sports nutritionist in your area, please visit the SportsMD "Find a Sports Nutritionist Near You" section (online at http://www.sportsmd.com/SportsMD_DoctorSearch/d/doctors.aspx).

References

Beals, K.A. (2004). *Disordered Eating Among Athletes: A Comprehensive Guide for Health Professionals*. Human Kinetics: Champaign, IL.

Epling W.P., Pierce, W.D. and Stefan, L. (1983). A theory of activity-based anorexia. *International Journal of Eating Disorders*, 3, 27–46.

Kaye, W.H. and Weltzin, T.E. (1991). Serotonin activity in anorexia and bulimia nervosa: Relationship to the modulation of feeding and mood. *Journal of Clinical Psychiatry* 52: 41–18.

Kettles, M., Cole, C.L., and Wright, B.S. (2006). *Women's Health and Fitness Guide*. Human Kinetics: Champaign, IL.

Thompson, R.A & Trattner Sherman, R. (1993). Helping Athletes with Eating Disorders. Human Kinetics: Champaign, IL.

www.dove.us. Campaign for Real Beauty. Accessed on September 21, 2010.

Chapter 6

Negative Body Image May Contribute To Eating Disorders

About Body Image

Is your body image positive or negative? If your answer is negative, you are not alone. Many women in the United States feel pressured to measure up to a certain social and cultural ideal of beauty, which can lead to poor body image. Women are constantly bombarded with "Barbie Doll-like" images. By presenting an ideal that is so difficult to achieve and maintain, the cosmetic and diet product industries are assured of growth and profits. It's no accident that youth is increasingly promoted, along with thinness, as an essential criterion of beauty. The message we're hearing is either "all women need to lose weight" or that the natural aging process is a "disastrous" fate.

Other pressures can come from the people in our lives.

- Family and friends can influence your body image with positive and negative comments.

- A doctor's health advice can be misinterpreted and affect how a woman sees herself and feels about her body.

About Eating Disorders

"Mirror, Mirror on the wall...who's the thinnest one of all?" According to the National Eating Disorders Association, the average American woman is 5 feet 4 inches tall and weighs 140 pounds. The average American model is 5 feet 11 inches tall and weighs 117 pounds. All too often, society associates being "thin" with "hard-working, beautiful, strong, and self-disciplined." On the other hand, being "fat" is associated with being "lazy, ugly, weak, and

About This Chapter: From "About Body Image" and "Body Image: Eating Disorders," Office on Women's Health (www.womenshealth.gov), September 2009.

lacking will-power." Because of these harsh critiques, rarely are women completely satisfied with their image. As a result, they often feel great anxiety and pressure to achieve and/or maintain an imaginary appearance.

Eating disorders are serious medical problems. Anorexia nervosa, bulimia nervosa, and binge-eating disorder are all types of eating disorders. Eating disorders frequently develop during adolescence or early adulthood, but can occur during childhood or later in adulthood. Females are more likely than males to develop an eating disorder.

Eating disorders are more than just a problem with food. Food is used to feel in control of other feelings that may seem overwhelming. For example, starving is a way for people with anorexia to feel more in control of their lives and to ease tension, anger, and anxiety. Purging and other behaviors to prevent weight gain are ways for people with bulimia to feel more in control of their lives and to ease stress and anxiety.

Body Image

Body image refers to the thoughts, impressions, and perceptions that one has about his/her body. Body image is constructed by the brain using a "body schema" that relies on physical and cognitive inputs. Negative or distorted body image is a very common symptom of an eating disorder, characterized by body dissatisfaction; that image is unduly influenced by weight, shape, and appearance and oftentimes the weight seen on the scale is the predominant determinant of body image and mood. Body image typically improves after weight restoration, but most eating disorder treatment involves the addressing of body image issues. Some patients suffer from a brain disorder independent of the malnourishment and experience a distorted body image that is seen and felt by the patient.

Body Image Distortion

Body image distortion is a brain condition where the person is unable to see himself or herself accurately in the mirror and perceives features and body size as distorted. Malnourishment is known to create this illusion, possibly an adaptation to famine where the person will continue to feel well-fed and pursue food for the community. The image the individual perceives may be huge despite an actual state of emaciation. The distortion affects touch as well; anorexics may physically feel that their arms, thighs, or stomachs are many times their actual size. Researchers have identified parts of the brain that appear to control or process body image information.

Source: Excerpted from "Eating Disorders Glossary," © 2012 Families Empowered and Supporting Treatment of Eating Disorders (www.feast-ed.org).

Learning To Love What You See In The Mirror

We all want to look our best, but a healthy body is not always linked to appearance. In fact, healthy bodies come in all shapes and sizes. Changing your body image means changing the way you think about your body. At the same time, healthy lifestyle choices are also key to improving body image.

- Healthy eating can promote healthy skin and hair, along with strong bones.
- Regular exercise has been shown to boost self-esteem, self-image, and energy levels.
- Plenty of rest is key to stress management.

Source: "About Body Image," Office on Women's Health, September 2009.

Although there is no single known cause of eating disorders, several things may contribute to the development of these disorders:

- **Culture:** In the United States extreme thinness is a social and cultural ideal, and women partially define themselves by how physically attractive they are.

- **Personal Characteristics:** Feelings of helplessness, worthlessness, and poor self-image often accompany eating disorders.

- **Other Emotional Disorders:** Other mental health problems, like depression or anxiety, occur along with eating disorders.

- **Stressful Events Or Life Changes:** Things like starting a new school or job or being teased and traumatic events like rape can lead to the onset of eating disorders.

- **Biology:** Studies are being done to look at genes, hormones, and chemicals in the brain that may have an effect on the development of, and recovery from, eating disorders.

- **Families:** Parents' attitudes about appearance and diet can affect their kids' attitudes. Also, if your mother or sister has bulimia, you are more likely to have it.

Over-Exercising

Too much of a good thing can be very bad for you. Just like eating disorders, societal pressures to be thin can also push women to exercise too much. Over-exercise is when someone engages in strenuous physical activity to the point that is unsafe and unhealthy. In fact, some studies indicate that young women who are compelled to exercise at excessive levels are at risk for developing eating disorders.

Eating disorders and over-exercising go hand-in-hand—they both can be a result of an unhealthy obsession with your body. The most dangerous aspect of over-exercising is the ease with which it can go unrecognized. The condition can be easily hidden by an emphasis on fitness or a desire to be healthy. Like bulimia and anorexia, in which persons deny themselves adequate nutrition by restrictive eating behaviors, over-exercising is a controlled behavior that denies the body the energy and nutrition needed to maintain a healthy weight.

According to the *American Journal of Sports Medicine*, a host of physical consequences can result from over-exercising—pulled muscles, stress fractures, knee trauma, shin splints, strained hamstrings, and ripped tendons.

Remember, fitness should be done within limits and integrated into your lifestyle, done in moderation like everything else in life. If exercising is getting in the way of your daily activities or relationships, you may need to slow down.

Chapter 7

Genetics And The Impact Of Culture On Eating Disorders

There is renewed interest and research into genetic influences on the development of eating disorders. This article looks at some of the assumptions underpinning this research.

Classical Views On Genes

Most of us are captured by the classical idea of genes as hereditary factors that control the characteristics of living things. With this view, to say that the gene or genes for a characteristic have been found, implies both that certain genes determine or control the characteristic and that they have been identified. Today's molecular biology brings us an understanding of genes that undermines this view. A gene is now understood to be a sequence of DNA containing the code to make a protein. Very few characteristics or diseases are the direct result of a single or even several such proteins. In spite of this, the classical view continues to affect the way that genetic influences are seen and discussed.

New Understanding Of Genes

While every analogy has its limits, here is one that might help explain this new understanding. A gene or set of genes might be compared to an idea or set of ideas for a novel. If the author never writes the novel, the ideas influence nothing. If the author proceeds to write the novel, the ideas have a very strong influence at the beginning of the writing process, but quite early in the process, the characters, setting, and plot may interact and develop according to principles not restricted by the original novel ideas, each influencing the other. J.K. Rowling, for example, recently described the death of a character in *Harry Potter and the Order of the Phoenix* as deeply upsetting to her, perhaps not something that had been part of her original idea, and yet consistent with the logic of the characters and events of the novel.

Suppose that our author's novel is published and eventually is to become a Hollywood movie. The screenwriter chosen to adapt the novel for the screen brings his or her own ideas to influence the story. The American studio system brings many other influences to bear as well: economics, ideology, censorship, star-promotion, and marketing to name a few. Each new level of operations brings new rules and principles to influence the end result. We may or may not recognize the original author's ideas in the movie version of the novel, however those ideas were involved in the development of the movie. We might say that they made the movie possible, but they definitely did not determine its content.

Similarly with genetic influences, the more complex a level of the organism's functioning we are concerned with, the less direct an influence any proteins coded by genes are likely to have. Eating disorders are complex conditions that involve physiological functioning; thinking processes; behaviors that have individual beneficial effects, like self-comforting; behavioral choices which have cultural value, like the benefits derived from being thin; and individual meanings, like demonstrating one's strength through self-denial, or communicating distress. There are extremely few diseases which are the result of a mutation to a single gene, as Huntington's disease is. In fact, this is one of the reasons that the classical view of genes was overthrown. While genes will be *involved* in eating disorders, like the author's initial ideas for a novel are involved in the movie based on it, we will not find a gene or mutation that *causes* eating disorders.

Susceptibility And Genes

Some researchers have suggested instead that we look for "susceptibility genes" for eating disorders. When an individual has susceptibility genes for a particular disease, he or she is at risk for the disease because it will manifest in a certain environment. Examples given by eating disorders researchers often include the risk of diabetes in people of Asian and Native American ancestry, which becomes manifest in an environment when food is abundant. With some such diseases, we know how to lower or eliminate the risk through environmental changes. For example, phenylketonuria is a hereditary disease caused by the lack of a liver enzyme required to digest phenylalanine, an amino acid most commonly found in protein-containing foods such as meat, cows' milk, and breast milk. This condition can cause brain damage in affected babies, which can be prevented by early detection and manipulation of the feeding environment, that is, eliminating phenylalanine from the child's diet. What these examples have in common is that the illness or disease can be completely defined in physical terms, that biochemical processes specific to the illness are candidates for locating genetic contributions, and that the manifesting environment is physical or biochemical, rather than interpersonal or sociocultural. Suggesting that these conditions are models for what we might find with eating disorders still plays on the classical idea of genes and fails to take into account their significant and qualitative differences from eating disorders.

Environment And Genes

The effects of genes that may be involved with eating disorders have not been established. Some possibilities researchers are investigating include genes that code for proteins involved in neurotransmitter variations (related to serotonin and dopamine, for instance) which differently affect mood, anxiety, and novelty-seeking; or genes that code for proteins involved in information processing tendencies; or those involved in "traits" like perfectionism or perseverance. No environment or set of environments in which genetic susceptibility would necessarily manifest has yet been specified. There is no reason to believe that either separately or together, the current candidate genetic influences would be specific to eating disorders, as we

Important Terms

Brain And Neurobiology Of Eating Disorders: A growing field of research in eating disorders is the use of brain imaging technologies to identify the pathways and structures involved in anorexia and bulimia.

Genes: Hereditary factors that are transmitted by parents to their children and that determine a wide range of characteristics.

Genetic Predisposition: Studies of twins have shown that 50–80% of the risk of developing an eating disorder is genetic. Continued research on the genetic and biological features of eating disorders may reveal additional factors which increase the risk for these conditions.

Neurotransmitters: Chemicals that transmit information from one cell to another in the brain. They effect hormone production and hypothalamic function. In recent studies, symptoms seen in anorexia and bulimia have been shown to correlate to neurotransmission dysfunction in key regions of the brain associated with weight, hunger and satiety, body image, and mood.

Source: Excerpted from "Eating Disorders Glossary," © 2012 Families Empowered and Supporting Treatment of Eating Disorders (www.feast-ed.org).

know them to be involved in other conditions, and we know that eating disorders often occur along with other conditions. We should be skeptical of the susceptibility model until genetics researchers show us, either directly or in relation to more relevant diseases or disorders, how that model would work with the level of physical, behavioral, interpersonal, and socio-cultural complexity at which eating disorders exist.

In some ways, all genes are susceptibility genes for damage, disease, or death given the "right" environmental condition or other. The most extreme example would be the genes that contribute to our needing to breathe oxygen to stay alive. Given an oxygen-deprived environment, the vast majority of us will sustain brain damage or die. The idea of "susceptibility genes" in this case becomes meaningless. It would probably be more accurate just to call the oxygen-deprived environment a poor or poisonous one for human beings. To meaningfully label some set of genes as susceptibility genes for a condition or illness, it should be possible to show that they are specifically connected to the illness or condition and that the environment in which the illness manifests is one that does not harm most people.

Sociocultural Environment

Over the past 30 to 35 years, our sociocultural environment has idealized a body shape for women that minimizes body fat to pre-pubertal levels. This is opposite to the most common genetically influenced direction of development for women's bodies, which is increasing body fat at puberty and later. Thus, girls see their bodies developing in ways that they have been socialized to find offensive. It is no wonder that the vast majority of females in our culture react to finding themselves becoming offensive by trying to change themselves to be more acceptable. Although not all develop diagnosable eating disorders, the vast majority are dissatisfied with their bodies, and persistently act on this dissatisfaction through a range of body and appetite controlling efforts. A culture that sets females at odds with their own development and which supports industries that exploit the insecurities arising from this (e.g., the diet industry), is arguably a poor or poisonous environment for females to live in.

A sociocultural environment does not exist at an abstract external level; rather, it permeates individuals' relationships with one another in institutions like schools and workplaces, in families, in peer groups, and in other interpersonal interactions. When an individual girl is harassed about her body shape, this is not just an individual experience: it is a socioculturally mediated one. Schoolboys can hurt a girl by telling her that she is fat, not because she is actually fat, but because they know it will bother her, giving them the upper hand. Boys doing so are playing on the culture's negative associations with fat, the fact that girls are conditioned to see their personal value as appearance-related, and the power males have in evaluating female bodies. The economic interests satisfied through this culture (and perhaps expanding it currently by creating intense insecurities in boys about their appearances) act as a conservative force against changing it. Sociocultural environments are not neutral; they privilege some people's interests while disadvantaging others and therefore have political implications.

Think about this in relation to a different issue: suppose there are high rates of a criminal behavior like stealing among males living in poverty conditions. We may try to prevent the development of stealing among boys living in poverty by educating them that theft is wrong, teaching them techniques to help them resist impulses to steal, providing them with medications to reduce their impulsive behaviors, and so on. At the same time, let's say we know that a small percentage of them are said to have genetic loading for impulsive behavior and novelty-seeking, and are therefore likely to steal, especially when their culture bombards them with images of consumables that others purchase with ease, and that their culture values men who have big purchasing power. Let's say we also know that in cultures that don't hold these values and in which families are protected from poverty, stealing among males is radically reduced. What would we think about providing millions of dollars for genetics research, while paying lip service to the cultural and poverty issues?

Potential Contributions Of Genetic Research

Researchers in the field of genes and eating disorders suggest a number of potentially helpful contributions from their research. While these are currently appropriately vague, they may become more precise if it becomes possible to specify the involvement of particular genes and particular environments in these disorders. So far, the focus seems to be on refining practices that we already have, or could have, for example developing medications that could more specifically target individuals' neurotransmitter differences; teaching parents how to recognize early signs of perfectionism or obsessiveness, and how to help themselves and their children to use these to their own advantage, rather than be dominated by them; and guiding children to choose activities that do not exacerbate the effects of traits like perfectionism. These efforts might increase someone's ability to resist an eating disorder, but they will not provide a genetic prevention or cure in the classical sense.

It is true that if we could specify the genetic influences, we could also learn about protective factors by finding people who have the genes but don't develop eating disorders. While some boys and men do develop eating disorders, being male remains a major protective factor. It is tempting to suggest that the most effective gene therapy for eating disorders would consist of adding a Y chromosome to all "susceptible" females. A modest proposal.

Chapter 8

Media And Eating Disorders

The media are held responsible for the supposed growth of eating disorders in the country. To what extent is this true? In this short article I would like to separate myth from fact, and to provide the reader with some articles that might help them decide which is the cause and which is effect.

What Is The Media?

The media is an important aspect of life in our culture. About 95% of people own a TV set and watch for an average of three to four hours per day. By the end of the last century over 60% of men and 50% of women read a newspaper each day, and nearly half of all girls, from the age of seven read a girls magazine each week. In addition, people interact with a wide variety of other media such as music delivered by CDs or videos and communications via personal computers.

Each form of medium has a different purpose and content. The media seek to inform us, persuade us, entertain us, and change us. The media also seeks to engage large groups of people so that advertisers can sell them products or services by making them desirable. Other institutions such as governments also engage the public via the media to make ideas and values desirable. Institutions from politics to corporations can use the media to influence our behavior. We can trace our involvement with the media back to the drum messages of the Indians, the shouts of the town crier. All that has changed are the multitudinous ways in which information passes to us and the increasing sophistication of the media providers.

About This Chapter: "The Media and Eating Disorders," by Deanne Jade, © 2009 National Centre For Eating Disorders (www.eatingdisorders.org.uk). Reprinted with permission.

The argument about whether the media shape society or merely reflect current or nascent trends is constantly under debate. Before the Second World War, it was believed that the media "injects" values and morals into society. However, social research in the 1960s showed that the audience is not a passive receiver of moral values. Society is constructed of many different subcultures, classified by factors such as race, social class, political outlook, adhesion to value systems such as "vegetarianism," or lifestyles (such as "cocooners" (Popcorn 1999 [term coined by Faith Popcorn]). These differing social groups select and filter information and reject messages that are not consistent with the values of that group. On the other hand, irrespective of social clusters, research has shown that it is those with low confidence and self esteem within each group who are most influenced by media communications.

So there have been many debates about the influence of the media and social behavior, for example sexual morality or violence. We recognize, as a result of these debates, that the interaction between message and response is complex and audience dependent. To quote the British Medical Association (BMA) report on eating disorders, body image and the media:

> "In a media saturated culture, the argument that long term exposure can help shape the world views of particular sections of the audience is one that merits consideration, however, the EXTENT to which the media contribute to the personal identity remains unclear and is subject to continuing academic debate....the media do not, by their very definition, provide pure experience of the world but channel our experience of it in particular ways."

In other words, all research into the media must take into account the different levels of attention, and interpretation of individuals with different motivations, personalities, immediate situations, and sociocultural contexts who bring different information processing strategies to the task.

The latest "postmodern" thinking on the role of media is that it provides learning that is incidental rather than direct, and it is a significant part of the acculturation process.

Now the battle centers on a new morality of food and eating. We accuse the media, by glorifying the culture of thinness, of causing an epidemic of eating distress, especially among young women. The media denies culpability, or at least responsibility for doing anything about it. Kelly Brownell, a U.S. expert in eating disorders, argues that the media contribute to a toxic environment in which eating disorders may be more likely to occur. This is because of the "Damaging Paradox" of modern society in which the media promotes, in a compelling manner, a low weight sculptured ideal body.

At the same time the environment provides an increasing array of foods high in fat and calories, with compelling pressures to consume these products. As a result we are getting heavier, and the gap between the ideal and normal body weight is giving rise to anxiety. We seek to reduce this anxiety by reducing our body weight, the preferred method being to go on a diet, since we believe that weight is under our control and, in addition we believe that once weight is lost it should not be regained. But dieting causes rebound binge eating and attempts to deal with this, by going on further diets, will lead many people into a disturbed relationships with food.

There are other dangers arising from this cultural paradox. The models and actors who promote consumption of these calorie laden foods are usually slim and attractive, which would not be possible in a real world if they actually ate these foods. This will add to the cultural confusion, which is said to nurture the onset of eating distress. To what extent are these accusations true?

Is There An Increase In Eating Disorders?

There is no doubt that the ideal body size, as reflected in the style icons promoted in the media, is getting thinner. This ideal body size epitomized by "Gerri Halliwell" "Posh Spice" or "Ally Mcbeal" is unrealistically thin, their body mass index (BMI) is on the borders of what a clinician would regard as anorexic. Due to the proliferation of food in our culture, people are getting bigger, fatter, and maturing younger and younger as the years pass by. The gap between actual body sizes and the cultural ideal is getting wider, and giving rise to anxiety among almost all women, although it is the most vulnerable who are most affected by this.

There is a lot of dieting going on as a result, because dieting is viewed as the solution to the problem of "excess weight," even if the excess is just all in the mind, as a result of faulty messages from "out there." There is evidence from dieting studies that twice as many people diet as need to; in other words' of all people who diet, half are not even overweight. However, dieting doesn't inevitably lead to anorexia. Anorexia is not a slimming disease.

To push the point home, there is no strong evidence of an increase in anorexia. There are more reported cases coming to the attention of services, but we believe that this is just because we now know so much more about the illness. Hence we are more likely to recognize it rather than hide it away. There are more services available so the anorexic person is identified rather than left to fight the illness on their own. It is hard therefore to justify an accusation that exposure to supermodels will cause our teenagers to develop anorexia.

Dieting behaviors are however a risk factor for the other eating disorders, compulsive eating and its variant, bulimia nervosa, an illness in which the sufferer, usually a young woman but many men suffer too—diets, experiences rebound binge eating due to food deprivation and then purges to rid herself of unwanted calories. Compulsive eating is a direct outcome of rebellion against food restraint, a behavior that can rapidly turn into a remorseless habit. On the other hand, bulimia is an illness which may start out as a useful strategy to control weight gain but rapidly develops into an addictive illness, which engulfs the sufferer and becomes a way of coping with emotional difficulties.

Studies of prevalence show that bulimia nervosa is on the increase, although again these figures may just reflect a growing awareness of the disorder or an increased provision of services. People are more likely to apply for help. Still, the link between the media and bulimia is tenuous. Women feel pressure from many sides to control their weight, from the media but also from their peers, from boyfriends, from parents, and from the fashion shops that carry clothes in ranges and sizes that suit only the smallest among them.

What Power Does The Media Actually Have

There is no doubt that the media provides significant content on body related issues to young women, over 50% of whom, (between the ages of 11–15 years) read fashion and beauty related magazines. The exposure to ideal images coincides with a period in their lives where self regard and self efficacy is in decline, where body image is at its most fragile due to physical changes of puberty, and where the tendency for social comparison is at its peak. Girls thus find themselves in a subculture of dieting, reflecting messages not only from the media but also from parents, peers, and members of the opposite sex, as well as the media.

Analysis of media content both provide a stream of articles on weight control, either through fitness or food control, and physical beauty, together with models whose curvaceousness has declined steadily over the period from 1959–1978 (Guillen and Barr [Eileen O. Guillen and Susan I. Barr, "Nutrition, dieting, and fitness messages in a magazine for adolescent women, 1970–1990," *Journal of Adolescent Health*, 15, 464–472, 1994. And D.M. Garner, P.E. Garfinkel, and D. Schwartz, "Cultural expectations of thinness in women," *Psychological Reports* 47:483–491, 1980.]). In all cases, the emphasis on diet or fitness was designed to help someone become more physically attractive and thus acquire status.

In the late 1990s, there was a fair degree of comment from the media about Sindy dolls sold to girls under the age of puberty, with an impossible bust to waist ratio and impossibly long, lean legs. The accusation was that Sindy dolls would "encourage anorexia" by providing young girls with an adult body shape that they would aspire to but never achieve. Various experts appeared on radio and TV accusing the manufacturer of social irresponsibility.

It must be pointed out however, that while it is true that growing and adult women are exposed to thin images and many article on diet and fitness, this fact tells us little about how these messages are received by the audience or by parts of it.

How Messages Are Received

There have been a number of studies, which attempted to combine analysis of the content of messages with studies of attitudes or behavior to assess the impact of images or messages.

However, we are warned to guard against the short-term view of media influence on body image or eating behaviors, rather than assess the long-term outcome of exposure to certain images and values, or even to assess the effect of exposure to any set of values independently of the "shifting sands" of social and technological change.

Some of these studies point to a measurable, short-term association between reduced self esteem, heightened anxiety or anger and depression, and exposure to culturally ideal body shapes, less among men and more among women. However there is no way to know how or if this anxiety persists over time or translates into future dieting or aberrant eating behaviors. One other study showed that there was no relationship between body dissatisfaction and the number of hours of TV watched per week, although there was a relationship between body anxiety and number of hours spent watching soap operas. Drive for thinness, a different construct, is related significantly to watching pop or music videos among adolescent girls. Women in a variety of studies consistently report that magazines influence their idea of what a good body shape is, and lead to determination to lose weight with subsequent dieting behaviors.

These findings must be interpreted against the fact that women tend to overestimate their body size, a feature that extents back to early days of puberty. Waller and Hamilton have an interesting view of the effects of the media in this respect. They claim that the media may act as a "negative reinforcer of body size overestimation, which may lead to eating disorder" [K. Hamilton and G. Waller, "Media influences on body size estimation in anorexia and bulimia. An experimental study," *British Journal of Psychiatry*, 62:837–40, June 1993.] In other words, the media doesn't make women feel a need to be thinner per se, but the media may assist them in feeling bigger than they already feel themselves to be. The starting position for many females is thus a built-in vulnerability, which is reinforced by the culture of the media. This view must be considered alongside other, parallel studies on body image. These show that the development of body image over time, a more useful predictor of protection from eating distress, is dynamic and affected by many variables, including exposure to traumatic events, body issues in childhood and general self esteem derived from core personality traits.

Cross Cultural Studies

Many cultures have conferred status on a slim body size, for example in China—and some have had a preference for large builds for both sexes, such as in Polynesia. Anne Becker, an anthropologist of Harvard Medical School, who has worked extensively with the Fiji population, has shown that exposure to western ideals of beauty have led to a high percentage of adolescents dieting within the last decade. It is hard to prove that it is exposure to TV images which have caused this change, although it is reasonable to assume that this is the case.

Media Influences On Body-Image, Eating Behavior, And Self Esteem

It is hard to evaluate the relationship between the media and eating disorder without considering the multifaceted impact of media messages on body size, on food consumption, on the desirability of certain foods and their consequent consumption, and other matters relating to personal identity and status.

The media can have many influences in relation to food and eating including:

1. It confers hidden meanings on food—nostalgia, sexiness, being a good housewife and mother, rewarding oneself, having uninhibited fun, etc., and creates unnatural drives for food.

2. The media can persuade us that wrong eating habits are right and natural. I cite the case of a MacDonald's advertisement recently in which a young boy persuades both his parents to take him for a burger and chips rather than a healthy outing at the zoo.

3. The media can create anxieties about being deprived if we don't have what "everyone else" is having.

4. The media presents us with an idealized shape which is invested with attributes of being attractive, desirable, successful, and loveable but which is unattainable without resorting to sinister or dangerous eating habits.

5. The media perpetuates the feeling in people who do not have the ideal shape that their life would be fine if they were slim.

What Is Body Image?

Body image is an important part of self-identity and self esteem. We all have a body image which is defined as the physical and cognitive representation of the body which includes values about how we should look along many dimensions (age, size, height, color, attractiveness, etc.) and emotional feelings connected to acceptance or rejection. Body image is closely connected to self-esteem. It is possible to have low self worth and a good body image if other aspects of functioning are important. On the other hand it is hard to maintain good self worth if one's body image is disturbed.

It is believed that women and men configure an internalized ideal body and compare their actual or perceived actual shape against the socially represented ideal (Myers and Biocca) [Philip N. Myers, Jr. and Frank A. Biocca, "The Elastic Body Image: The Effects of Television Advertising and Programming on Body Image Distortions on Young Women," *Journal of Communications* 1–26, 1992.] This presents a body image which is elastic in that it will feel different at different times and in different contexts, such as being on a beach in a swimsuit.

We have already explained both that the ideal body has become smaller, thinner, and differently shaped over the past 20 years. The ideal body is now sculptured, pared of fat (with a BMI that would place most models firmly in the anorexic category), with narrow hips, a small waist, and rounded breasts, a stature which can only be achieved by most women with the help of surgery since under conditions of weight loss breast tissue tends to shrink.

This may explain two factors:

1. Why women consistently overestimate their weight, and

2. Why dieting behaviors are so prevalent. Over half of all dieters are not overweight, which means that of all people currently dieting, one in every two doesn't need to. Dieters, especially young ones, tend not to be responsible in their eating habits. We define this as "normative discontent," referring to the fact that poor body image is normal among women in today's society. But what is worrying is that, responding to this low level of body dissatisfaction; women may be harming themselves with their responses. On a study of 869 Australian diets in 1998, one third were using extreme methods such as fasting, crash dieting, smoking, or drugs, in the belief that these methods would be harmless.

It would seem that the media doesn't simply make the ideal body desirable, these dieting behaviors spring from an epidemic of low esteem, stress, guilt, and depression about having a body that falls short of the cultural ideal. People who diet believe that they look bad, and that this will affect their ability to get a good job or attract members of the opposite sex unless they are thinner. This is true to a certain extent. Research shows clearly that overweight women suffer in a number of important respects. They are less likely to be accepted into higher education, they have lower salaries; they are less likely to date in adolescence and are less likely to be married in adult life. Conversely, graduate career women are more likely to feel guilty about eating than any other target group.

This finding reflects the conflicting pressures on women of today which are reflected in media. Women are supposed to be thin, attractive, and successful in the workplace and in academia, while maintaining feminine characteristics of nurturing, maternal, warm, socially engaging, and givers. It is thought that women who cannot reconcile these roles and who feel out of control of their lives may turn to the control of weight to regain a sense of coping. However this is just a hypothesis.

The Media As Risk Factors For Eating Disorders

It is hard to separate the influence of the media in the development of eating disorders. Various studies point to the correlation between low self-esteem in young girls and high scores on eating distress measures as they grow. Self-esteem is a dynamic construct, like body image, which is influenced by a whole variety of factors such as parenting, childhood experiences, core personality, and body image especially in girls. It follows thus by logical reduction that influences on body image will affect self esteem and promote the risk of developing an eating disorder as a person turns to the control of their body in order to feel acceptable. In this respect the media may contribute to low self-esteem by promoting slenderness as the pathway to gaining love, acceptance, and respect while at the same time reflecting a trend in society to demonize fat. When women are asked what they fear most in life, most will cite the possibility of gaining weight. When women are asked what they least like about themselves most will describe a part of their body (usually stomach, thighs, legs) rather than no physical attributes like laziness or low confidence. Men conversely are more likely to mention nonphysical attributes. When women are asked what men find attractive in them, most mention physical appearance. Women thus feel judged by their looks rather than their other resources.

Esteem isn't the only risk factor for an eating disorder. Traumatic childhood experiences, timing of puberty, family functioning, emotional resilience, exposure to unhealthy eating patterns in other people, family concerns about weight, fear of growing up, sexuality problems, bullying, loss, and history of dieting, all may have an influence on a person's relationship with food. So we can conclude that the media may both steer and reflect our cultural obsession with how we look and what we put into our mouths.

Advertising Policies And The Counter Argument

Some institutions in government, psychology, and the media industry itself, are becoming concerned about the use of thin models to promote goods and service. There was a government [UK] "thin summit" in 2000 to which moguls of the magazine industry were invited. In a similar vein, the Independent Television Commission has issued guidelines stating that it is desirable to ensure that advertising does not stimulate unhealthy attitudes to eating and that is must not imply that being underweight is desirable.

Illness-Denying Risks

Pro-Ana: Refers to a sub-culture of individuals, mainly on-line, who believe that being anorexic is a lifestyle choice rather than an eating disorder/illness that requires treatment. The term is often shortened to "ana." There are various online organizations that differ in their stances, but most maintain that they exist to provide a safe and non-judgmental environment for individuals with anorexia to turn in order to discuss their illness, situation, and support those that chose to leave and seek recovery. Some deny that eating disorders are illnesses and discourage individuals from seeking treatment, provide tips and strategies on how to hide the symptoms, alter weight, or engage in symptoms, i.e. tricks for avoiding eating around family members, ways to alter your weight at doctors' appointments, how to dress to hide weight loss, etc. There are many dangers associated with individuals with eating disorders going to such sites or being involved in such organizations:

- They normalize the illness leading to minimization of symptoms/consequences.
- Negative influences are present that teach individuals who are already sick and vulnerable new "tricks."
- They fuel preoccupation with the illness leading to over-identification with the illness.
- They contribute to further isolation from available sources of support by providing pseudo online support.
- They promote unhealthy motivation called "thinspiration" and comradery in losing weight and staying sick.

Thinspiration: Any form of media, print, online, pictures, videos, etc. that are utilized in an unhealthy manner to promote continued weight loss. This information can take the form of images of slim celebrities, individuals afflicted with an eating disorder or emaciated models and is often exchanged amongst members of online pro-eating disorder communities (pro-ana, pro-mia). Reverse thinspiraton can include posting pictures of oneself at a high weight on mirrors or in the kitchen in attempts to induce guilt and prevent eating or pictures of morbidly obese individuals to facilitate disgust and motivate weight loss. Thinspiration can also include poems, music lyrics, quotes, sayings, etc. that encourage weight loss, promote the eating disorder, and endorse it as being a life style and choice rather than an illness.

Source: Excerpted from "Eating Disorders Glossary," © 2012 Families Empowered and Supporting Treatment of Eating Disorders (www.feast-ed.org).

Good in theory, but this is a policy which has not had significant impact on the sizes of models in magazines, nor of the size of girls in music bands. Celebrities continue to attract attention for their weight loss rather than their accomplishments, and the greater the furor about their size the more attention they receive. The new "celebrity anorexia" may be creating more ripples in society than any former use of models in fashion shoots.

As a direct repose to "do-gooders" in some sections of the media, a wristwatch manufacturer used an excessively thin model to advertise his watch. Many publishers, while paying lip service to a policy of self acceptance at any weight, continue to print pictures of slim models, run articles about dieting and fitness, and promote all sorts of esoteric eating plans. It is felt that the new wave of articles on healthy eating is just dieting in another guise, the objective being to manage health through control of weight thereby undermining such defenses as may exist against dieting per se. These new wave articles are so compelling, that, viewed against a background of increasing confusion about what is good or bad to eat, they are creating a new eating disorder known as "orthorexia." This is a condition where the sufferer becomes wedded to stringent eating plans (such as food combining or anti-allergy plans) which imply weight loss and which mask a profound unhealthy relationship with food.

Some style setters in the media frankly refuse to adjust their policies, they say, not unreasonably, that women like to look at perfect bodies, they won't buy magazines with pictures of ordinary people, and that they are not quite as silly to believe that these fantasy figures, photographically enhanced in many cases, are bodies that they should aspire to. This is to a certain extent confirmed by my own discussions with teenage girls in schools who are fully aware that diet and exercise would not be enough to get you looking like a model in a magazine.

The Media And The Obesity Epidemic

There is one aspect of media policy which has largely been ignored, because of over concern with thin images. This is the use of media to promote unhealthy eating attitudes which may be contributing to a national epidemic of obesity, which in itself will provoke damaging eating strategies as our ever-expanding nation seeks to control its weight. An individual watching television for two hours per day will see over 20,000 food advertisements in one year, most promoting foods high in sugar and fat, mainly urging us to eat for reasons that have little to do with survival. The problem is ever worse for children. During child-friendly broadcasting hours, they are exposed to a continual stream of advertisements for sweets, chocolate, and sugar-laden cereals. This aspect of media functioning supports the food industry in contributing to a significant effect on future problems with eating and with weight.

Positive Media Influences

The media does not influence eating patterns or self-esteem in an exclusively negative fashion. Broadcast and written media can be a source of valuable information on health and well-being. In addition, awareness of eating disorders, through magazines, articles, and television programs may educate people about the danger of abusing food, and may help to make sufferers aware that they have a problem and they are not alone.

In this respect the media may have two useful roles: the first in health promotion for the public at large, the second, in the arena of primary prevention. Health promotion seeks to promote healthful behaviors or attitudes to the public at large. Primary prevention is defined as an activity designed to eliminate or render ineffective, factors involved in the causation of a disorder and an activity designed to strengthen the host against noxious influences.

From this definition it can be seen that the media both opposes and contributes to health promotion and primary prevention.

It has been suggested that the media might respond to its critics in the following ways:

1. Present a greater variety of body shapes and sizes in photos, in the music industry, as television presenters, etc.

2. Should discourage dieting

3. Should assist people with an influence on young people (such as parents, teachers) from making weight an issue

4. Provide positive fat role models

5. Should not glamorize celebrities who lose weight

It is expected that such changes, if they were put in place, would take a while to filter down through society before any significant shift in attitudes could be achieved.

Can The Media Change Attitudes Against Current Trends?

Would all this work anyway? My personal view is that it would not. There is a larger dynamic behind cultural trends, which drive behaviors, cultural values, and attitudes. Such changes would be swimming against the tide. I do believe, therefore, that the media is sensitive to these emerging trends and brings them to the surface. In this respect they are seen to be trend creators, yet they are just mirrors of patterns which already exist.

In addition we are not isolated, but are part of a global culture. The trends cross the entire developed world are consistent in their glamorization of slenderness and youth as a feminine, and increasingly a masculine ideal.

The media would find it hard to convince the national psyche, therefore, that thinness is not a desirable ideal. By promoting sensible messages, however, they may impact on those individuals in society who are vulnerable and who may otherwise filter unhealthy messages, which will lead them into a path towards developing eating disorders.

Chapter 9

Eating Disorders Statistics

General

- Almost 50% of people with eating disorders meet the criteria for depression.

- Only 1 in 10 men and women with eating disorders receive treatment. Only 35% of people that receive treatment for eating disorders get treatment at a specialized facility for eating disorders.

- Up to 24 million people of all ages and genders suffer from an eating disorder (anorexia, bulimia, and binge eating disorder) in the U.S.

- Eating disorders have the highest mortality rate of any mental illness.

Students

- 91% of women surveyed on a college campus had attempted to control their weight through dieting. 22% dieted "often" or "always."

- 86% report onset of eating disorder by age 20; 43% report onset between ages of 16 and 20.

- Anorexia is the third most common chronic illness among adolescents.

- 95% of those who have eating disorders are between the ages of 12 and 25.

- 25% of college-aged women engage in bingeing and purging as a weight-management technique.

About This Chapter: "Eating Disorder Statistics," © 2012 National Association of Anorexia Nervosa and Associated Disorders (www.anad.org). All rights reserved. Reprinted with permission. The complete text of this document including references is available at http://www.anad.org.

- The mortality rate associated with anorexia nervosa is 12 times higher than the death rate associated with all causes of death for females 15–24 years old.

- Over one-half of teenage girls and nearly one-third of teenage boys use unhealthy weight control behaviors such as skipping meals, fasting, smoking cigarettes, vomiting, and taking laxatives.

- In a survey of 185 female students on a college campus, 58% felt pressure to be a certain weight, and of the 83% that dieted for weight loss, 44% were of normal weight.

Men

- An estimated 10–15% of people with anorexia or bulimia are male.

- Men are less likely to seek treatment for eating disorders because of the perception that they are "woman's diseases."

- Among gay men, nearly 14% appeared to suffer from bulimia and over 20% appeared to be anorexic.

Media, Perception, Dieting

- 95% of all dieters will regain their lost weight within five years.

- 35% of "normal dieters" progress to pathological dieting. Of those, 20–25% progress to partial or full-syndrome eating disorders.

- The body type portrayed in advertising as the ideal is possessed naturally by only 5% of American females.

- 47% of girls in 5th–12th grade reported wanting to lose weight because of magazine pictures.

- 69% of girls in 5th–12th grade reported that magazine pictures influenced their idea of a perfect body shape.

- 42% of 1st–3rd grade girls want to be thinner.

- 81% of 10 year olds are afraid of being fat.

For Women

- Women are much more likely than men to develop an eating disorder. Only an estimated 5 to 15 percent of people with anorexia or bulimia are male.

- An estimated 0.5 to 3.7 percent of women suffer from anorexia nervosa in their lifetime. Research suggests that about 1 percent of female adolescents have anorexia.

- An estimated 1.1 to 4.2 percent of women have bulimia nervosa in their lifetime.

- An estimated 2 to 5 percent of Americans experience binge-eating disorder in a six-month period.

- About 50 percent of people who have had anorexia develop bulimia or bulimic patterns.

- 20% of people suffering from anorexia will prematurely die from complications related to their eating disorder, including suicide and heart problems.

Mortality Rates

Although eating disorders have the highest mortality rate of any mental disorder, the mortality rates reported on those who suffer from eating disorders can vary considerably between studies and sources. Part of the reason why there is a large variance in the reported number of deaths caused by eating disorders is because those who suffer from an eating disorder may ultimately die of heart failure, organ failure, malnutrition, or suicide. Often, the medical complications of death are reported instead of the eating disorder that compromised a person's health.

According to a study done by colleagues at the *American Journal of Psychiatry* (2009), crude mortality rates were:

- 4% for anorexia nervosa

- 3.9% for bulimia nervosa

- 5.2% for eating disorder not otherwise specified

Athletes

- Risk Factors: In judged sports—sports that score participants—prevalence of eating disorders is 13% (compared with 3% in refereed sports).

- Significantly higher rates of eating disorders found in elite athletes (20%), than in a female control group (9%).

- Female athletes in aesthetic sports (for example, gymnastics, ballet, figure skating) found to be at the highest risk for eating disorders.

- A comparison of the psychological profiles of athletes and those with anorexia found these factors in common: perfectionism, high self-expectations, competitiveness, hyperactivity, repetitive exercise routines, compulsiveness, drive, tendency toward depression, body image distortion, pre-occupation with dieting and weight.

Part Two
Understanding Eating Disorders
And Body Image Disorders

Chapter 10

Anorexia Nervosa

What is anorexia nervosa?

A person with anorexia nervosa, often called anorexia, has an intense fear of gaining weight. Someone with anorexia thinks about food a lot and limits the food she or he eats, even though she or he is too thin. Anorexia is more than just a problem with food. It's a way of using food or starving oneself to feel more in control of life and to ease tension, anger, and anxiety. Most people with anorexia are female. An anorexic often has these characteristics:

- Has a low body weight for her or his height
- Resists keeping a normal body weight
- Has an intense fear of gaining weight
- Thinks she or he is fat even when very thin
- Misses three menstrual periods in a row (for girls/women who have started having their periods)

Who becomes anorexic?

While anorexia mostly affects girls and women (85–95 percent of anorexics are female), it can also affect boys and men. It was once thought that women of color were shielded from eating disorders by their cultures, which tend to be more accepting of different body sizes. It is not known for sure whether African American, Latina, Asian/Pacific Islander, and American Indian and Alaska Native people develop eating disorders because American culture values

About This Chapter: From "Anorexia Nervosa Fact Sheet," Office on Women's Health (www.womenshealth.gov), June 2009.

thin people. People with different cultural backgrounds may develop eating disorders because it's hard to adapt to a new culture (a theory called "culture clash"). The stress of trying to live in two different cultures may cause some minorities to develop their eating disorders.

What causes anorexia?

There is no single known cause of anorexia. Eating disorders are real, treatable medical illnesses with causes in both the body and the mind. Some of these things may play a part:

- **Culture:** Women in the U.S. are under constant pressure to fit a certain ideal of beauty. Seeing images of flawless, thin females everywhere makes it hard for women to feel good about their bodies. More and more, women are also feeling pressure to have a perfect body.

- **Families:** If you have a mother or sister with anorexia, you are more likely to develop the disorder. Parents who think looks are important, diet themselves, or criticize their children's bodies are more likely to have a child with anorexia.

- **Life Changes Or Stressful Events:** Traumatic events (like rape) as well as stressful things (like starting a new job), can lead to the onset of anorexia.

- **Personality Traits:** Someone with anorexia may not like her or himself, hate the way she or he looks, or feel hopeless. She or he often sets hard-to-reach goals for her or himself and tries to be perfect in every way.

- **Biology:** Genes, hormones, and chemicals in the brain may be factors in developing anorexia.

What are signs of anorexia?

Someone with anorexia may look very thin. She or he may use extreme measures to lose weight by doing the following:

- Making herself or himself throw up

- Taking pills to urinate or have a bowel movement

- Taking diet pills

- Not eating or eating very little

- Exercising a lot, even in bad weather or when hurt or tired

- Weighing food and counting calories

- Eating very small amounts of only certain foods

- Moving food around the plate instead of eating it

Someone with anorexia may also have a distorted body image, shown by thinking she or he is fat, wearing baggy clothes, weighing her or himself many times a day, and fearing weight gain.

Anorexia can also cause someone to not act like her or himself. She or he may talk about weight and food all the time, not eat in front of others, be moody or sad, or not want to go out with friends. People with anorexia may also have other psychiatric and physical illnesses, including the following:

- Depression
- Anxiety
- Obsessive behavior
- Substance abuse
- Issues with the heart and/or brain
- Problems with physical development

What happens to your body with anorexia?

With anorexia, your body doesn't get the energy from foods that it needs, so it slows down. Look at the picture in Figure 10.1 to find out how anorexia affects your health.

Can someone with anorexia get better?

Yes. Someone with anorexia can get better. A health care team of doctors, nutritionists, and therapists will help bring the person back to a normal weight, treat any psychological issues related to anorexia, and help the person get rid of any actions or thoughts that cause the eating disorder. These three steps will prevent relapse (relapse means to get sick again, after feeling well for a while).

Some research suggests that the use of medicines—such as antidepressants, antipsychotics, or mood stabilizers—may sometimes work for anorexic patients. It is thought that these medicines help the mood and anxiety symptoms that often co-exist with anorexia. Other recent studies, however, suggest that antidepressants may not stop some patients with anorexia from relapsing. Also, no medicine has shown to work 100 percent of the time during the important first step of restoring a patient to healthy weight. So, it is not clear if and how medications can help anorexic patients get better, but research is still ongoing.

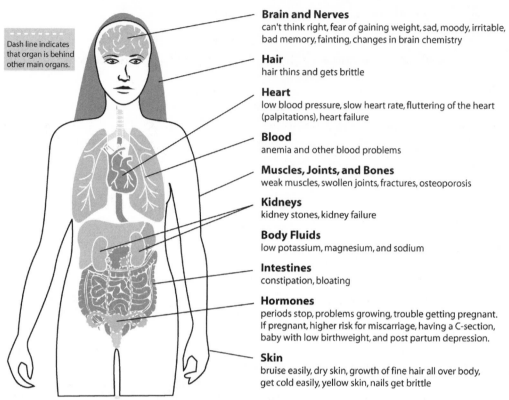

Brain and Nerves
can't think right, fear of gaining weight, sad, moody, irritable, bad memory, fainting, changes in brain chemistry

Hair
hair thins and gets brittle

Heart
low blood pressure, slow heart rate, fluttering of the heart (palpitations), heart failure

Blood
anemia and other blood problems

Muscles, Joints, and Bones
weak muscles, swollen joints, fractures, osteoporosis

Kidneys
kidney stones, kidney failure

Body Fluids
low potassium, magnesium, and sodium

Intestines
constipation, bloating

Hormones
periods stop, problems growing, trouble getting pregnant. If pregnant, higher risk for miscarriage, having a C-section, baby with low birthweight, and post partum depression.

Skin
bruise easily, dry skin, growth of fine hair all over body, get cold easily, yellow skin, nails get brittle

Dash line indicates that organ is behind other main organs.

Figure 10.1. Anorexia Affects Your Whole Body.

Some forms of psychotherapy can help make the psychological reasons for anorexia better. Psychotherapy is sometimes known as talk therapy. It uses different ways of communicating to change a patient's thoughts or behavior. This kind of therapy can be useful for treating eating disorders in young patients who have not had anorexia for a long time.

Individual counseling can help someone with anorexia. If the patient is young, counseling may involve the whole family. Support groups may also be a part of treatment. In support groups, patients, and families meet and share what they've been through.

Some researchers point out that prescribing medicines and using psychotherapy designed just for anorexic patients works better at treating anorexia than just psychotherapy alone. Whether or not a treatment works, though, depends on the person involved and his or her situation. Unfortunately, no one kind of psychotherapy always works for treating adults with anorexia.

Is it safe for young people to take antidepressants for anorexia?

It may be safe for young people to be treated with antidepressants. However, drug companies who make antidepressants are required to post a black box warning label on the medication. A black box warning is the most serious type of warning on prescription drugs. It may be possible that antidepressants make children, adolescents, and young adults more likely to think about suicide or commit suicide. The latest information from the U.S. Food and Drug Administration (FDA)—including what drugs are included in this warning and things to look for—can be found on the FDA website at http://www.fda.gov.

What is outpatient care for anorexia treatment and how is it different from inpatient care?

With outpatient care, the patient receives treatment through visits with members of their health care team. Often this means going to a doctor's office. Outpatients usually live at home.

Some patients may need partial hospitalization. This means that the person goes to the hospital during the day for treatment, but sleeps at home at night.

Sometimes, the patient goes to a hospital and stays there for treatment. This is called inpatient care. After leaving the hospital, the patient continues to get help from her health care team and becomes an outpatient.

What should I do if I think someone I know has anorexia?

If someone you know is showing signs of anorexia, you may be able to help.

1. Set a time to talk. Set aside a time to talk privately with your friend. Make sure you talk in a quiet place where you won't be distracted.

2. Tell your friend about your concerns. Be honest. Tell your friend about your worries about her or his not eating or over exercising. Tell your friend you are concerned and that you think these things may be a sign of a problem that needs professional help.

3. Ask your friend to talk to a professional. Your friend can talk to a counselor or doctor who knows about eating issues. Offer to help your friend find a counselor or doctor and make an appointment, and offer to go with her or him to the appointment.

4. Avoid conflicts. If your friend won't admit that she or he has a problem, don't push. Be sure to tell your friend you are always there to listen if she or he wants to talk.

5. Don't place shame, blame, or guilt on your friend. Don't say, "You just need to eat." Instead, say things like, "I'm concerned about you because you won't eat breakfast or lunch." Or, "It makes me afraid to hear you throwing up."

6. Don't give simple solutions. Don't say, "If you'd just stop, then things would be fine!"

7. Let your friend know that you will always be there no matter what.

(These tips were adapted from "What Should I Say? Tips for Talking to a Friend Who May Be Struggling with an Eating Disorder" from the National Eating Disorders Association.)

Chapter 11

Bulimia Nervosa

What is bulimia?

Bulimia nervosa, often called bulimia, is a type of eating disorder. A person with bulimia eats a lot of food in a short amount of time (binging) and then tries to prevent weight gain by getting rid of the food (purging). Purging might be done by making oneself throw up or by taking laxatives (pills or liquids that speed up the movement of food through your body and lead to a bowel movement).

A person with bulimia feels he or she cannot control the amount of food eaten. Also, bulimics might exercise a lot, eat very little or not at all, or take pills to pass urine often to prevent weight gain.

Unlike anorexia, people with bulimia can fall within the normal range for their age and weight. But like people with anorexia, bulimics fear gaining weight, want desperately to lose weight, and are very unhappy with their body size and shape.

Who becomes bulimic?

Many people think that eating disorders affect only young, upper-class white females. It is true that most bulimics are women (around 85–90%). But bulimia affects people from all walks of life, including males, women of color, and even older women. It is not known for sure whether African American, Latina, Asian/Pacific Islander, and American Indian and Alaska Native people develop eating disorders because American culture values thin people. People with different cultural backgrounds may develop eating disorders because it's hard to adapt to a new culture (a theory called "culture clash"). The stress of trying to live in two different cultures may cause some minorities to develop eating disorders.

About This Chapter: From "Bulimia Nervosa Fact Sheet," Office on Women's Health (www.womenshealth.gov), June 2009.

Impaired Brain Activity Underlies Impulsive Behaviors In Women With Bulimia

Women with bulimia nervosa (BN), when compared with healthy women, showed different patterns of brain activity while doing a task that required self-regulation. This abnormality may underlie binge eating and other impulsive behaviors that occur with the eating disorder, according to an article published in the January 2009 issue of the *Archives of General Psychiatry*.

Background

In the first study of its kind, Rachel Marsh, Ph.D., Columbia University, and colleagues assessed self-regulatory brain processes in women with BN without using disorder-specific cues, such as pictures of food.

In this study, 20 women with BN and 20 healthy controls viewed a series of arrows presented on a computer screen. Their task was to identify the direction in which the arrows were pointing while the researchers observed their brain activity using functional magnetic resonance imaging (fMRI).

People generally complete such tasks easily when the direction of the arrow matches the side of the screen it is on—an arrow on the left side pointing to the left—but respond more slowly and with more errors when the two do not match. In such cases, healthy adults activate self-regulatory processes in the brain to prevent automatic responses and to focus greater attention on resolving the conflicting information.

What causes bulimia?

Bulimia is more than just a problem with food. A binge can be triggered by dieting, stress, or uncomfortable emotions, such as anger or sadness. Purging and other actions to prevent weight gain are ways for people with bulimia to feel more in control of their lives and ease stress and anxiety. There is no single known cause of bulimia, but there are some factors that may play a part:

- **Culture:** Women in the U.S. are under constant pressure to fit a certain ideal of beauty. Seeing images of flawless, thin females everywhere makes it hard for women to feel good about their bodies.

- **Families:** If you have a mother or sister with bulimia, you are more likely to also have bulimia. Parents who think looks are important, diet themselves, or criticize their children's bodies are more likely to have a child with bulimia.

Results Of The Study

Women with BN tended to be more impulsive during the task, responding faster and making more mistakes when presented with conflicting information, compared with healthy controls.

Patterns in brain activity also differed between the two groups. Even when they answered correctly to conflicting information, women with BN generally did not show as much activity in brain areas involved in self-regulation as healthy controls did. Women with the most severe cases of the disorder showed the least amount of self-regulatory brain activity and made the most errors on the task.

Significance

Altered patterns of brain activity may underlie impaired self-regulation and impulse control problems in women with BN. These findings increase the understanding of causes of binge eating and other impulsive behaviors associated with BN and may help researchers to develop better-targeted treatments.

What's Next

The researchers are currently conducting further studies on brain functioning in teens with BN, which would offer a closer look at the beginnings of the illness. They also recommend studying people in remission from an eating disorder. Comparison studies with impulsive people who have healthy weight and eating habits could also provide more information about which patterns of brain activity are most directly related to eating disorders.

From "Impaired Brain Activity Underlies Impulsive Behaviors in Women with Bulimia," National Institute of Mental Health (www.nimh.nih.gov), September 10, 2010.

- **Life Changes Or Stressful Events:** Traumatic events (like rape), as well as stressful things (like starting a new job), can lead to bulimia.

- **Personality Traits:** A person with bulimia may not like herself, hate the way she looks, or feel hopeless. She may be very moody, have problems expressing anger, or have a hard time controlling impulsive behaviors.

- **Biology:** Genes, hormones, and chemicals in the brain may be factors in developing bulimia.

What are signs of bulimia?

A person with bulimia may be thin, overweight, or have a normal weight. Also, bulimic behavior, such as throwing up, is often done in private because the person with bulimia feels shame or disgust. This makes it hard to know if someone has bulimia. But there are warning signs to look out for. Someone with bulimia may use extreme measures like these to lose weight:

- Using diet pills, or taking pills to urinate or have a bowel movement

- Going to the bathroom all the time after eating (to throw up)

- Exercising a lot, even in bad weather or when hurt or tired

Someone with bulimia may show signs of throwing up, such as the following:

- Swollen cheeks or jaw area

- Calluses or scrapes on the knuckles (if using fingers to induce vomiting)

- Teeth that look clear

- Broken blood vessels in the eyes

People with bulimia often have other mental health conditions, including depression, anxiety, or substance abuse problems.

Someone with bulimia may also have a distorted body image, shown by thinking she or he is fat, hating her or his body, and fearing weight gain.

Bulimia can also cause someone to not act like her or himself. She or he may be moody or sad, or may not want to go out with friends.

What happens to someone who has bulimia?

Bulimia can be very harmful to the body. Look at the picture in Figure 11.1 to find out how bulimia affects your health.

Can someone with bulimia get better?

Yes. Someone with bulimia can get better. A health care team of doctors, nutritionists, and therapists will help the patient recover. They will help the person learn healthy eating patterns and cope with their thoughts and feelings. Treatment for bulimia uses a combination of options. Whether or not the treatment works depends on the patient. To stop a person from binging and purging, a doctor may recommend the patient receive nutritional advice and psychotherapy, especially cognitive behavioral therapy (CBT) and be prescribed medicine.

CBT is a form of psychotherapy that focuses on the important role of thinking in how we feel and what we do. CBT that has been tailored to treat bulimia has shown to be effective in changing binging and purging behavior and eating attitudes. Therapy for a person with bulimia may be one-on-one with a therapist or group-based.

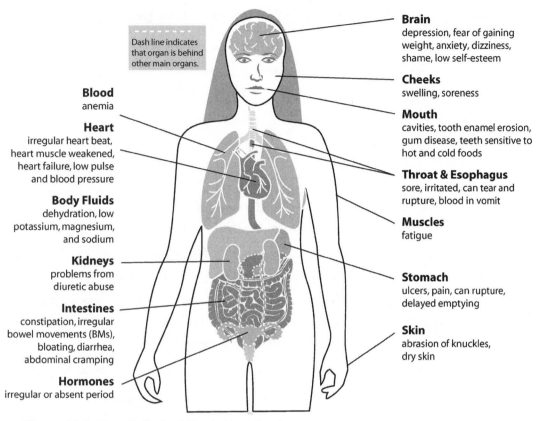

Figure 11.1. How Bulimia Affects Your Body.

Some antidepressants, such as fluoxetine (Prozac), which is the only medication approved by the U.S. Food and Drug Administration (FDA) for treating bulimia, may help patients who also have depression and/or anxiety. It also appears to help reduce binge-eating and purging behavior, reduces the chance of relapse, and improves eating attitudes. ("Relapse" means to get sick again, after feeling well for a while.)

Is it safe for young people to take antidepressants for bulimia?

Drug companies who make antidepressants are required to post a black box warning—the most serious type of warning on prescription medicines—on the medication. It may be possible that antidepressants make children, adolescents, and young adults more likely to think about suicide or commit suicide. The U.S. Food and Drug Administration (FDA) offers the latest information through their website at http://www.fda.gov.

What should I do if I think someone I know has bulimia?

If someone you know is showing signs of bulimia, you may be able to help.

1. Set a time to talk. Set aside a time to talk privately with your friend. Make sure you talk in a quiet place where you won't be distracted.

2. Tell your friend about your concerns. Be honest. Tell your friend about your worries about his or her eating or exercising habits. Tell your friend you are concerned and that you think these things may be a sign of a problem that needs professional help.

3. Ask your friend to talk to a professional. Your friend can talk to a counselor or doctor who knows about eating issues. Offer to help your friend find a counselor or doctor and make an appointment, and offer to go with him or her to the appointment.

4. Avoid conflicts. If your friend won't admit that he or she has a problem, don't push. Be sure to tell your friend you are always there to listen if he or she wants to talk.

5. Don't place shame, blame, or guilt on your friend. Don't say, "You just need to eat." Instead, say things like, "I'm concerned about you because you won't eat breakfast or lunch." Or, "It makes me afraid to hear you throwing up."

6. Don't give simple solutions. Don't say, "If you'd just stop, then things would be fine!"

7. Let your friend know that you will always be there no matter what.

(These tips were adapted from "What Should I Say? Tips for Talking to a Friend Who May Be Struggling with an Eating Disorder" from the National Eating Disorders Association.)

Chapter 12

Binge Eating Disorder

What is binge eating disorder (BED)?

Individuals with binge eating disorder (BED) engage in binge eating, but in contrast to people with bulimia nervosa (BN) they do not regularly use inappropriate compensatory weight control behaviors such as fasting or purging to lose weight. Binge eating, by definition, is eating that is characterized by rapid consumption of a large amount of food by social comparison and experiencing a sense of the eating being out of control. Binge eating is often accompanied by uncomfortable fullness after eating, and eating large amounts of food when not hungry, and distress about the binge eating. There is no specific caloric amount that qualifies an eating episode as a binge. A binge may be ended by abdominal discomfort, social interruption, or running out of food. Some who have placed strict restrictions on what and when it is OK to eat might feel like they have binged after only a small amount of food (like a cookie). Since this is not an objectively large amount of food by social comparison, it is called a subjective binge and is not part of binge eating disorder.

When the binge is over, the person often feels disgusted, guilty, and depressed about overeating. For some individuals, BED can occur together with other psychiatric disorders such as depression, substance abuse, anxiety disorders, or self-injurious behavior. The person suffering from BED often feels caught up in a vicious cycle of negative mood followed by binge eating, followed by more negative mood. Over time, individuals with BED tend to gain weight due to overeating; therefore, BED is often, but not always, associated with overweight and obesity. Previous terms used to describe these problems included compulsive overeating, emotional eating, or food addiction.

When identifying and diagnosing BED, doctors and mental health professionals refer to the criteria in the *Diagnostic and Statistical Manual IV* (*DSM-IV*) which says, a person must have had, on average, a minimum of two binge-eating episodes a week for at least six months. Although this is a somewhat arbitrary criterion and any amount of binge eating should be attended to.

What are binge eating disorder and binge eating episodes?

Binge eating disorder (BED) is characterized by recurrent episodes of binge eating but without the characteristic compensatory purging behaviors of bulimia nervosa such as vomiting, use of laxatives or excessive exercise.

Binge eating episodes are associated with: eating much more rapidly than normal, eating until feeling uncomfortably full, a sense of being out of control, dissociation, eating large amounts of food when not feeling physically hungry, eating alone due to embarrassment about how much one is eating, feeling disgusted, depressed, or guilty following overeating. Binges can also occur secondary to restrictive eating and as a result of starvation.

Source: Excerpted from "Eating Disorders Glossary," © 2012 Families Empowered and Supporting Treatment of Eating Disorders (www.feast-ed.org).

Who develops BED?

[BED is officially classified as an eating disorder not otherwise specified (EDNOS).] EDNOS is the most commonly diagnosed disorder among individuals seeking professional help for an eating disorder. Estimates vary about the prevalence of BED; however, recent statistics indicate that in the United States BED affects an estimated three and one-half percent of females and two percent of males at some point in their lifetime (compared to anorexia nervosa [AN], for example, which affects an estimated one-half to one percent of the population). The prevalence of BED among obese individuals is even higher (approximately five percent to eight percent). The average age of onset for BED is in young adulthood (early 20s) and slightly later in life compared to BN and AN. Although, recognition of binge eating in children is increasing.

How do people with BED control their weight?

Unlike people with anorexia nervosa and bulimia nervosa, people with BED do not engage in repeated attempts to control their weight by vomiting, using drugs to stimulate bowel movements and urination, and exercising excessively. As a result, many individuals who binge eat take in more calories than they burn for energy, and they become overweight and remain so as long as they continue to binge eat. Some individuals may attempt to overly restrict their food intake after a binge episode but this can backfire and lead to increased hunger and lead to more binge eating. Individuals with BED can get stuck in a vicious cycle of weight gain, depression, dieting, and binge eating.

What are the common signs of BED?

Most people who suffer from BED tend to do so in secret. They tend to limit their binge episodes to when they are alone, thus it is not easy to identify someone with BED. Weight gain is a common sign, but not everyone who gains weight does so because they binge eat. Many people with BED struggle with depressed and/or anxious mood. Some individuals with BED can develop strict rules about what foods are "good" vs. "bad" to eat. In turn, they become preoccupied with enforcing these rules as a means for distracting from their painful feelings, tension, and anxiety. In the end, this preoccupation only serves to perpetuate the need for these rigid rule-based behaviors.

Are there any serious medical complications?

The most common medical complications associated with BED are related to the weight gain and other metabolic disturbances that occur. In some cases, individuals can become obese and develop nutritional problems and type 2 diabetes. In rare instances, binge eating can cause the stomach to rupture. Studies suggest that there are medical and psychiatric correlates of binge BED that are independent of obesity including insomnia, increased pain, and decreased quality of life.

What are compensatory behaviors?

Compensatory behaviors are behaviors meant to compensate or "un-do" eating. They are utilized to relieve guilt associated with eating and consuming more calories than intended or discomfort for a patient; or to relieve anxiety that may not be directly correlated with food/eating but provides physical and/or emotional relief. Examples include: purging via self-induced vomiting, misuse of laxatives, enemas, colonics or diuretics, fasting or restricting intake for a period of time following consumption, use of diet pills, chewing and spitting, or over-exercising.

Source: Excerpted from "Eating Disorders Glossary," © 2012 Families Empowered and Supporting Treatment of Eating Disorders (www.feast-ed.org).

Do we know what causes BED?

BED has been shown to aggregate in families and it is believed to be influenced by both genetic and environmental factors. Although no specific genetic variants have yet been identified, several studies are underway to identify genes that influence risk for binge eating.

BED is influenced by a combination of background factors that increase vulnerability to binge eating and by current triggers that are thought to play key roles in the initiation of binge episodes. For example, overweight individuals, particularly those with a high degree of body dissatisfaction, will often restrict food intake in an attempt to lose weight. Unfortunately, caloric deprivation only can increase the likelihood of subsequent binge eating. In addition, many individuals who suffer from binge eating experience marked increases in depressed and/or anxious mood prior to bingeing. Another key trigger seems to be cravings for sweets and simple carbohydrates, which are frequently found in patients with eating- and mood-related disorders. Some people with BED are highly reactive to food cues in the environment and have difficulty refraining from eating when confronted with high risk cues such as the sights and smells of potential binge foods.

Is treatment available for persons with BED?

Treatment for binge eating disorder targets both the elimination of binge eating and the development and maintenance of a healthy weight. Most people with BED can benefit from psychotherapy based on cognitive-behavioral principles and/or medication. Usually hospitalization is not required but admission to an eating disorders treatment program could be helpful in interrupting severe binge eating cycles.

Group therapy is especially effective for college-aged and young adult women because of the understanding of the group members. In group therapy they can talk with peers who have similar experiences. Additionally, support groups can be helpful as they can be attended for as long as necessary, have flexible schedules, and generally have no charge. Support groups, however, do not take the place of treatment. Sometimes a person with an eating disorder is unable to benefit from group therapy or support groups without the encouragement of a personal therapist.

Cognitive behavioral therapy (CBT), either in a group setting or individual therapy session, has been shown to benefit many persons with BED. It focuses on self-monitoring of eating behaviors, identifying binge triggers, and changing distorted thinking patterns about food and negative thinking patterns about oneself. CBT can help reduce binge frequency and promote binge abstinence. Certain medications, particularly antidepressants, have been shown to help some individuals reduce binge behaviors, improve mood, and lose small amounts of weight. A comprehensive treatment strategy that combines CBT with medication and nutritional counseling may be recommended. Abstinence rates from binge eating across studies have ranged from 20–60%. When seeking this type of treatment it is important to remember to review the possible risks and benefits with your doctor and to never stop your medication without a doctor's consultation.

Treatment plans should be adjusted to meet the needs of the individual concerned, but usually a comprehensive treatment plan involving a variety of experts and approaches is best. It is important to take an approach that involves developing support for the person with an eating disorder from the family environment or within the patient's community environment (support groups or other socially supportive environments). Consultation with a dietitian is a valuable component of treatment to help establish a healthy eating plan and appreciation of appropriate portion sizes.

What about prevention?

Because a history of repeated dieting, concerns about body shape, and negative mood, and self-esteem may be precursors the development of binge eating and BED, efforts are needed to reduce the media's influence through its damaging articles from teen magazines on "dieting" and the importance of "being thin." In addition, creating more opportunities for young people to talk about their binge eating experiences in less judgmental/threatening environments may help bring BED out in the open. Using technology, such as web-based chat rooms for discussing BED and text messaging for monitoring binge eating behavior may prove helpful in bringing BED out of the shadows and reducing the shame and secrecy associated with this disorder.

Resources

Berkman ND, Bulik CM, Brownley KA, Lohr KN, Sedway JA, Rooks A, Gartlehner G. *Management of eating disorders.* Evid Rep Technol Assess (Full Rep). 2006 Apr;(135):1–166. Review. PMID: 17628126

Brownley KA, Berkman ND, Sedway JA, Lohr KN, Bulik CM. Binge eating disorder treatment: a systematic review of randomized controlled trials. *Int J Eat Disord.* 2007 May;40(4):337–48. Review. PMID: 17370289

Chapter 13

Emotional Eating

Imagine you've had a fight with your best friend. It's a stupid fight, something you'll both get over. But right now you're upset. When you walk in the door, your mom asks what's wrong. How are you most likely to respond?

- Tell your mom what happened and have a long, comforting talk about it.

  Or—

- Tell your mom, "Everything's fine" and head to the freezer for the ice cream.

But can that pint of Rocky Road really help you feel better—or just make you feel sickeningly full?

What Is Emotional Eating?

Emotional eating is when people use food as a way to deal with feelings instead of to satisfy hunger. We've all been there, finishing a whole bag of chips out of boredom or downing cookie after cookie while cramming for a big test. But when done a lot—especially without realizing it—emotional eating can affect weight, health, and overall well-being.

Not many of us make the connection between eating and our feelings. But understanding what drives emotional eating can help people take steps to change it.

About This Chapter: ""Emotional Eating," February 2010, reprinted with permission from www.kidshealth.org. This information was provided by KidsHealth®, one of the largest resources online for medically reviewed health information written for parents, kids, and teens. For more articles like this, visit www.KidsHealth.org, or www.TeensHealth.org. Copyright © 1995-2012 The Nemours Foundation. All rights reserved.

One of the biggest myths about emotional eating is that it's prompted by negative feelings. Yes, people often turn to food when they're stressed out, lonely, sad, anxious, or bored. But emotional eating can be linked to positive feelings too, like the romance of sharing dessert on Valentine's Day or the celebration of a holiday feast.

Sometimes emotional eating is tied to major life events, like a death or a divorce. More often, though, it's the countless little daily stresses that cause someone to seek comfort or distraction in food.

Emotional eating patterns can be learned: A child who is given candy after a big achievement may grow up using candy as a reward for a job well done. A kid who is given cookies as a way to stop crying may learn to link cookies with comfort.

It's not easy to "unlearn" patterns of emotional eating. But it is possible. And it starts with an awareness of what's going on.

"Comfort" Foods

We all have our own comfort foods. Interestingly, they may vary according to moods and gender. One study found that happy people seem to want to eat things like pizza, while sad people prefer ice cream and cookies. Bored people crave salty, crunchy things, like chips. Researchers also found that guys seem to prefer hot, homemade comfort meals, like steaks and casseroles. Girls go for chocolate and ice cream.

This brings up a curious question: Does no one take comfort in carrots and celery sticks? Researchers are looking into that, too. What they're finding is that high-fat foods, like ice cream, may activate certain chemicals in the body that create a sense of contentment and fulfillment. This almost addictive quality may actually make you reach for these foods again when feeling upset.

Physical Hunger Vs. Emotional Hunger

We're all emotional eaters to some extent (who hasn't suddenly found room for dessert after a filling dinner?). But for some people, emotional eating can be a real problem, causing serious weight gain or cycles of binging and purging.

The trouble with emotional eating (aside from the health issues) is that once the pleasure of eating is gone, the feelings that cause it remain. And you often may feel worse about eating the amount or type of food you did. That's why it helps to know the differences between physical hunger and emotional hunger.

Next time you reach for a snack, check in and see which type of hunger is driving it.

Table 13.1. Physical Hunger Vs. Emotional Hunger

Physical Hunger	vs.	Emotional Hunger
Tends to come on gradually and can be postponed		Feels sudden and urgent
Can be satisfied with any number of foods		Causes very specific cravings (say, for pizza or ice cream)
Once full, you're likely to stop eating		You tend to eat more than you normally would
Doesn't cause feelings of guilt		Can cause guilt afterwards

Questions To Ask Yourself

You can also ask yourself these questions about your eating:

- Have I been eating larger portions than usual?

- Do I eat at unusual times?

- Do I feel a loss of control around food?

- Am I anxious over something, like school, a social situation, or an event where my abilities might be tested?

- Has there been a big event in my life that I'm having trouble dealing with?

- Am I already overweight or obese, or has there recently been a big jump in my weight or body mass index (BMI)?

- Do other people in my family use food to soothe their feelings too?

If you answered yes to many of these questions, then it's possible that eating has become a coping mechanism instead of a way to fuel your body.

Diets Aren't The Answer

If you go for fad diets that leave your body starved for energy, you may be more likely to give into emotional eating.

Breaking The Cycle

Managing emotional eating means finding other ways to deal with the situations and feelings that make someone turn to food.

For example, do you come home from school each day and automatically head to the kitchen? Stop and ask yourself, "Am I really hungry?" Is your stomach growling? Are you having difficulty concentrating or feeling irritable? If these signs point to hunger, choose something light and healthy to take the edge off until dinner.

Not really hungry? If the post-school food foraging has just become part of your routine, think about why.

Tips To Try

These three techniques can help:

1. Explore why you're eating and find a replacement activity. For example:

    *   If you're bored or lonely, call or text a friend or family member.

    *   If you're stressed out, try a yoga routine. Or listen to some feel-good tunes and let off some steam by jogging in place, doing jumping jacks, or dancing around your room until the urge to eat passes.

    *   If you're tired, rethink your bedtime routine. Tiredness can feel a lot like hunger, and food won't help if sleepless nights are causing daytime fatigue.

    *   If you're eating to procrastinate, open those books and get that homework over with. You'll feel better afterwards (honestly).

2. Write down the emotions that trigger your eating. One of the best ways to keep track is with a mood and food journal. Write down what you ate, how much, and how you felt as you ate (for example: bored, happy, worried, sad, mad) and whether you were really hungry or just eating for comfort.

    *   Through journaling, you'll start to see patterns emerging between what you feel and what you eat. You'll be able to use this information to make better choices (like choosing to clear your head with a walk around the block instead of a bag of Doritos).

3. Pause and "take 5" before you reach for food. Too often, we rush through the day without really checking in with ourselves. We're so stressed, overscheduled, and plugged-in that we lose out on time to reflect.

- Instead of eating when you get in the door, take a few minutes to transition from one part of your day to another. Go over the things that happened that day. Acknowledge how they made you feel: Happy? Grateful? Excited? Angry? Worried? Jealous? Left out?

Getting Help

Even when we understand what's going on, many of us still need help breaking the cycle of emotional eating. It's not easy—especially when emotional eating has already led to weight and self-esteem issues. So don't go it alone when you don't have to.

Take advantage of expert help. Counselors and therapists can help you deal with your feelings. Nutritionists can help you identify your eating patterns and get you on track with a better diet. Fitness experts can get your body's feel-good chemicals firing through exercise instead of food.

If you're worried about your eating, talk to your doctor. He or she can make sure you reach your weight-loss goals safely and put you in touch with professionals who can put you on a path to a new, healthier relationship with food.

Chapter 14

Night Eating And Sleep Eating Syndromes

Eating disorders do not typically follow clear daily, time-related cycles; however, there are several recognized disorders that involve unusual patterns of eating exclusively during the evening and night hours. Recognizing their unique characteristics may improve diagnosis and treatment.

Night Eating Syndrome

Night eating syndrome (NES), which is also sometimes called nocturnal eating syndrome, is a distinct but only recently recognized disorder. It differs from most other eating disorders in that its symptoms specifically relate to times of the day. Unlike binge eating disorder, in which excessive eating can occur at any time of day, people with NES eat abnormally in very specific patterns.

People with NES typically have little or no appetite in the mornings, and generally do not eat breakfast. They will eat significant amounts in the evening—at least 25% of their daily calories—after the dinner meal. Commonly, people with NES will awaken from sleep to eat during the night and feel unable to fall asleep again without eating. People with NES are aware of their behavior, and suffer distress or impairment in functioning as a result.

Recognition and treatment of NES is important because NES can significantly worsen obesity. Some studies suggest that obese people with NES have greater difficulty losing weight than those without NES. While cause-and-effect has not been firmly worked out, there is evidence that suggests that NES may precede obesity, and may lead to the development of obesity.

About This Chapter: "Night Eating Syndrome and Sleep-Related Eating Disorder," by David A. Cooke, MD, FACP, © 2012 Omnigraphics.

The cause of NES is not known. It tends to occur during periods of increased stress, which may indicate relationships to the factors that underlie mood and anxiety disorders. It is believed that abnormalities in the internal timers that govern sleep-wake cycles are involved. Small studies have suggested that people with NES have abnormal levels and release patterns of brain chemicals involved in sleep, appetite, and mood.

NES is estimated to affect about 1.5% of the general population, but, it appears to be much more common in certain subgroups. It has been reported that about 5–15% of obese patients have NES, and as much as 42% of people considered for weight loss surgery. It is strongly associated with other psychiatric disorders, particularly depression and anxiety. NES may also coexist with other eating disorders. In contrast to most other eating disorders, it appears to affect men and women equally.

Several medications have been tried for NES, with varying degrees of success. The best studied therapies have been selective serotonin re-uptake inhibitor (SSRI) antidepressants such as paroxetine and fluvoxamine, which have shown improvement in some trials. Not all studies have seen success, however. For example, a study of another SSRI, escitalopram, showed no significant benefit in NES. An antiseizure medication, topiramate, has also been reported to be effective in NES.

Data on non-medication therapy are much more limited. There have been individual case reports of success in NES using psychotherapy. There have also been case reports of improvement with bright light therapy. Neither approach has been studied in trials with large numbers of patients, so it is unknown how effective they are, or how they compare with medical therapy.

There is also very limited data suggesting that weight loss surgery may be effective for NES. More studies are required before this can be widely recommended as treatment for NES.

Sleep-Related Eating Disorder

Despite some superficial similarities, sleep-related eating disorder (SRED) is a quite different condition than NES, both in terms of symptom pattern and underlying causes.

By definition, the nocturnal eating in SRED occurs while the person is asleep. In contrast, patients with NED may leave their bed order to eat, but they are fully awake while they consume food.

SRED is considered a parasomnia. Parasomnias are a class of neurologic disorders that occur during sleep and the transition from wakefulness to sleep. Other disorders of this type include sleep walking, sleep talking, and night terrors.

People with SRED will rise from sleep in a semi-conscious state and proceed to eat or drink. Frequently, they will consume large quantities of food and may open packages or cook while asleep. Some people with SRED eat foods during sleep that they would not eat while awake or make very odd food choices. For example, one patient consumed a potato with mayonnaise and Coca Cola sauce, while another was reported to have drunk vinegar. In some cases, patients may even eat non-food items or poisonous substances.

People with SRED typically have no memory of their eating episodes, and they may only learn of them when they wake in the morning and find themselves uncomfortably full and the kitchen in disarray. Sleep partners and family members will sometimes observe the episodes and make the patient aware of them.

SRED can be a chronic disorder, and can actually lead to significant weight gain in some cases. The disorder does appear to be more common among the obese, although only a small fraction of obese people are affected.

The cause of SRED is unknown, but is presumed to result in a failure of normal brain mechanisms that prevent active movement during sleep. In keeping with this theory, people with SRED are significantly more likely to sleepwalk or have other types of parasomnias.

The ideal treatment for SRED is not clear; however, several medications including topiramate, pramipexole, and clonazepam have been reported to be effective.

Hypnosedative Induced Complex Behaviors

In recent years, it has been recognized that certain sedatives can cause sleep behaviors that closely resemble SRED. Affected persons may engage in complex sleep behaviors after taking medication for sleep, including preparing meals, cooking, eating, and even driving. While this looks very much like SRED, these medication-induced cases probably represent a different disorder.

It appears that only a very small proportion of people who take sleep medications develop unusual sleep behaviors. Nevertheless, the widespread use of these medications led the U.S. Food and Drug Administration to require warning labels regarding these effects on a number of sleep medications.

The largest number of case reports of unusual sleep behavior have involved zolpidem (Ambien). It is unclear whether zolpidem is particularly likely to cause abnormal sleep behaviors or if this is simply due to the drug's popularity and heavy prescribing. Other drugs reported to cause similar behaviors during sleep include zaleplon (Sonata), triazolam (Halcion), temazepam (Restoril), and ramelteon (Rozerem).

It is unknown why certain people develop abnormal sleep behaviors with these medications, when most do not. Data suggest that the abnormal behaviors may relate to high blood levels of the drugs, either due to taking higher than usual doses or taking other medications that may raise levels of the sleep drug.

In contrast to SREM, abnormal behaviors typically stop when the responsible medication is stopped; however, this can be difficult in patients who are highly dependent on sleeping medications.

Chapter 15

Orthorexia

Those who are obsessed with healthy eating may be suffering from *orthorexia nervosa*, a term which means literally "fixation on righteous eating." Orthorexia starts out as an innocent attempt to eat more healthfully, but the orthorexic becomes fixated on food quality and purity. They become more and more consumed with what and how much to eat, and how to deal with "slip-ups." An iron-clad will is needed to maintain this rigid eating style. Every day is a day to eat right, be "good," rise above others in dietary prowess, and self-punish if temptation wins (usually stricter eating, fasts, and exercise). Self-esteem becomes wrapped up in the purity of their diet and they often feel superior to others, especially in regards to food intake.

Eventually food choices become so restrictive, with both variety and calories, that health suffers—an ironic twist for a person so completely dedicated to healthy eating. Eventually, the obsession with healthy eating can crowd out other activities and interests, impair relationships, and become physically dangerous.

Is Orthorexia An Eating Disorder?

Orthorexia is a term coined by Steven Bratman, MD, to describe his own experience with food and eating. It is not an officially recognized disorder, but is similar to other eating disorders—those with anorexia nervosa or bulimia nervosa obsess about calories and weight while orthorexics obsess about healthy eating (not about being "thin" and losing weight).

About This Chapter: "Orthorexia Nervosa," reprinted with permission from the National Eating Disorders Association, © 2006. All rights reserved. For more information, visit www.nationaleatingdisorders.org. Reviewed by David A. Cooke, M.D., FACP, August 2012.

Why Does Someone Get Orthorexia?

Orthorexia appears to be motivated by health, but there are underlying motivations, which can include safety from poor health, compulsion for complete control, escape from fears, wanting to be thin, improving self-esteem, searching for spirituality through food, and using food to create an identity.

Do I Have Orthorexia?

Consider the following questions. The more "yes" responses, the more likely you are dealing with orthorexia:

- Do you wish that occasionally you could just eat and not worry about food quality?

- Do you ever wish you could spend less time on food and more time on living and loving?

- Does it sound beyond your ability to eat a meal prepared with love by someone else—one single meal—and not try to control what is served?

- Are you constantly looking for the ways foods are unhealthy for you?

- Do love, joy, play, and creativity take a backseat to having the perfect diet?

- Do you feel guilt or self-loathing when you stray from your diet?

- Do you feel in control when you eat the correct diet?

- Have you positioned yourself on a nutritional pedestal and wonder how others can possibly eat the food they eat?

So What's The Big Deal?

The diet of the orthorexic can actually be unhealthy, with the nutritional problems dependent on the specific diet the person has imposed upon him or herself. Social problems are more obvious. An orthorexic may be socially isolated, often because they plan their life around food. They may have little room in life for anything other than thinking about and planning food intake. Orthorexics lose the ability to eat intuitively—to know when they are hungry, how much they need, and when they are full. The orthorexic never learns how to eat naturally and is destined to keep "falling off the wagon" and thus feeling shameful, similar to any other diet mentality.

When Orthorexia Becomes All Consuming

Dr. Bratman, who went through orthorexia, states, "I pursued wellness through healthy eating for years, but gradually I began to sense that something was going wrong. The poetry of my life was disappearing. My ability to carry on normal conversations was hindered by intrusive thoughts of food. The need to obtain meals free of meat, fat, and artificial chemicals had put nearly all social forms of eating beyond my reach. I was lonely and obsessed. ... I found it terribly difficult to free myself. I had been seduced by righteous eating. The problem of my life's meaning had been transferred inexorably to food, and I could not reclaim it" (Source: www.orthorexia.com).

Are You Telling Me It's Unhealthy To Follow A Healthy Diet?

Following a healthy diet does not mean you are orthorexic, and nothing is wrong with eating healthfully. Unless, however, 1) it is taking up an inordinate amount of time and attention in your life; 2) deviating from that diet is met with guilt and self-loathing; and/or 3) it is used to avoid life issues.

What Is The Treatment For Orthorexia?

Society pushes healthy eating and thinness, so it is easy for many to not realize how problematic this behavior can become. Even more difficult is that the person doing the healthy eating can hide behind the thought that they are simply eating well (and that others do not). Further complicating treatment is the fact that motivation behind orthorexia is multi-faceted. First, the orthorexic must admit there is a problem, then identify what caused the obsession. They must also become more flexible and less dogmatic with their eating. There will be deeper emotional issues, and working through them will make the transition to normal eating easier.

While orthorexia is not a condition your doctor will diagnose, recovery can require professional help. A practitioner skilled at treating those with eating disorders is the best choice. This text can be used to help the professional understand more about orthorexia.

Recovery

The recovered orthorexic will still eat healthfully, but there will be a different understanding of what healthy eating is. They will realize that food will not make them a better person and that basing their self-esteem on the quality of their diet is irrational. Their identity will shift from "the person who eats health food" to a broader definition of who they are—a person who loves, who works, who is fun. They will find that while food is important, it is one small aspect of life and, often, there are things that are more important.

Reference

The Orthorexia Home Page. (2003). Retrieved February 8, 2006, from http://www.ortho rexia.com.

Chapter 16

Eating Disorders Not Otherwise Specified (EDNOS)

What is eating disorder not otherwise specified (EDNOS)?

The *Diagnostic and Statistical Manual—4th Edition* (*DSM-IV*) recognizes two distinct eating disorder types, anorexia nervosa and bulimia nervosa. If a person is struggling with eating disorder thoughts, feelings, or behaviors, but does not have all the symptoms of anorexia or bulimia, that person may be diagnosed with eating disorder not otherwise specified (EDNOS). The following section lists examples of how an individual may have a profound eating problem and not have anorexia nervosa or bulimia nervosa.

- A female patient could meet all of the diagnostic criteria for anorexia nervosa except she is still having her periods.

- A person could meet all of the diagnostic criteria for anorexia nervosa are met except that, despite significant weight loss the individual's current weight is in the normal range.

- A person could meet all of the diagnostic criteria for bulimia nervosa are met except that the binge eating and inappropriate compensatory mechanisms occur at a frequency of less than twice a week or for duration of less than three months.

- The person could use inappropriate compensatory behavior by an individual of normal body weight after eating small amounts of food (for example, self-induced vomiting after the consumption of two cookies). This variant is often called purging disorder.

- The person could be repeatedly chewing and spitting out, but not swallowing, large amounts of food.

- Binge-eating disorder is also officially an EDNOS category: recurrent episodes of binge eating in the absence of the regular use of inappropriate compensatory behaviors characteristic of bulimia nervosa (see separate chapter for information about BED).

The examples provided above illustrate the variety of ways in which disordered eating can look when a person has EDNOS, but this list of examples does not provide a complete picture of the many different ways that eating disorder symptoms can occur.

The "not otherwise specified" label often suggests to people that these disorders are not as important, as serious, or as common as anorexia or bulimia nervosa. This is not true. Far more individuals suffer from EDNOS than from bulimia and anorexia combined, and the risks associated with having EDNOS are often just as profound as with anorexia or bulimia because many people with EDNOS engage in the same risky, damaging behaviors seen in other eating disorders.

Individuals with EDNOS who are losing weight and restricting their caloric intake often report the same fears and obsessions as patients with anorexia. They may be overly driven to be thin, have very disturbed body image, restrict their caloric intake to unnatural and unhealthy limits, and may eventually suffer the same psychological, physiological, and social consequences of anorexic people. Those who binge, purge, or binge and purge typically report the same concerns as people with bulimia, namely, that they feel they need to purge to control their weight, that they are afraid of getting out of control with their eating, and that binging and/or purging often turn into a very addictive, yet ineffective coping strategy that they feel they can not do without. In all meaningful ways, people with EDNOS are very similar to those with anorexia or bulimia, and are just as likely to require extensive, specialized, multidisciplinary treatment.

Who develops EDNOS?

Eating disorders NOS typically begin in adolescence or early adulthood although they can occur at any time throughout the lifespan. Like anorexia nervosa and bulimia, EDNOS is far more common in females; however, among those individuals whose primary symptom is binge eating, the number of males and females is more even. Because EDNOS has not been studied as extensively as anorexia and bulimia, it is harder to gauge an exact prevalence, but estimates suggest that EDNOS accounts for almost three quarters of all community treated eating disorder cases.

What are the common signs of EDNOS?

Signs of EDNOS are the same signs you would look for in anorexia and bulimia nervosa. Constant concern about food and weight is a primary sign, as are behaviors designed to restrict eating or compensate for eating (such as exercise or purging). For individuals who binge, most notable is the disappearance of large amounts of food, long periods of eating, or noticeable blocks of time when the individual is alone. Individuals who restrict often find the need to eat by the end of the day and the urge is so strong that it results in a binge. This binge can lead to guilt and shame that leads to purging, which may prompt the individual to promise to "do better tomorrow" by restricting. Cycles like this are consistent with EDNOS and bulimia, and can become very intractable if not addressed. Characteristically, these individuals have many rules about food—for example, good foods, bad foods—and can be entrenched in these rules and particular thinking patterns. This preoccupation and these behaviors allow the person to shift their focus from painful feelings and reduce tension and anxiety perpetuating the need for these behaviors appropriately.

Are there any serious medical complications?

Individuals with EDNOS are at risk for many of the medical complications of anorexia or bulimia, depending on the symptoms they have. Those who binge and purge run risks similar to bulimia in that they can severely damage their bodies. Electrolyte imbalance and dehydration can occur and may cause cardiac complications and, occasionally, sudden death. In rare instances, binge eating can cause the stomach to rupture, and purging can result in heart failure due to the loss of vital minerals like potassium. Persons with EDNOS who are restricting may have low blood pressure, slower heart rate, disruption of hormones, bone growth, and significant mental and emotional disturbance.

Do we know what causes EDNOS?

As with other eating disorders that have been more widely studied, the cause of EDNOS is most likely a combination of environmental and biological factors that contribute to the development and expression of these disorders. While each individual may feel that they developed these behaviors "on their own" they are often amazed to find that other people have the same obsessions, irrational fears, and self-loathing. They are not alone, and they are not to blame for having this problem.

Is treatment available for persons with EDNOS?

Unfortunately, treatment studies specifically for EDNOS are rare. Cognitive behavioral therapy, either in a group setting or individual therapy session, has been shown to benefit many people with bulimia and would logically be applicable to those with EDNOS who binge or purge. It focuses on self-monitoring of eating and purging behaviors as well as changing the distorted thinking patterns associated with the disorder. Cognitive behavioral therapy is often combined with nutritional counseling and/or antidepressant medications such as fluoxetine (Prozac).

Treatment plans should be adjusted to meet the needs of the individual concerned, but usually a comprehensive treatment plan involving a variety of experts and approaches is best. It is important to take an approach that involves developing support for the person with an eating disorder from the family environment or within the patient's community environment (support groups or other socially supportive environments).

What about prevention?

Prevention research is increasing as scientists study the known "risk factors" for these disorders. Given that EDNOS and other eating disorders are multi-determined and often affect young people, there is preliminary information on the role and extent such factors as self esteem, resilience, family interactions, peer pressure, the media, and dieting might play in its development. Eating disorders and body image is commonly seen as a problem affecting women, but men are also touched by media influence. Steroid abuse and body image to create the strong, cut male physic results in many short and long term effects, but falls off under the radar in terms of indicating distorted body image and eating disorders. Advocacy groups are also engaged in prevention through efforts such as removing damaging articles from teen magazines on "dieting" and the importance of "being thin."

Chapter 17

Pica

Many young kids put nonfood items in their mouths at one time or another. They're naturally curious about their environment and might, for instance, eat some dirt out of the sandbox.

Kids with pica, however, go beyond this innocent exploration of their surroundings. Between 10% and 30% of kids ages of one to six years have the eating disorder pica, which is characterized by persistent and compulsive cravings (lasting one month or longer) to eat nonfood items.

About Pica

The word pica comes from the Latin word for magpie, a bird known for its large and indiscriminate appetite.

Pica is most common in people with developmental disabilities, including autism and mental retardation, and in children between the ages of two and three. Pica also may surface in children who've had a brain injury affecting their development. It can also be a problem for some pregnant women, as well as people with epilepsy.

People with pica frequently crave and consume nonfood items such as:

- dirt
- clay
- paint chips

About This Chapter: "Pica," January 2011, reprinted with permission from www.kidshealth.org. This information was provided by KidsHealth®, one of the largest resources online for medically reviewed health information written for parents, kids, and teens. For more articles like this, visit www.KidsHealth.org, or www.TeensHealth .org. Copyright © 1995-2012 The Nemours Foundation. All rights reserved.

- plaster
- chalk
- cornstarch
- laundry starch
- baking soda
- coffee grounds

- cigarette ashes
- burnt match heads
- cigarette butts
- feces
- ice
- glue

- hair
- buttons
- paper
- sand
- toothpaste
- soap

Although consumption of some items may be harmless, pica is considered to be a serious eating disorder that can sometimes result in serious health problems such as lead poisoning and iron-deficiency anemia.

Signs Of Pica

Warning signs that a child may have pica include:

- Repetitive consumption of nonfood items, despite efforts to restrict it, for a period of at least one month or longer

- The behavior is considered inappropriate for the child's age or developmental stage (older than 18 to 24 months)

- The behavior is not part of a cultural, ethnic, or religious practice

Why Do Some People Eat Nonfood Items?

The specific causes of pica are unknown, but certain conditions and situations can increase a person's risk:

- Nutritional deficiencies, such as iron or zinc, that may trigger specific cravings (however, the nonfood items craved usually don't supply the minerals lacking in the person's body)

- Dieting—people who diet may attempt to ease hunger by eating nonfood substances to get a feeling of fullness

- Malnutrition, especially in underdeveloped countries, where people with pica most commonly eat soil or clay

- Cultural factors—in families, religions, or groups in which eating nonfood substances is a learned practice

- Parental neglect, lack of supervision, or food deprivation—often seen in children living in poverty

- Developmental problems, such as mental retardation, autism, other developmental disabilities, or brain abnormalities

- Mental health conditions, such as obsessive-compulsive disorder (OCD) and schizophrenia

- Pregnancy, but it's been suggested that pica during pregnancy occurs more frequently in women who exhibited similar practices during their childhood or before pregnancy or who have a history of pica in their family

Eating earth substances such as clay or dirt is a form of pica known as geophagia, which can cause iron deficiency. One theory to explain pica is that in some cultures, eating clay or dirt may help relieve nausea (and therefore, morning sickness), control diarrhea, increase salivation, remove toxins, and alter odor or taste perception.

Some people claim to enjoy the taste and texture of dirt or clay, and eat it as part of a daily habit (much like smoking is a daily routine for others). And some psychological theories explain pica as a behavioral response to stress or an indication that the individual has an oral fixation (is comforted by having things in his or her mouth).

Another explanation is that pica is a cultural feature of certain religious rituals, folk medicine, and magical beliefs. For example, some people in various cultures believe that eating dirt will help them incorporate magical spirits into their bodies.

None of these theories, though, explains every form of pica. A doctor must treat each case individually to try to understand what's causing the condition.

When To Call The Doctor

If you think you are at risk for pica, talk to your doctor. If you or someone else has consumed a harmful substance, seek medical care immediately. If you think you or someone else has ingested something poisonous, call Poison Control at 800-222-1222.

A child who continues to consume nonfood items may be at risk for serious health problems, including:

- Lead poisoning (from eating paint chips in older buildings with lead-based paint)

- Bowel problems (from consuming indigestible substances like hair, cloth, etc.)

- Intestinal obstruction or perforation (from eating objects that could get lodged in the intestines)

- Dental injury (from eating hard substances that could harm the teeth)

- Parasitic infections (from eating dirt or feces)

Medical emergencies and death can occur if the craved substance is toxic or contaminated with lead or mercury, or if the item forms an indigestible mass blocking the intestines. Pica involving lead-containing substances during pregnancy may be associated with an increase in both maternal and fetal lead levels.

What Will The Doctor Do?

When a child has pica, the doctor will play an important role in helping parents manage and prevent pica-related behaviors, educating them on teaching their child about acceptable and unacceptable food substances. The doctor will also work with them on ways to restrict the nonfood items the child craves (i.e., using child-safety locks and high shelving, and keeping household chemicals and medications out of reach).

Some kids require behavioral intervention and families may need to work with a psychologist or other mental health professional.

Depending on a child's age and developmental stage, doctors will work with kids to teach them ways to eat more appropriately. Medication may also be prescribed if pica is associated with significant behavioral problems not responding to behavioral treatments.

The child's doctor may check for anemia or other nutritional deficiencies, if indicated. A child who has ingested a potentially harmful substance, such as lead, will be screened for lead and other toxic substances and might undergo stool testing for parasites. In some cases, x-rays or other imaging may be helpful to identify what was eaten or to look for bowel problems, such as an obstruction.

Fortunately, pica is usually a temporary condition that improves as kids get older or following pregnancy. But for individuals with developmental or mental health issues, pica can be a more prolonged concern.

Following treatment, if a child's pica behavior continues beyond several weeks despite attempts to intervene, additional treatment may be necessary. Remember that patience is key in treating pica because it can take time for some kids to stop wanting to eat nonfood items.

Chapter 18

Substances Abused
In Eating Disorders

Diet Pills

Both prescription and over-the-counter (OTC) diet pills are one of the most dangerous and unhealthy ways to lose weight. The scariest aspect of OTC diet pills is that they are readily available in grocery stores, pharmacies, gas stations, health food stores, etc. to everyone, including children and teens. Similar to other addictions, individuals will start to take the pills as recommended, but will completely start abusing them and become dependent on them. Natural (herbal) diet pills are just as dangerous and are not regulated by the Food and Drug Administration.

Some adverse side effects of diet pill abuse include:

- Headaches
- Heart palpitations
- Dizziness
- Vomiting
- Shallow breathing
- Blurred vision

- Hallucinations
- Convulsions/seizures
- Fatigue
- Chest pains
- High blood pressure

About This Chapter: The main text of this chapter includes "Diet Pills," "Diuretics," and "Laxatives," reprinted with permission from the Alliance for Eating Disorders Awareness, © 2012. All rights reserved. For more information, visit www.allianceforeatingdisorders.com. Additional material is cited separately within the chapter.

Eating Disorders And Substance Abuse

Anorexia nervosa and bulimia are disorders involving food, either radical restriction or extreme consumption. It is also not unusual for women and girls struggling with eating disorders to either abuse or become dependent on substances. These include, but are not limited to, the following:

Alcohol

Typically those with restricting anorexia do not consume alcohol, due to its high calorie content. However, for those with bulimia and a sub-group of those with anorexia who also binge and purge, alcohol is frequently consumed, then eliminated through vomiting.

Caffeine

This stimulant is often used by those with eating disorders. It is consumed in the form of black coffee or diet drinks to fill the stomach and stave off hunger. Caffeine also serves as a diuretic, and people with eating disorders confuse temporary fluid loss with actual weight loss. In addition, liquids in general are used by those with bulimia because self-induced vomiting is easier when the stomach is full of fluid.

Amphetamines And Cocaine

These drugs are more commonly used by those with bulimia, but also used at times by those with anorexia. These substances are used because they suppress appetite and provide energy in the absence of adequate food intake.

Nicotine

Nicotine is an appetite suppressant that can increase metabolism in females as much as 10%. It is not unusual for girls with eating disorders to take up smoking to control appetite in an effort to lose unwanted pounds.

Source: "Eating Disorders and Substance Abuse," © 2012 Remuda Ranch. All rights reserved. Reprinted with permission. For additional information, visit www.remudaranch.com.

Diuretics

Diuretics come in a pill form, as do stimulant laxatives, and they are used to rid the body of fluid. They act on the kidneys to increase the flow of urine. They are NOT intended for weight loss. Actually, it only reduces the amount of water in the body, and water in the body is vital for the appropriate functioning of all systems. Individuals use them as a "quick fix," an attempt to control weight, or to lose weight. However, if diuretics are misused, there is a high risk of developing several serious side effects.

Adverse side effects (may include):

- Headaches
- Dizziness
- Dehydration
- Muscle weakness
- Potassium deficiency
- Electrolyte imbalance
- Kidney damage
- Cardiac arrhythmia
- Heart palpitations
- Fluid retention
- Nausea
- Death

Ipecac Syrup

Ipecac Syrup is an over-the-counter emetic; it induces vomiting by both gastric irritation and central stimulation of the chemoreceptor trigger zone. The intended use is to induce vomiting in the early management of certain oral poisonings; individuals with eating disorders abuse it in attempts to induce vomiting when otherwise "unsuccessful." Toxicity can result from overuse and overdose. Adverse effects include: myopathy, muscle weakness and pain, stiffness, hypotension, and severe cardiac complications resulting in death. Abusers of Ipecac are given an EKG immediately to assess cardiac functioning.

Source: Excerpted from "Eating Disorders Glossary," © 2012 Families Empowered and Supporting Treatment of Eating Disorders (www.feast-ed.org).

Laxatives

Laxative abuse is defined as a use (or overuse) of laxatives over a long period of time, and used a means of weight control. Laxative abuse is most common among those struggling from bulimia (although not exclusive) as a way of purging. There are two main types of laxatives, stimulant laxatives and bulk-forming laxatives. Stimulant laxatives irritate the colon to induce bowel movements (and are not recommended for use longer than one week) and bulk-forming laxatives add mass and volume to the bowel movement. Continual overstimulation of the intestines from laxative abuse can eventually cause the bowels to become non-responsive.

Over a period of time, laxatives lose their effectiveness and actually start working against you. Some of the adverse side effects of laxative abuse include:

Health Complications (May Include)

- SEVERE abdominal pain and cramping
- Diarrhea (which can occur while sleeping in extreme abuse situations)
- Dehydration
- Stomach ulcers

- Constipation

- Fluid retention/bloating (especially in your hands, feet, ankles, face, and stomach)

- Development of blood in stools which leads to anemia

- Renal stones

- Severe electrolyte, fluid and mineral imbalances

- Fatigue and lethargy

- Malabsorption (which can cause deformed bone development)

More Facts About Laxative, Diuretic, And Over-The-Counter Diet Pill Abuse

Laxatives and diuretics, like so many over-the-counter medications, are intended to address a specific medical need during a delimited time-frame. And although laxatives and diuretics are not often considered drugs of abuse or dependence, individuals can become dependent on them. With prolonged use, these people develop both tolerance and withdrawal, and can experience serious medical consequences, including death. A study in 2003 found that in a sample of 200 bulimics, 31% used diuretics.

It may be a surprise to many people, including some healthcare providers, that over-the-counter products and supplements for dieting purposes are frequently abused by those with eating disorders. But, in fact they are. For example, in the study mentioned above, a full 64% of eating disorder patients abused diet pills. The health consequences of diet pill abuse are enormous and include high blood pressure, abnormal heart rhythms, tremors, thickening of the heart muscle, and kidney damage.

Source: "Eating Disorders and Substance Abuse," © 2012 Remuda Ranch. All rights reserved. Reprinted with permission. For additional information, visit www.remudaranch.com.

Chapter 19

Compulsive Exercise

Rachel and her cheerleading team practice three to five times a week. Rachel feels a lot of pressure to keep her weight down—as head cheerleader, she wants to set an example to the team. So she adds extra daily workouts to her regimen. But lately, she's been feeling worn out, and she has a hard time just making it through a regular team practice.

You may think you can't get too much of a good thing, but in the case of exercise, a healthy activity can sometimes turn into an unhealthy compulsion. Rachel is a good example of how an overemphasis on physical fitness or weight control can become unhealthy. Read on to find out more about compulsive exercise and its effects.

Too Much Of A Good Thing?

We all know the benefits of exercise, and it seems that everywhere we turn, we hear that we should exercise more. The right kind of exercise does many great things for your body and soul: It can strengthen your heart and muscles, lower your body fat, and reduce your risk of many diseases.

Many teens who play sports have higher self-esteem than their less active pals, and exercise can even help keep the blues at bay because of the endorphin rush it can cause. Endorphins are chemicals that naturally relieve pain and lift mood. These chemicals are released in your body during and after a workout and they go a long way in helping to control stress.

So how can something with so many benefits have the potential to cause harm?

About This Chapter: "Compulsive Exercise," October 2010, reprinted with permission from www.kidshealth .org. This information was provided by KidsHealth®, one of the largest resources online for medically reviewed health information written for parents, kids, and teens. For more articles like this, visit www.KidsHealth.org, or www.TeensHealth.org. Copyright © 1995-2012 The Nemours Foundation. All rights reserved.

Why Do People Over-Exercise?

Lots of people start working out because it's fun or it makes them feel good, but exercise can become a compulsive habit when it is done for the wrong reasons.

Some people start exercising with weight loss as their main goal. Although exercise is part of a safe and healthy way to control weight, many people may have unrealistic expectations. We are bombarded with images from advertisers of the ideal body: young and thin for women; strong and muscular for men. To try to reach these unreasonable ideals, people may turn to diets, and for some, this may develop into eating disorders such as anorexia and bulimia. And some people who grow frustrated with the results from diets alone may over-exercise to speed up weight loss.

Some athletes may also think that repeated exercise will help them to win an important game. Like Rachel, they add extra workouts to those regularly scheduled with their teams without consulting their coaches or trainers. The pressure to succeed may also lead these people to exercise more than is healthy. The body needs activity but it also needs rest. Over-exercising can lead to injuries like fractures and muscle strains.

Are You A Healthy Exerciser?

Fitness experts recommend that teens do at least 60 minutes of moderate to vigorous physical activity every day. Most young people exercise much less than this recommended amount (which can be a problem for different reasons), but some—such as athletes—do more.

Experts say that repeatedly exercising beyond the requirements for good health is an indicator of compulsive behavior. Some people need more than the average amount of exercise, of course—such as athletes in training for a big event. But several workouts a day, every day, when a person is not in training is a sign that the person is probably overdoing it.

People who are exercise dependent also go to extremes to fit activity into their lives. If you put workouts ahead of friends, homework, and other responsibilities, you may be developing a dependence on exercise.

Signs Of Compulsive Exercise

If you are concerned about your own exercise habits or a friend's, ask yourself the following questions. Do you:

• force yourself to exercise, even if you don't feel well?

• prefer to exercise rather than being with friends?

- become very upset if you miss a workout?

- base the amount you exercise on how much you eat?

- have trouble sitting still because you think you're not burning calories?

- worry that you'll gain weight if you skip exercising for a day?

If the answer to any of these questions is yes, you or your friend may have a problem. What should you do?

How To Get Help

The first thing you should do if you suspect that you are a compulsive exerciser is get help. Talk to your parents, doctor, a teacher or counselor, a coach, or another trusted adult. Compulsive exercise, especially when it is combined with an eating disorder, can cause serious and permanent health problems, and in extreme cases, death.

Because compulsive exercise is closely related to eating disorders, help can be found at community agencies specifically set up to deal with anorexia, bulimia, and other eating problems. Your school's health or physical education department may also have support programs and nutrition advice available. Ask your teacher, coach, or counselor to recommend local organizations that may be able to help.

You should also schedule a checkup with a doctor. Because our bodies go through so many important developments during the teen years, guys and girls who have compulsive exercise problems need to see a doctor to make sure they are developing normally. This is especially true if the person also has an eating disorder. Girls who overexercise and restrict their eating may stop having periods and develop osteoporosis (weakening of the bones), a condition called female athlete triad. Medical help is necessary to resolve the physical problems associated with over-exercising before they cause long-term damage to the body.

Make A Positive Change

Girls and guys who exercise compulsively may have a distorted body image and low self-esteem. They may see themselves as overweight or out of shape even when they are actually a healthy weight.

Compulsive exercisers need to get professional help for the reasons described above. But there are also some things that you can do to help you take charge again:

- Work on changing your daily self-talk. When you look in the mirror, make sure you find at least one good thing to say about yourself. Be more aware of your positive attributes.

- When you exercise, focus on the positive, mood-boosting qualities.

- Give yourself a break. Listen to your body and give yourself a day of rest after a hard workout.

- Control your weight by exercising and eating moderate portions of healthy foods. Don't try to change your body into an unrealistically lean shape. Talk with your doctor, dietitian, coach, athletic trainer, or other adult about what a healthy body weight is for you and how to develop healthy eating and exercise habits.

Exercise and sports are supposed to be fun and keep you healthy. Working out in moderation will do both.

Chapter 20

Female Athlete Triad

Hannah joined the track team her freshman year and trained hard to become a lean, strong sprinter. When her coach told her losing a few pounds would improve her performance, she immediately started counting calories and increased the duration of her workouts. She was too busy with practices and meets to notice that her period had stopped—she was more worried about the stress fracture in her ankle slowing her down.

Although Hannah thinks her intense training and disciplined diet are helping her performance, they may actually be hurting her—and her health.

What Is Female Athlete Triad?

Sports and exercise are part of a balanced, healthy lifestyle. People who play sports are healthier; get better grades; are less likely to experience depression; and use alcohol, cigarettes, and drugs less frequently than people who aren't athletes. But for some girls, not balancing the needs of their bodies and their sports can have major consequences.

Some girls who play sports or exercise intensely are at risk for a problem called female athlete triad. Female athlete triad is a combination of three conditions: disordered eating, amenorrhea, and osteoporosis. A female athlete can have one, two, or all three parts of the triad.

About This Chapter: "Female Athlete Triad," February 2010, reprinted with permission from www.kidshealth .org. This information was provided by KidsHealth®, one of the largest resources online for medically reviewed health information written for parents, kids, and teens. For more articles like this, visit www.KidsHealth.org, or www.TeensHealth.org. Copyright © 1995-2012 The Nemours Foundation. All rights reserved.

Triad Factor #1: Disordered Eating

Most girls with female athlete triad try to lose weight as a way to improve their athletic performance. The disordered eating that accompanies female athlete triad can range from avoiding certain types of food the athlete thinks are "bad" (such as foods containing fat) to serious eating disorders like anorexia nervosa or bulimia nervosa.

Triad Factor #2: Amenorrhea

Exercising intensely and not eating enough calories can lead to decreases in estrogen, the hormone that helps to regulate the menstrual cycle. As a result, a girl's periods may become irregular or stop altogether. Of course, it's normal for teens to occasionally miss periods, especially in the first year. A missed period does not automatically mean female athlete triad. It could mean something else is going on, like pregnancy or a medical condition. If you are having sex and miss your period, talk to your doctor.

Some girls who participate intensively in sports may never even get their first period because they've been training so hard. Others may have had periods, but once they increase their training and change their eating habits, their periods may stop.

Triad Factor #3: Osteoporosis

Low estrogen levels and poor nutrition, especially low calcium intake, can lead to osteoporosis, the third aspect of the triad. Osteoporosis is a weakening of the bones due to the loss of bone density and improper bone formation. This condition can ruin a female athlete's career because it may lead to stress fractures and other injuries.

Usually, the teen years are a time when girls should be building up their bone mass to their highest levels—called peak bone mass. Not getting enough calcium now can also have a lasting effect on how strong a woman's bones are later in life.

Who Gets Female Athlete Triad?

Many girls have concerns about the size and shape of their bodies. But being a highly competitive athlete and participating in a sport that requires you to train extra hard can increase that worry.

Girls with female athlete triad often care so much about their sports that they would do almost anything to improve their performance. Martial arts and rowing are examples of sports that classify athletes by weight class, so focusing on weight becomes an important part of the training program and can put a girl at risk for disordered eating.

Participation in sports where a thin appearance is valued can also put a girl at risk for female athlete triad. Sports such as gymnastics, figure skating, diving, and ballet are examples of sports that value a thin, lean body shape. Some athletes may even be told by coaches or judges that losing weight would improve their scores.

Even in sports where body size and shape aren't as important, such as distance running and cross-country skiing, girls may be pressured by teammates, parents, partners, and coaches who mistakenly believe that "losing just a few pounds" could improve their performance.

The truth is, losing those few pounds generally doesn't improve performance at all. People who are fit and active enough to compete in sports generally have more muscle than fat, so it's the muscle that gets starved when a girl cuts back on food. Plus, if a girl loses weight when she doesn't need to, it interferes with healthy body processes such as menstruation and bone development.

In addition, for some competitive female athletes, problems such as low self-esteem, a tendency toward perfectionism, and family stress place them at risk for disordered eating.

What Are The Signs And Symptoms?

If a girl has risk factors for female athlete triad, she may already be experiencing some symptoms and signs of the disorder, such as:

- weight loss
- no periods or irregular periods
- fatigue and decreased ability to concentrate
- stress fractures (fractures that occur even if a person hasn't had a significant injury)
- muscle injuries

Girls with female athlete triad often have signs and symptoms of eating disorders, such as:

- continued dieting in spite of weight loss
- preoccupation with food and weight
- frequent trips to the bathroom during and after meals
- using laxatives
- brittle hair or nails
- dental cavities because in girls with bulimia tooth enamel is worn away by frequent vomiting

- sensitivity to cold

- low heart rate and blood pressure

- heart irregularities and chest pain

How Doctors Help

An extensive physical examination is a crucial part of diagnosing female athlete triad. A doctor who thinks a girl has female athlete triad will probably ask questions about her periods, her nutrition and exercise habits, any medications she takes, and her feelings about her body. This is called the medical history.

Poor nutrition can also affect the body in many ways, so a doctor might order blood tests to check for anemia and other problems associated with the triad. The doctor also will check for medical reasons why a girl may be losing weight and missing her periods. Because osteoporosis can put someone at higher risk for bone fractures, the doctor may also request tests to measure bone density.

Tips For Female Athletes

Here are a few tips to help teen athletes stay on top of their physical condition:

- **Keep Track Of Your Periods:** It's easy to forget when you had your last visit from Aunt Flo, so keep a calendar in your gym bag and mark down when your period starts and stops and if the bleeding is particularly heavy or light. That way, if you start missing periods, you'll know right away and you'll have accurate information to give to your doctor.

- **Don't Skip Meals Or Snacks:** If you're constantly on the go between school, practice, and competitions you may be tempted to skip meals and snacks to save time. But eating now will improve performance later, so stock your locker or bag with quick and easy favorites such as bagels, string cheese, unsalted nuts and seeds, raw vegetables, granola bars, and fruit.

- **Visit A Dietitian Or Nutritionist Who Works With Teen Athletes:** He or she can help you get your dietary game plan into gear and find out if you're getting enough key nutrients such as iron, calcium, and protein. And if you need supplements, a nutritionist can recommend the best choices.

- **Do It For You:** Pressure from teammates, parents, or coaches can turn a fun activity into a nightmare. If you're not enjoying your sport, make a change. Remember: It's your body and your life. You—not your coach or teammates—will have to live with any damage you do to your body now.

Doctors don't work alone to help a girl with female athlete triad. Coaches, parents, physical therapists, pediatricians and adolescent medicine specialists, nutritionists and dietitians, and mental health specialists can all work together to treat the physical and emotional problems that a girl with female athlete triad faces.

It might be tempting to shrug off several months of missed periods, but getting help right away is important. In the short term, female athlete triad may lead to muscle weakness, stress fractures, and reduced physical performance. Over the long term, it can cause bone weakness, long-term effects on the reproductive system, and heart problems.

A girl who is recovering from female athlete triad might work with a dietitian to help reach and maintain a healthy weight while eating enough calories and nutrients for health and good athletic performance. Depending on how much the girl is exercising, she may have to reduce the length of her workouts. Talking to a psychologist or therapist can help her deal with depression, pressure from coaches or family members, or low self-esteem and can help her find ways to deal with her problems other than restricting food intake or exercising excessively.

Some girls may need to take hormones to supply their bodies with estrogen to help prevent further bone loss. Calcium and vitamin D supplementation can also help when someone has bone loss as the result of female athlete triad.

What If I Think Someone I Know Has It?

It's tempting to ignore female athlete triad and hope it goes away. But it requires help from a doctor and other health professionals. If a friend, sister, or teammate has signs and symptoms of female athlete triad, discuss your concerns with her and encourage her to seek treatment. If she refuses, you may need to mention your concern to a parent, coach, teacher, or school nurse.

You might worry about seeming nosy when you ask questions about a friend's health, but you're not: Your concern is a sign that you're a caring friend. Lending an ear may be just what your friend needs.

Chapter 21

Body Dysmorphic Disorder And Bigorexia

Focusing On Appearance

Most of us spend time in front of the mirror checking our appearance. Some people spend more time than others, but taking care of our bodies and being interested in our appearance is natural.

How we feel about our appearance is part of our body image and self-image. Many people have some kind of dissatisfaction with their bodies. This can be especially true during the teen years when our bodies and appearance go through lots of changes.

Although many people feel dissatisfied with some aspect of their appearance, these concerns usually don't constantly occupy their thoughts or cause them to feel tormented. But for some people, concerns about appearance become quite extreme and upsetting.

Some people become so focused on imagined or minor imperfections in their looks that they can't seem to stop checking or obsessing about their appearance. Being constantly preoccupied and upset about body imperfections or appearance flaws is called body dysmorphic disorder.

What Is Body Dysmorphic Disorder?

Body dysmorphic disorder (BDD) is a condition that involves obsessions, which are distressing thoughts that repeatedly intrude into a person's awareness. With BDD, the distressing thoughts are about perceived appearance flaws.

About This Chapter: "Body Dysmorphic Disorder," October 2010, reprinted with permission from www.kidshealth .org. This information was provided by KidsHealth®, one of the largest resources online for medically reviewed health information written for parents, kids, and teens. For more articles like this, visit www.KidsHealth.org, or www.TeensHealth.org. Copyright © 1995-2012 The Nemours Foundation. All rights reserved.

People with BDD might focus on what they think is a facial flaw, but they can also worry about other body parts, such as short legs, breast size, or body shape. Just as people with eating disorders obsess about their weight, those with BDD become obsessed over an aspect of their appearance. They may worry their hair is thin, their face is scarred, their eyes aren't exactly the same size, their nose is too big, or their lips are too thin.

BDD has been called "imagined ugliness" because the appearance issues the person is obsessing about usually are so small that others don't even notice them. Or, if others do notice them, they consider them minor. But for someone with BDD, the concerns feel very real, because the obsessive thoughts distort and magnify any tiny imperfection.

Because of the distorted body image caused by BDD, a person might believe that he or she is too horribly ugly or disfigured to be seen.

Behaviors That Are Part of BDD

Besides obsessions, BDD also involves compulsions and avoidance behaviors.

A compulsion is something a person does to try to relieve the tension caused by the obsessive thoughts. For example, someone with obsessive thoughts that her nose is horribly ugly might check her appearance in the mirror, apply makeup, or ask someone many times a day whether her nose looks ugly. These types of checking, fixing, and asking are compulsions.

Somebody with obsessions usually feels a strong or irresistible urge to do compulsions because they can provide temporary relief from the terrible distress. The compulsions seem like the only way to escape bad feelings caused by bad thoughts. Compulsive actions often are repeated many times a day, taking up lots of time and energy.

Avoidance behaviors are also a part of BDD. A person might stay home or cover up to avoid being seen by others. Avoidance behaviors also include things like not participating in class or socializing, or avoiding mirrors.

With BDD, a pattern of obsessive thoughts, compulsive actions, and avoidance sets in. Even though the checking, fixing, asking, and avoiding seem to relieve terrible feelings, the relief is just temporary. In reality, the more someone performs compulsions or avoids things, the stronger the pattern of obsessions, compulsions, and avoidance becomes.

After a while, it takes more and more compulsions to relieve the distress caused by the bad thoughts. A person with BDD doesn't want to be preoccupied with these thoughts and behaviors, but with BDD it can seem impossible to break the pattern.

Facts About Body Dysmorphic Disorder

Body dysmorphic disorder (BDD) is a serious illness in which a person is preoccupied with minor or imaginary physical flaws, usually of the skin, hair, and nose. A person with BDD tends to have cosmetic surgery, and even if the surgery is successful, does not think it was and is unhappy with the outcome.

Symptoms Of BDD

- Being preoccupied with minor or imaginary physical flaws, usually of the skin, hair, and nose, such as acne, scarring, facial lines, marks, pale skin, thinning hair, excessive body hair, large nose, or crooked nose.

- Having a lot of anxiety and stress about the perceived flaw and spending a lot of time focusing on it, such as frequently picking at skin, excessively checking appearance in a mirror, hiding the imperfection, comparing appearance with others, excessively grooming, seeking reassurance from others about how they look, and getting cosmetic surgery.

- Getting cosmetic surgery can make BDD worse. They are often not happy with the outcome of the surgery. If they are, they may start to focus attention on another body area and become preoccupied trying to fix the new "defect." In this case, some patients with BDD become angry at the surgeon for making their appearance worse and may even become violent towards the surgeon.

Treatment For BDD

- **Medications:** Serotonin reuptake inhibitors or SSRIs are antidepressants that decrease the obsessive and compulsive behaviors.

- **Cognitive Behavioral Therapy:** This is a type of therapy with several steps: The therapist asks the patient to enter social situations without covering up her "defect." The therapist helps the patient stop doing the compulsive behaviors to check the defect or cover it up. This may include removing mirrors, covering skin areas that the patient picks, or not using make-up. The therapist helps the patient change their false beliefs about their appearance.

Source: Excerpted from "Body Image: Cosmetic Surgery," Office on Women's Health (www.womenshealth.gov), September 22, 2009.

What Causes BDD?

Although the exact cause of BDD is still unclear, experts believe it is related to problems with serotonin, one of the brain's chemical neurotransmitters. Poor regulation of serotonin also plays a role in obsessive compulsive disorder (OCD) and other anxiety disorders, as well as depression.

Some people may be more prone to problems with serotonin balance, including those with family members who have problems with anxiety or depression. This may help explain why some people develop BDD but others don't.

Cultural messages can also play a role in BDD by reinforcing somebody's concerns about appearance. Critical messages or unkind teasing about appearance as someone is growing up may also contribute to a person's sensitivity to BDD. But while cultural messages, criticism, and teasing might harm someone's body image, these things alone usually do not result in BDD.

It's hard to know exactly how common BDD is because most people with BDD are unwilling to talk about their concerns or seek help. But compared with those who feel somewhat dissatisfied with their appearance, very few people have true BDD. BDD usually begins in the teen years, and if it's not treated, can continue into adulthood.

How BDD Can Affect A Person's Life

Sometimes people with BDD feel ashamed and keep their concerns secret. They may think that others will consider them vain or superficial.

Other people might become annoyed or irritated with somebody's obsessions and compulsions about appearance. They don't understand BDD or what the person is going through. As a result, those with BDD may feel misunderstood, unfairly judged, or alone. Because they avoid contact with others, they may have few friends or activities to enjoy.

It's extremely upsetting to be tormented by thoughts about appearance imperfections. These thoughts intrude into a person's awareness throughout the day and are hard to ignore. People with mild to moderate symptoms of BDD usually spend a great deal of time grooming themselves in the morning. Throughout the day, they may frequently check their appearance

Bigorexia Or Muscle Dysmorphia

Muscle dysmorphia (also called reverse anorexia or bigorexia) is a form of body dysmorphic disorder that affects males and females. Sufferers develop a pathological preoccupation with their muscularity, believing themselves to be small and weak, no matter how large their muscles. Like anorexics, they may also see themselves as fat and develop a range of eating rituals. One method of treatment is cognitive behavior therapy (CBT).

Source: Excerpted from "Eating Disorders Glossary," © 2012 Families Empowered and Supporting Treatment of Eating Disorders (www.feast-ed.org).

in mirrors or windows. In addition, they may repeatedly seek reassurance from people around them that they look OK.

Although people with mild BDD usually continue to go to school, the obsessions can interfere with their daily lives. For example, someone might measure or examine the "flawed" body part repeatedly or spend large sums of money and time on makeup to cover the problem.

Some people with BDD hide from others, and avoid going places because of fear of being seen. Spending so much time and energy on appearance concerns robs a person of pleasure and happiness, and of opportunities for fun and socializing.

People with severe symptoms may drop out of school, quit their jobs, or refuse to leave their homes. Many people with BDD also develop depression. Those with the most severe BDD might even consider or attempt suicide.

Many people with BDD seek the help of a dermatologist or cosmetic surgeon to try to correct appearance flaws. But dermatology treatments or plastic surgery don't change the BDD. Those who find cosmetic surgeons willing to perform surgery are often not satisfied with the results. They may find that even though their appearance has changed, the obsessive thinking is still present, and they begin to focus on some other imperfection.

Getting Help For BDD

If you or someone you know has BDD, the first step is recognizing what might be causing the distress. Many times, people with BDD are so focused on their appearance that they believe the answer lies in correcting how they look, not with their thoughts.

The real problem with BDD lies in the obsessions and compulsions, which distort body image, making someone feel ugly. Because people with BDD believe what they're perceiving is true and accurate, sometimes the most challenging part of overcoming the disorder is being open to new ideas about what might help.

BDD can be treated by an experienced mental health professional. Usually, the treatment involves a type of talk therapy called cognitive behavioral therapy. This approach helps to correct the pattern that's causing the body image distortion and the extreme distress.

In cognitive behavioral therapy, a therapist helps a person to examine and change faulty beliefs, resist compulsive behaviors, and face stressful situations that trigger appearance concerns. Sometimes doctors prescribe medication along with the talk therapy.

Treatment for BDD takes time, hard work, and patience. It helps if a person has the support of a friend or loved one. If someone with BDD is also dealing with depression, anxiety, feeling isolated or alone, or other life situations, the therapy can address those issues, too.

Body dysmorphic disorder, like other obsessions, can interfere with a person's life, robbing it of pleasure and draining energy. An experienced psychologist or psychiatrist who is knowledgeable about BDD can help break the grip of the disorder so that a person can fully enjoy life.

Part Three
Medical Consequences And Co-Occurring Concerns

Chapter 22

Complications Of Eating Disorders

Complications Of Bulimia

Effects Of Bulimic Behavior On The Body

Many medical problems are directly associated with bulimic behavior, including:

- Tooth erosion, cavities, and gum problems

- Water retention, swelling, and abdominal bloating

- Acute stomach distress

- Fluid loss with low potassium levels (due to excessive vomiting or laxative use; can lead to extreme weakness, near paralysis, or lethal heart rhythms)

- Irregular menstrual periods

- Swallowing problems and esophagus damage

Forced vomiting can cause:

- Rupture of the esophagus

- Weakened rectal walls (a rare but serious condition that requires surgery)

About This Chapter: Excerpted from "Eating Disorders: In-Depth Report," © 2012 A.D.A.M., Inc. Reprinted with permission.

Self-Destructive Behavior

A number of self-destructive behaviors occur with bulimia:

- **Smoking:** Many teenage girls with eating disorders smoke because they believe it will help prevent weight gain.

- **Impulsive Behaviors:** Women with bulimia may be at higher-than-average risk for dangerous impulsive behaviors, such as sexual promiscuity, self-cutting, and kleptomania.

- **Alcohol And Substance Abuse:** Many patients with bulimia abuse alcohol, drugs, or both. Women with bulimia also frequently abuse over-the-counter medications, such as laxatives, appetite suppressants, diuretics, and drugs that induce vomiting (ipecac).

Complications Of Anorexia

Anorexia nervosa is a very serious illness that has a wide range of effects on the body and mind. It is frequently associated with a number of other medical problems, ranging from frequent infections and general poor health to life-threatening conditions.

Psychological Effects And Substance Abuse

Adolescents with eating behaviors associated with anorexia are at high risk for anxiety and depression in young adulthood. Patients with anorexia are at risk for suicidal behavior or attempts. Alcohol and drug abuse are also common in patients with anorexia nervosa.

Hormonal Changes

One of the most serious effects of anorexia nervosa is hormonal changes, which can have severe health consequences.

- Reproductive hormones, including estrogen and dehydroepiandrosterone (DHEA), are lower. Estrogen is important for healthy hearts and bones. DHEA, a weak male hormone, may also be important for bone health and for other functions.

- Thyroid hormones are lower.

- Stress hormones are higher.

- Growth hormones are lower. Children and adolescents with anorexia may experience retarded growth.

Consequences Of Eating Disorders

Psychosocial

Eating disorders can have a profoundly negative impact on an individual's quality of life. Self-image, interpersonal relationships, financial status, and job performance are often negatively affected. The extent to which these problems are an inherent part of the disorders or are secondary to it is unclear. The range of the negative effects does, however, highlight the critical importance of treatment.

Eating disorders are also associated with high rates of other co-existing psychiatric disorders, particularly mood disorders, and anxiety disorders. Bulimia nervosa may be particularly associated with alcohol and/or drug abuse problems.

Medical

Semi-starvation in anorexia nervosa can affect most organ systems. Physical signs and symptoms (in addition to the lack of menstrual periods in women) can include constipation, cold intolerance, abnormally low heart rate, abdominal distress, dryness of skin, hypotension, and fine body hair (lanugo). Anorexia nervosa causes anemia, kidney dysfunction, cardiovascular problems, changes in brain structure, and osteoporosis (i.e., inadequate bone calcium).

Self-induced vomiting seen in both anorexia nervosa and bulimia nervosa can lead to swelling of salivary glands, electrolyte and mineral disturbances, and dental enamel erosion. Use of ipecac to induce vomiting can lead to extreme muscle weakness, including heart muscle weakness. Laxative abuse can lead to long lasting disruptions of normal bowel functioning. Rarer complications are tearing the esophagus, rupturing of the stomach, and life-threatening irregularities of the heart rhythm.

Source: "Consequences of Eating Disorders," © 2012 Academy for Eating Disorders (www.aedweb.org); reprinted with permission.

The result of many of these hormonal abnormalities in women is long-term, irregular, or absent menstruation (amenorrhea). This can occur early on in anorexia, even before severe weight loss. Over time this causes infertility, bone density loss, and other problems.

Heart Disease

Heart disease is the most common medical cause of death in people with severe anorexia nervosa. The effects of anorexia on the heart are:

- Dangerous heart rhythms, including slow rhythms known as bradycardia, may develop. Such abnormalities can show up even in teenagers with anorexia.

- Blood flow is reduced.

- Blood pressure may drop.

- The heart muscles starve, losing size.

A primary danger to the heart is from imbalances of minerals, such as potassium, calcium, magnesium, and phosphate, which are normally dissolved in the body's fluid. The dehydration and starvation that occurs with anorexia can reduce fluid and mineral levels and produce a condition known as electrolyte imbalance. Certain electrolytes (especially calcium and potassium) are critical for maintaining the electric currents necessary for a normal heartbeat. An imbalance in these electrolytes can be very serious and even life threatening unless fluids and minerals are replaced. Heart problems are a particular risk when anorexia is compounded by bulimia and the use of ipecac, a drug that causes vomiting.

Starvation Syndrome

The effects of starvation on the human body are well documented. When starved of calories, the human body responds in a way known as *starvation syndrome*. People with anorexia nervosa suffer from starvation as a result of severely restricting their calorie intake. In bulimia nervosa, purging and restricting behavior can also result in a depletion of caloric absorption, which can therefore lead to self-starvation.

The Minnesota Experiment

In the 1940s, there was an experiment involving a group of fit young men who had been drafted into the U.S. army. They were conscientious objectors to military service and they had volunteered to be in a humanitarian program.

The Minnesota Experiment required them to reduce their calorie intake by half. After six months of this planned starvation, the men experienced not only the expected physical changes, but mental changes too:

- Decrease in physical strength

- Giddiness and momentary blackouts

- Pale, cold, dry, and marked skin

- Tiredness

- Decrease in mental alertness

- Hair that is thin, dry, and/or falling out

- Preoccupation with food, including persistent thoughts and dreams about food

Effect On Fertility And Pregnancy

After treatment and an increase in weight, estrogen levels are usually restored and periods resume. In severe anorexia, however, even after treatment, normal menstruation never returns in some patients.

- If a woman with anorexia becomes pregnant before regaining normal weight, she faces a higher risk for miscarriage, cesarean section, and for having an infant with low birth weight or birth defects. She may also be at higher risk for postpartum depression.

- Women with anorexia who seek fertility treatments have lower chances for success.

- Change in mealtime behaviors. This can include toying with food, or being ritualistic about the way in which food is eaten.
- Decrease in self-discipline
- Decrease in comprehension
- Loss in concentration
- Apathy
- Depression
- A loss of ambition
- Moodiness and irritability

These symptoms are experienced by anyone who is starved of calories. *If you recognize these symptoms in your own life, it is important to remember that they all stem from one thing: starvation.*

Recovery From Starvation

The men in the Minnesota Experiment recovered from their physical and mental symptoms when they began to eat again.

The physical and mental changes you have experienced will also be reversed when you increase your food intake and supply your body with the energy it needs.

Through regular and healthy eating, your body can regain its strength and fight these symptoms of starvation. You may need to consult a medical practitioner or other health professional for support with this.

Effect On Bones And Growth

Almost 90% of women with anorexia experience osteopenia (loss of bone calcium), and 40% have osteoporosis (more advanced loss of bone density). Up to two-thirds of children and adolescent girls with anorexia fail to develop strong bones during their critical growing period. Boys with anorexia also suffer from stunted growth. The less the patient weighs, the more severe the bone density loss. Women with anorexia who also binge-purge face an even higher risk for bone density loss.

Bone density loss in women is mainly due to low estrogen levels that occur with anorexia. Other biologic factors in anorexia also may contribute to bone density loss, including high levels of stress hormones (which impair bone growth) and low levels of calcium, certain growth factors, and DHEA (a weak male hormone). Weight gain, unfortunately, does not completely restore bone. Only achieving regular menstruation as soon as possible can protect against permanent bone density loss. The longer the eating disorder persists the more likely the bone density loss will be permanent.

Testosterone levels decline in boys as they lose weight, which also can affect their bone density. In young boys with anorexia, weight restoration produces some catch-up growth, but it may not produce full growth.

Neurological Problems

People with severe anorexia may suffer nerve damage that affects the brain and other parts of the body. The following nerve-related conditions have been reported:

- Seizures
- Disordered thinking
- Numbness or odd nerve sensations in the hands or feet (peripheral neuropathy)

Brain scans indicate that parts of the brain undergo structural changes and abnormal activity during anorexic states. Some of these changes return to normal after weight gain, but some damage may be permanent.

Blood Problems

Anemia (low number of red blood cells) is a common result of anorexia and starvation. A particularly serious blood problem is caused by severely low levels of vitamin B12. If anorexia becomes extreme, the bone marrow dramatically reduces its production of blood cells, a life-threatening condition called pancytopenia.

Gastrointestinal Problems

Bloating and constipation are both very common problems in people with anorexia.

Multiorgan Failure

In very late stages of anorexia, the organs simply fail. The main warning sign is high blood levels of liver enzymes, which require immediate administration of calories.

Complications In Adolescents With Type 1 Diabetes

Eating disorders are particularly serious for young people with type 1 diabetes.

Low blood sugar, for example, is a danger for anyone with anorexia, but it is a particularly dangerous risk for those with diabetes. If patients do not take their insulin, high blood sugar, which is also very dangerous, can occur. Unfortunately, patients with eating disorders may skip or reduce their daily insulin in order to decrease their intake of calories. Extremely high blood sugar levels can cause diabetic ketoacidosis, a condition in which acidic chemicals (ketones) accumulate in the body. This condition can lead to coma and death.

Chapter 23

Obesity And Its Consequences

The terms *overweight* and *obesity* refer to a person's overall body weight and whether it's too high. Overweight is having extra body weight from muscle, bone, fat, and/or water. Obesity is having a high amount of extra body fat.

The most useful measure of overweight and obesity is body mass index (BMI). BMI is based on height and weight and is used for adults, children, and teens.

Overview

Millions of Americans and people worldwide are overweight or obese. Being overweight or obese puts you at risk for many diseases and conditions. The more body fat that you have and the more you weigh, the more likely you are to develop these conditions:

- Coronary heart disease (also called coronary artery disease)
- High blood pressure
- Type 2 diabetes
- Gallstones
- Breathing problems
- Certain cancers

Your weight is the result of many factors. These factors include environment, family history and genetics, metabolism (the way your body changes food and oxygen into energy), behavior

About This Chapter: Excerpted from "What Are Overweight And Obesity," National Heart Lung And Blood Institute, November 2010.

or habits, and more. You can't change some factors, such as family history. However, you can change other factors, such as your lifestyle habits.

You can take steps to prevent or treat overweight or obesity. Follow a healthy eating plan and keep your calorie needs in mind. Do physical activity regularly and try to limit the amount of time that you're inactive.

Weight-loss medicines and surgery also are options for some people who need to lose weight if lifestyle changes aren't enough.

Outlook

Reaching and staying at a healthy weight is a long-term challenge for people who are overweight or obese. But it also can be a chance to lower your risk of other serious health problems. With the right treatment and motivation, it's possible to lose weight and lower your long-term disease risk.

What Causes Overweight And Obesity?

Lack Of Energy Balance

A lack of energy balance most often causes overweight and obesity. Energy balance means that your *energy in* equals your *energy out*. Energy in is the amount of energy or calories you get from food and drinks. Energy out is the amount of energy your body uses for things like breathing, digesting, and being physically active.

To maintain a healthy weight, your energy in and out don't have to balance exactly every day. It's the balance over time that helps you maintain a healthy weight.

- The same amount of energy in and energy out over time: weight stays the same

- More energy in than energy out over time: weight gain

- More energy out than energy in over time: weight loss

Overweight and obesity happen over time when you take in more calories than you use.

An Inactive Lifestyle

Many Americans aren't very physically active. One reason for this is that many people spend hours in front of TVs and computers doing work, schoolwork, and leisure activities. In fact, more than two hours a day of regular TV viewing time has been linked to overweight and obesity.

Other reasons for not being active include: relying on cars instead of walking, fewer physical demands at work or at home because of modern technology and conveniences, and lack of physical education classes in schools for children.

People who are inactive are more likely to gain weight because they don't burn up the calories that they take in from food and drinks. An inactive lifestyle also raises your risk of coronary heart disease, high blood pressure, diabetes, colon cancer, and other health problems.

Environment

Our environment doesn't support healthy lifestyle habits; in fact, it encourages obesity. These are some of the reasons:

- **Lack Of Neighborhood Sidewalks And Safe Places For Recreation:** Not having area parks, trails, sidewalks, and affordable gyms makes it hard for people to be physically active.

- **Work Schedules:** People often say that they don't have time to be physically active because of long work hours and time spent commuting.

- **Oversized Food Portions:** Americans are surrounded by huge food portions in restaurants, fast food places, gas stations, movie theaters, supermarkets, and even home.

- **Some Of These Meals And Snacks Can Feed Two Or More People:** Eating large portions means too much energy in. Over time, this will cause weight gain if it isn't balanced with physical activity.

- **Lack Of Access To Healthy Foods:** Some people don't live in neighborhoods that have supermarkets that sell healthy foods, such as fresh fruits and vegetables. Or, for some people, these healthy foods are too costly.

- **Food Advertising:** Americans are surrounded by ads from food companies. Often children are the targets of advertising for high-calorie, high-fat snacks and sugary drinks. The goal of these ads is to sway people to buy these high-calorie foods, and often they do.

Genes And Family History

Studies of identical twins who have been raised apart show that genes have a strong influence on a person's weight. Overweight and obesity tend to run in families. Your chances of being overweight are greater if one or both of your parents are overweight or obese.

Your genes also may affect the amount of fat you store in your body and where on your body you carry the extra fat. Because families also share food and physical activity habits, a link exists between genes and the environment.

Children adopt the habits of their parents. A child who has overweight parents who eat high-calorie foods and are inactive will likely become overweight too. However, if the family adopts healthy food and physical activity habits, the child's chance of being overweight or obese is reduced.

Health Conditions

Some hormone problems may cause overweight and obesity, such as underactive thyroid (hypothyroidism), Cushing syndrome, and polycystic ovarian syndrome (PCOS).

Underactive thyroid is a condition in which the thyroid gland doesn't make enough thyroid hormone. Lack of thyroid hormone will slow down your metabolism and cause weight gain. You'll also feel tired and weak.

Cushing syndrome is a condition in which the body's adrenal glands make too much of the hormone cortisol. Cushing syndrome also can develop if a person takes high doses of certain medicines, such as prednisone, for long periods. People who have Cushing syndrome gain weight, have upper-body obesity, a rounded face, fat around the neck, and thin arms and legs.

PCOS is a condition that affects about 5–10 percent of women of childbearing age. Women who have PCOS often are obese, have excess hair growth, and have reproductive problems and other health issues due to high levels of hormones called androgens.

Medicines

Certain medicines may cause you to gain weight. These medicines include some corticosteroids, antidepressants, and seizure medicines.

These medicines can slow the rate at which your body burns calories, increase your appetite, or cause your body to hold on to extra water. All of these factors can lead to weight gain.

Emotional Factors

Some people eat more than usual when they're bored, angry, or stressed. Over time, overeating will lead to weight gain and may cause overweight or obesity.

Smoking

Some people gain weight when they stop smoking. One reason is that food often tastes and smells better after quitting smoking.

Another reason is because nicotine raises the rate at which your body burns calories, so you burn fewer calories when you stop smoking. However, smoking is a serious health risk, and quitting is more important than possible weight gain.

Age

As you get older, you tend to lose muscle, especially if you're less active. Muscle loss can slow down the rate at which your body burns calories. If you don't reduce your calorie intake as you get older, you may gain weight.

Midlife weight gain in women is mainly due to aging and lifestyle, but menopause also plays a role. Many women gain around five pounds during menopause and have more fat around the waist than they did before.

Pregnancy

During pregnancy, women gain weight so that their babies get proper nourishment and develop normally. After giving birth, some women find it hard to lose the weight. This may lead to overweight or obesity, especially after a few pregnancies.

Lack Of Sleep

Studies find that the less people sleep, the more likely they are to be overweight or obese. People who report sleeping five hours a night, for example, are much more likely to become obese compared with people who sleep seven to eight hours a night.

People who sleep fewer hours also seem to prefer eating foods that are higher in calories and carbohydrates, which can lead to overeating, weight gain, and obesity over time.

Hormones that are released during sleep control appetite and the body's use of energy. For example, insulin controls the rise and fall of blood sugar levels during sleep. People who don't get enough sleep have insulin and blood sugar levels that are similar to those in people who are likely to have diabetes.

Also, people who don't get enough sleep regularly seem to have high levels of a hormone called ghrelin (which causes hunger) and low levels of a hormone called leptin (which normally helps curb hunger).

Overweight And Obesity-Related Health Problems In Children And Teens

Overweight and obesity also increase the health risks for children and teens. Type 2 diabetes once was rare in American children, but an increasing number of children are developing the disease. Also, overweight children are more likely to become overweight or obese as adults, with the same disease risks.

Who Is At Risk For Overweight And Obesity?

Overweight and obesity affect Americans of all ages, sexes, and racial/ethnic groups. This serious health problem has been growing over the last 30 years.

Children And Teens

Children also have become heavier. In the past 30 years, obesity has more than doubled among children ages 2–5, has tripled among children ages 6–11, and has more than tripled among adolescents ages 12–19.

According to the National Health and Nutrition Examination Survey (NHANES) 2007–2008, about one in six American children ages 2–19 are obese. The survey also suggests that overweight and obesity are having a greater effect on minority groups, including African Americans and Hispanics.

How Are Overweight And Obesity Diagnosed?

The most common way to find out whether you're overweight or obese is to figure out your body mass index (BMI). BMI is an estimate of body fat, and it's a good gauge of your risk for diseases that occur with more body fat. The higher your BMI, the higher your risk of disease. BMI is calculated from your height and weight.

Body Mass Index For Children And Teens

Overweight is defined differently for children and teens than it is for adults. Children are still growing and boys and girls mature at different rates. BMIs for children and teens compare their heights and weights against growth charts that take age and sex into account. This is called BMI-for-age percentile. A child or teen's BMI-for-age percentile shows how his or her BMI compares with other boys and girls of the same age (see Figures 23.1 and 23.2).

Table 23.1. What Does The BMI-for-Age Percentile Mean?

Less than 5th percentile	Underweight
5th percentile to less than the 85th percentile	Healthy weight
85th percentile to less than the 95th percentile	Risk of overweight
95th percentile or greater	Overweight

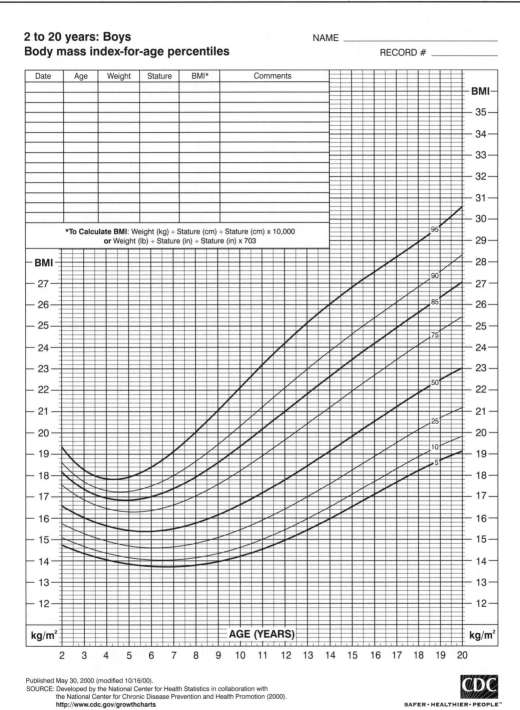

2 to 20 years: Boys
Body mass index-for-age percentiles

NAME _____

RECORD # _____

Figure 23.1. Body Mass Index: Boys Aged 2–20

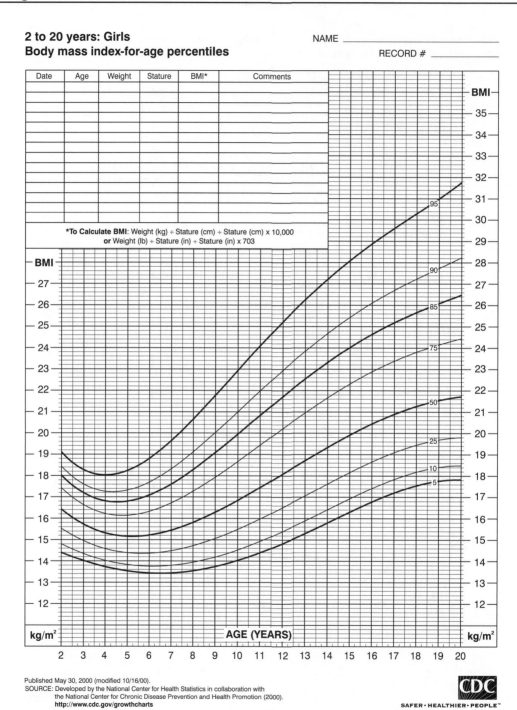

Figure 23.2. Body Mass Index: Girls Aged 2–20

Specialists Involved

A pediatrician will assess your BMI, waist measurement, and overall health risk. If you're overweight or obese, or have a large waist size, your doctor should explain the health risks and find out whether you're interested and willing to lose weight.

If you are, you and your doctor can work together to create a treatment plan. The plan may include weight-loss goals and treatment options that are realistic for you.

Your doctor may send you to other health care specialists, such as those listed below, if you need expert care:

- An endocrinologist if you need to be treated for type 2 diabetes or a hormone problem, such as an underactive thyroid
- A registered dietitian or nutritionist to work with you on ways to change your eating habits
- An exercise physiologist or trainer to figure out your level of fitness and show you how to do physical activities suitable for you
- A bariatric surgeon if weight-loss surgery is an option for you
- A psychiatrist, psychologist, or clinical social worker to help treat depression or stress

How Are Overweight And Obesity Treated?

Successful weight-loss treatments include setting goals and making lifestyle changes, such as eating fewer calories and doing physical activity regularly. Medicines and weight-loss surgery also are options for some people if lifestyle changes aren't enough.

Realistic Goals For Children And Teens

Setting realistic weight-loss goals is an important first step to losing and maintaining weight. If you are overweight or at risk of being overweight, your goals will be to maintain your current weight and to focus on eating healthy and being physically active. Ideally, these goals should be part of a family effort to make lifestyle changes. If you are overweight and have a health condition related to overweight or obesity, your doctor may refer you to a pediatric obesity treatment center.

Lifestyle Changes

For long-term weight-loss success, it's important for you and your family to make lifestyle changes:

- Focus on balancing energy in (calories from food and drinks) and energy out (physical activity).

- Follow a healthy eating plan.

- Learn how to adopt healthy lifestyle habits.

Over time, these changes will become part of your everyday life.

Calories

For overweight children or teens, it's important to slow the rate of weight gain. However, reduced-calorie diets aren't advised unless you talk with a health care provider.

Healthy Eating Plan

A healthy eating plan gives your body the nutrients it needs every day. It has enough calories for good health, but not so many that you gain weight.

A healthy eating plan also will lower your risk of heart disease and other conditions. A healthy eating plan is low in saturated fat, trans fat, cholesterol, sodium (salt), and added sugar.

Obesity And Its Consequences

Research has shown that as weight increases to reach the levels referred to as *overweight* and *obesity*, the risks for the following conditions also increases:

- Coronary heart disease
- Type 2 diabetes
- Cancers (endometrial, breast, and colon)
- Hypertension (high blood pressure)
- Dyslipidemia (for example, high total cholesterol or high levels of triglycerides)
- Stroke
- Liver and gallbladder disease
- Sleep apnea and respiratory problems
- Osteoarthritis (a degeneration of cartilage and its underlying bone within a joint)
- Gynecological problems (abnormal menses, infertility)

In adults, overweight is defined as a body mass index (BMI) of 25 or higher; obesity is defined as a BMI of 30 or higher.

From "The Health Effects of Overweight and Obesity," Centers For Disease Control And Prevention, August 2011.

Here are some examples of healthy foods:

- Fat-free and low-fat milk and milk products, such as low-fat yogurt, cheese, and milk

- Lean meat, fish, poultry, cooked beans, and peas

- Whole-grain foods, such as whole-wheat bread, oatmeal, and brown rice. Other grain foods include pasta, cereal, bagels, bread, tortillas, couscous, and crackers.

- Fruits, which can be canned (in juice or water), fresh, frozen, or dried

- Vegetables, which can be canned (without salt), fresh, frozen, or dried

Canola and olive oils, and soft margarines made from these oils, are heart healthy. However, you should use them in small amounts because they're high in calories.

You also can include unsalted nuts, like walnuts and almonds, in your diet as long as you limit the amount you eat (nuts also are high in calories).

Foods To Limit

Foods that are high in saturated and trans fats and cholesterol raise blood cholesterol levels and also may be high in calories. These fats raise the risk of heart disease, so they should be limited.

Saturated fat mainly is found in these types of foods:

- Fatty cuts of meat, such as ground beef, sausage, and processed meats (for example, bologna, hot dogs, and deli meats)

- Poultry with the skin

- High-fat milk and milk products like whole-milk cheeses, whole milk, cream, butter, and ice cream

- Lard, coconut, and palm oils, which are found in many processed foods

Trans fat mainly is found in these kinds of products:

- Foods with partially hydrogenated oils, such as many hard margarines and shortening

- Baked products and snack foods, such as crackers, cookies, doughnuts, and breads

- Foods fried in hydrogenated shortening, such as french fries and chicken

Cholesterol mainly is found in these types of foods:

- Egg yolks

- Organ meats, such as liver

- Shrimp

- Whole milk or whole milk products, such as butter, cream, and cheese

Limiting foods and drinks with added sugars, like high-fructose corn syrup, is important. Added sugars will give you extra calories without nutrients like vitamins and minerals. Added sugars are found in many desserts, canned fruit packed in syrup, fruit drinks, and non-diet drinks.

Check the list of ingredients on food packages for added sugars like high-fructose corn syrup. Drinks that contain alcohol also will add calories, so it's a good idea to limit your alcohol intake.

Portion Size

A portion is the amount of food that you choose to eat for a meal or snack. It's different from a serving, which is a measured amount of food and is noted on the Nutrition Facts label on food packages.

Anyone who has eaten out lately is likely to notice how big the portions are. In fact, they're oversized. These growing portion sizes have changed what we think of as a normal portion. Cutting back on portion size is a good way to help you eat fewer calories and balance your energy in.

Food Weight

Studies have shown that we all tend to eat a constant weight of food. Ounce for ounce, our food intake is fairly consistent. Knowing this, you can lose weight if you eat foods that are lower in calories and fat for a given amount of food.

For example, replacing a full-fat food product that weighs two ounces with a low-fat product that weighs the same helps you cut back on calories. Another helpful practice is to eat foods that contain a lot of water, such as vegetables, fruits, and soups.

Physical Activity

Being physically active and eating fewer calories will help you lose weight and keep weight off over time. Physical activity also will benefit you in these other ways:

- Lowering your risk of heart disease, heart attack, diabetes, and cancers (such as breast, uterine, and colon cancers)

- Strengthening your heart and help your lungs work better

- Strengthening your muscles and keep your joints in good condition

- Slowing bone loss

- Giving you more energy

- Helping you to relax and cope better with stress

- Allowing you to fall asleep more quickly and sleep more soundly

- Giving you an enjoyable way to share time with friends and family

The four main types of physical activity are aerobic, muscle-strengthening, bone strengthening, and stretching. You can do physical activity with light, moderate, or vigorous intensity. The level of intensity depends on how hard you have to work to do the activity.

People vary in the amount of physical activity they need to control their weight. Many people can maintain their weight by doing 150 to 300 minutes (two hours and 30 minutes to five hours) of moderate-intensity activity per week, such as brisk walking.

People who want to lose a large amount of weight (more than five percent of their body weight) may need to do more than 300 minutes of moderate-intensity activity per week. This also may be true for people who want to keep off weight that they've lost.

You don't have to do the activity all at once. You can break it up into short periods of at least 10 minutes each.

If you have a heart problem or chronic disease, such as heart disease, diabetes, or high blood pressure, talk with your doctor about what types of physical activity are safe for you. You also should talk with your doctor about safe physical activities if you have symptoms such as chest pain or dizziness.

Children should get at least 60 minutes or more of physical activity every day. Most physical activity should be moderate-intensity aerobic activity. Activity should vary and be a good fit for the child's age and physical development.

Many people lead inactive lives and may not be motivated to do more physical activity. When starting a physical activity program, some people may need help and supervision to avoid injury.

If you're obese, or if you haven't been active in the past, start physical activity slowly and build up the intensity a little at a time.

When starting out, one way to be active is to do more everyday activities, such as taking the stairs instead of the elevator and doing household chores and yard work. The next step is to start walking, biking, or swimming at a slow pace, and then build up the amount of time you exercise or the intensity level of the activity.

To lose weight and gain better health, it's important to get moderate-intensity physical activity. Choose activities that you enjoy and that fit into your daily life.

A daily, brisk walk is an easy way to be more active and improve your health. Use a pedometer to count your daily steps and keep track of how much you're walking. Try to increase the number of steps you take each day. Other examples of moderate-intensity physical activity include dancing, gardening, and water aerobics.

For greater health benefits, try to step up your level of activity or the length of time you're active. For example, start walking for 10 to 15 minutes three times a week, and then build up to brisk walking for 60 minutes, five days a week.

Behavioral Changes

Changing your behaviors or habits related to food and physical activity is important for losing weight. The first step is to understand which habits lead you to overeat or have an inactive lifestyle. The next step is to change these habits.

Below are some simple tips to help you adopt healthier habits.

Change Your Surroundings

You may be more likely to overeat when watching TV, when treats are easily available, or when you're with a certain friend. You also may find it hard to motivate yourself to do physical activity regularly. However, you can change these habits.

- Instead of watching TV, dance to music in your living room or go for a walk.

- Bring a change of clothes to school. Head straight to an exercise class on the way home.

- Put a note on your calendar to remind yourself to take a walk or go to your exercise class.

Keep A Record

A record of your food intake and the amount of physical activity that you do each day will help inspire you. You also can keep track of your weight. For example, when the record shows that you've been meeting your physical activity goals, you'll want to keep it up. A record also is an easy way to track how you're doing, especially if you're working with a registered dietitian or nutritionist.

Seek Support

Ask for help or encouragement from your friends, family, and health care provider. You can get support in person, through e-mail, or by talking on the phone. You also can join a support group.

Reward Success

Reward your success for meeting your weight-loss goals or other achievements with something you would like to do, not with food. Choose rewards that you'll enjoy, such as a movie, music CD, a massage, or personal time.

How Can Overweight And Obesity Be Prevented?

Following a healthy lifestyle can help you prevent overweight and obesity. Many lifestyle habits begin during childhood. Thus, everyone in the family should encourage other family members to make healthy choices, such as following a healthy diet and doing enough physical activity. Here are some tips for helping your family follow a healthy lifestyle:

- Follow a healthy eating plan. Make healthy food choices, keep your calorie needs and your family's calorie needs in mind, and focus on the balance of energy in and energy out.

- Focus on portion size. Watch the portion sizes in fast food and other restaurants. The portions served often are enough for two or three people. Children's portion sizes should be smaller than those for adults. Cutting back on portion size will help you balance energy in and energy out.

- Be active. Make personal and family time active. Find activities that everyone will enjoy. For example, go for a brisk walk, bike or rollerblade, or train together for a walk or run.

- Reduce screen time. Limit the use of TVs, computers, DVDs, and videogames because they limit time for physical activity. Health experts recommend two hours or less a day of screen time that's not work or homework related.

- Keep track of your weight, body mass index, and waist circumference.

Chapter 24

Oral Health Consequences Of Eating Disorders

Eating Disorders And Oral Health

- The oral effects of an eating disorder are hard to hide from a dental professional.

- Telltale signs appear early in the mouth and despite the secretive nature of the disease a dental professional may be the first to know and encourage a patient to get help.

- The most common eating disorders that cause problems in the mouth are bulimia nervosa and anorexia nervosa. Although there are other types of eating disorders these tend to cause the most damage to the teeth and mouth.

Bulimia And Oral Health

Bulimia is an eating disorder that involves eating more food at one time that you think you should, called binge eating, and then trying to get rid of that food by purging—self-induced vomiting, use of laxatives, fasting, diuretics, diet pills or over exercising. Bulimia is dangerous to your overall health and especially harmful to your teeth:

- When repeated vomiting is used to purge food from the body, the strong acids in the digestive system erode tooth enamel and weaken fillings and teeth become worn and translucent.

About This Chapter: This chapter begins with "Eating Disorders and Oral Health," produced by the Colorado Department of Public Health and Environment—Oral Health Program, August 2006. You can contact them for additional information (http://www.cde.state.co.us). The chapter continues with "Steps to a Healthy Mouth," excerpted from "Oral Health" produced by the Office on Women's Health (www.womenshealth.gov), November 2008. Reviewed by David A. Cooke, MD, FACP, August 2012.

- Your mouth, throat, and salivary glands become swollen and tender.

- Repeatedly vomiting can cause sores in the corners of the mouth and bad breath.

About 1% of female adolescents have anorexia and 4% of college-aged women have bulimia according to Anorexia Nervosa and Related Eating Disorders Inc.

Anorexia And Oral Health

Anorexia is a psychological disorder that involves a distortion of body image, an intense fear of weight gain, and the desire to be thinner. Anorexia often involves self-induced starvation, purging, and over-exercising the same as bulimia.

Anorexia nervosa may produce some of the same oral symptoms as bulimia.

The Dental Professional

- May encourage you to seek professional help for the eating disorder.

- May create a mouth guard that covers the teeth to help protect them from further erosion by stomach acid.

- Restore damaged teeth, but not until after you get treatment for the eating disorder.

- Provide you with fluoride treatments to help protect your teeth.

Steps To A Healthy Mouth

Use Good Oral Hygiene

- Drink fluoridated water.

Protect Your Teeth

In order to neutralize the effects of stomach acid on your teeth you should:

- Immediately after purging, do not brush, but rinse the mouth with baking soda mixed in water, or sugar-free, alcohol-free mouth rinse, or with plain water if nothing else is available.

- Brush and floss daily

Source: Colorado Department of Public Health and Environment Oral Health Program, 2006. Reviewed by David A. Cooke, MD, FACP, August 2012.

Dental Complications

A complication of purging is the erosion of tooth enamel, caused by repeated regurgitation of gastric acids during vomiting. Perimylolysis refers to erosion of the enamel on the surface of the teeth near the tongue from acid in vomit. Vomiting is also associated with an increase in dental cavities, gum inflammation, temperature sensitivity, and other periodontal disease. Malnutrition associated with all eating disorders can contribute to serious general dental complications including gum disease and tooth extractions.

Gum disease, a complication of self-induced vomiting, is caused by regurgitated stomach acids and enzymes. Other facets of an eating disorder may also cause gum disease: lack of vitamin D and calcium, hormonal imbalance, and general malnutrition.

Source: Excerpted from "Eating Disorders Glossary," © 2012 Families Empowered and Supporting Treatment of Eating Disorders (www.feast-ed.org).

- Brush your teeth at least twice each day with fluoride toothpaste. Look for the American Dental Association's (ADA) Seal of Acceptance.

- Floss daily.

- Gently brush all sides of your teeth with a soft bristled brush and toothpaste. Circular and short back-and-forth strokes work best.

- Take time to brush along the gum line. Brush your tongue lightly.

- Change your toothbrush when the bristles spread out, or at least every three months.

Choose A Healthy Lifestyle

- Don't use tobacco. It raises your risk of getting gum disease, oral and throat cancers, and oral fungal infections.

- Teens should not drink alcohol and adults should limit alcohol use. Heavy alcohol use raises your risk of oral and throat cancers.

- Using alcohol and tobacco together raise your risk of oral cancer even more than using one alone.

- Eat a well-balanced diet and healthy snacks.

- Limit soft drinks. Even diet sodas contain acid that can erode tooth enamel.

Have Regular Checkups

Have an oral exam once or twice a year. Your dentist may recommend more or fewer visits depending on your oral health. At most routine visits, you will be treated by the dentist and a dental hygienist. A thorough checkup includes:

- A health history and oral exam of your teeth and gums. You will be examined for changes, problems, signs of oral cancer or other diseases, and overall oral health.

- Teeth cleaning and polishing to remove hardened plaque and stains.

- X-rays of the teeth and mouth to look for cavities, injury, and problems below the gum-line. How often you need x-rays depends on your health, age, disease risk, and symptoms. Radiation risk is very low.

See your dentist right away if:

- Your gums bleed often.

- You see red or white patches on the gums, tongue, or floor of the mouth that last more than one to two weeks.

- You have mouth or jaw pain that does not go away.

- You have mouth sores that do not heal within two weeks.

- You have problems swallowing or chewing.

Chapter 25

The Link Between Osteoporosis And Anorexia

What Is Anorexia Nervosa?

Anorexia nervosa is an eating disorder characterized by an irrational fear of weight gain. People with anorexia nervosa believe that they are overweight even when they are extremely thin. According to the National Institute of Mental Health, an estimated 0.5–3.7% of females have anorexia nervosa. Although the majority of people with anorexia are female, an estimated 5–15% of people with anorexia are male.

Individuals with anorexia become obsessed with food and severely restrict their dietary intake. The disease is associated with several health problems and, in rare cases, even death. The disorder may begin as early as the onset of puberty. The first menstrual period is typically delayed in girls who have anorexia when they reach puberty. For girls who have already reached puberty when they develop anorexia, menstrual periods are often infrequent or absent.

What Is Osteoporosis?

Osteoporosis is a condition in which the bones become less dense and more likely to fracture. Fractures from osteoporosis can result in significant pain and disability. Osteoporosis is a major health threat for an estimated 44 million Americans, 68 percent of whom are women.

Risk factors for developing osteoporosis include the following:

- Thinness or small frame
- Family history of the disease

About This Chapter: From "What People with Anorexia Nervosa Need to Know about Osteoporosis," National Institute of Arthritis and Musculoskeletal and Skin Diseases (www.niams.nih.gov), January 2011.

- Being postmenopausal and particularly having had early menopause

- Abnormal absence of menstrual periods (amenorrhea)

- Prolonged use of certain medications, such as those used to treat lupus, asthma, thyroid deficiencies, and seizures

- Low calcium intake

- Lack of physical activity

- Smoking

- Excessive alcohol intake

Osteoporosis often can be prevented. It is known as a silent disease because, if undetected, bone loss can progress for many years without symptoms until a fracture occurs. Osteoporosis has been called a childhood disease with old age consequences because building healthy bones in youth helps prevent osteoporosis and fractures later in life.

The Link Between Anorexia Nervosa And Osteoporosis

Anorexia nervosa has significant physical consequences. Affected individuals can experience nutritional and hormonal problems that negatively impact bone density. Low body weight in females causes the body to stop producing estrogen, resulting in a condition known as amenorrhea, or absent menstrual periods. Low estrogen levels contribute to significant losses in bone density.

In addition, individuals with anorexia often produce excessive amounts of the adrenal hormone cortisol, which is known to trigger bone loss. Other problems, such as a decrease in the production of growth hormone and other growth factors, low body weight (apart from the estrogen loss it causes), calcium deficiency, and malnutrition, contribute to bone loss in girls and women with anorexia. Weight loss, restricted dietary intake, and testosterone deficiency may be responsible for the low bone density found in males with the disorder.

Studies suggest that low bone mass (osteopenia) is common in people with anorexia and that it occurs early in the course of the disease. Girls with anorexia are less likely to reach their peak bone density and therefore may be at increased risk for osteoporosis and fracture throughout life.

Osteoporosis Management Strategies

Up to one-third of peak bone density is achieved during puberty. Anorexia is typically identified during mid to late adolescence, a critical period for bone development. The longer the duration of the disorder, the greater the bone loss and the less likely it is that bone mineral density will ever return to normal.

The primary goal of medical therapy for individuals with anorexia is weight gain and, in females, the return of normal menstrual periods. However, attention to other aspects of bone health is also important.

Nutrition

A well-balanced diet rich in calcium and vitamin D is important for healthy bones. Good sources of calcium include low-fat dairy products; dark green, leafy vegetables; and calcium-fortified foods and beverages. Supplements can help ensure that people get adequate amounts of calcium each day, especially in people with a proven milk allergy. The Institute of Medicine recommends a daily calcium intake of 1,000 mg (milligrams) for men and women up to age 50. Women over age 50 and men over age 70 should increase their intake to 1,200 mg daily.

Vitamin D plays an important role in calcium absorption and bone health. Food sources of vitamin D include egg yolks, saltwater fish, and liver. Many people may need vitamin D supplements to achieve the recommended intake of 600 to 800 International Units (IU) each day.

Exercise

Like muscle, bone is living tissue that responds to exercise by becoming stronger. The best activity for your bones is weight-bearing exercise that forces you to work against gravity. Some examples include walking, climbing stairs, lifting weights, and dancing.

Although walking and other types of regular exercise can help prevent bone loss and provide many other health benefits, these potential benefits need to be weighed against the risk of fractures, delayed weight gain, and exercise-induced amenorrhea in people with anorexia and those recovering from the disorder.

Healthy Lifestyle

Smoking is bad for bones as well as the heart and lungs. In addition, smokers may absorb less calcium from their diets. Alcohol also can have a negative effect on bone health. Those who drink heavily are more prone to bone loss and fracture, because of both poor nutrition and increased risk of falling.

Bone Density Test

A bone mineral density (BMD) test measures bone density in various parts of the body. This safe and painless test can detect osteoporosis before a fracture occurs and can predict one's chances of fracturing in the future. The BMD test can help determine whether medication should be considered.

Medication

There is no cure for osteoporosis. However, medications are available to prevent and treat the disease in postmenopausal women, men, and both women and men taking glucocorticoid medication. Some studies suggest that there may be a role for estrogen preparations among girls and young women with anorexia. However, experts agree that estrogen should not be a substitute for nutritional support.

Chapter 26

Eating Disorders Impact Fertility And Pregnancy

Although most teens are not actively planning pregnancies, this information on how eating disorders can impact fertility, pregnancy, and infant health will help readers better understand the far-reaching health consequences of eating disorders.

Eating disorders affect approximately seven million American women each year and tend to peak during childbearing years. Pregnancy is a time when body image concerns are more prevalent, and for those who are struggling with an eating disorder, the nine months of pregnancy can cause disorders to become more serious.

Two of the most common types of eating disorders are anorexia and bulimia. Anorexia involves obsessive dieting or starvation to control weight gain. Bulimia involves binge eating and vomiting or using laxatives to rid the body of excess calories. Both types of eating disorders may negatively affect the reproductive process and pregnancy.

How Do Eating Disorders Affect Fertility?

Eating disorders, particularly anorexia, affect fertility by reducing your chances of conceiving. Most women with anorexia do not have menstrual cycles, and approximately 50% of women struggling with bulimia do not have regular menstrual cycles. The absence of menstruation is caused by reduced calorie intake, excessive exercise, and/or psychological stress. If a woman is not having regular periods, getting pregnant can be very challenging.

About This Chapter: "Eating Disorders during Pregnancy," © 2011 American Pregnancy Association (www .americanpregnancy.org). Reprinted with permission.

How Do Eating Disorders Affect Pregnancy?

Eating disorders affect pregnancy in a number of ways. The following complications are associated with eating disorders during pregnancy:

- Premature labor

- Low birth weight

- Stillbirth or fetal death

- Increased risk of cesarean birth

- Delayed fetal growth

- Respiratory problems

- Gestational diabetes

- Complications during labor

- Depression

- Miscarriage

- Preeclampsia

Women who are struggling with bulimia will often gain excess weight, which places them at risk for hypertension. Women with eating disorders have higher rates of postpartum depression and are more likely to have problems with breastfeeding.

The laxatives, diuretics, and other medications taken may be harmful to the developing baby. These substances take away nutrients and fluids before they are able to feed and nourish the baby. It is possible they may lead to fetal abnormalities as well, particularly if they are used on a regular basis.

Reproductive Recommendations For Women With Eating Disorders

If you are struggling with an eating disorder, getting help to overcome it is the best thing you can do for your reproductive and pregnancy health. The majority of women with eating disorders can have healthy babies if they have normal weight gain throughout pregnancy.

Here are some suggested guidelines for women with eating disorders who are trying to conceive or have discovered that they are pregnant:

Prior To Pregnancy

- Achieve and maintain a healthy weight.

- Avoid purging.

- Consult your health care provider for a pre-conception appointment.

- Meet with a nutritionist and start a healthy pregnancy diet, which may include prenatal vitamins.

- Seek counseling to address your eating disorder and any underlying concerns; seek both individual and group therapy.

During Pregnancy

- Schedule a prenatal visit early in your pregnancy and inform your health care provider that you have been struggling with an eating disorder.

- Strive for healthy weight gain.

- Eat well-balanced meals with all the appropriate nutrients.

- Find a nutritionist who can help you with healthy and appropriate eating.

- Avoid purging.

- Seek counseling to address your eating disorder and any underlying concerns; seek both individual and group therapy.

After Pregnancy

- Continue counseling to improve physical and mental health.

- Inform your safe network (health care provider, spouse, and friends) of your eating disorder and the increased risk of postpartum depression; ask them to be available after the birth.

- Contact a lactation consultant to help with early breastfeeding.

- Find a nutritionist who can help work with you to stay healthy, manage your weight, and invest in your baby.

Chapter 27

The Impact Of Other Conditions On Eating Disorder Symptoms And Treatment

Each patient, and each patient's family, is unique. Each individual brings strengths, skills, and experiences to tackling the problems of life, including a biologically based illness like an eating disorder. When an eating disorder is diagnosed, the clinical team will also be looking for other factors which may impact the illness and recovery. When two illnesses are present at the same time, it is called "co-morbidity" or "dual diagnosis." Some of these conditions are worsened by the symptoms of the eating disorder, some make recovery more difficult, some put the patient at risk of relapse. But there is good news as well: successful diagnosis and treatment of co-morbid illnesses can offer benefits in treating the eating disorder and quality of life after recovery.

Anxiety

One of the most common conditions found along with an eating disorder is anxiety. Anxiety disorders, in fact, are often found in families and relatives of eating disorder patients. Most patients who go on to develop anorexia, in particular, have a history of anxiety and "obsessionality."

Anxiety does not always look like the classic stereotype of a nervous person. Anxiety often looks to others like irritability, anger, shyness, or rigidity. A young person who finds benign issues unbearable, or a child who avoids situations for what seem to be irrational reasons, for example, may be suffering from crippling anxiety.

Obsessionality is also often misunderstood. People are often admired for the same traits that with examination are discovered to be things the person "has to" do rather than "wants to" do. A very diligent student who won't stop studying even when peers are exhausted is an example. Or the athlete who "lives for" her sport and works harder than all her teammates, even to the point of injury.

Since anxiety disorders often become apparent during puberty, the same time eating disorders usually begin, it can be hard to discover which came first. Young people are often unable to articulate the strong anxiety they are feeling, and the rapid changes of that developmental phase confound clear delineation between conditions.

The behaviors of an eating disorder are often experienced by young people as anxiety relievers; restricting, binging, and purging feel better than the intolerable level of anxiety they feel every day. For those with this predisposition, restricting calories reduces physiological sensations of anxiety. This means even low levels of malnutrition can keep a person in a state of lowered anxiety just at a time when they normally would be learning skills of emotional regulation and tolerating distress. Binging and purging also provide physiological effects which blunt or temporarily reduce anxiety for certain people.

Recovery from an eating disorder often requires treatment for underlying anxiety issues. For some this will mean psychotherapy (usually cognitive behavioral therapy or dialectical behavioral therapy) to learn techniques and skills to cope with stress and anxiety and avoid use of eating disorder behaviors. Some patients have underlying anxiety disorders that will need treatment through psychotherapy or drugs.

Depression

Another common co-morbid condition is depression. Like anxiety, it can be hard to discover what came first—the eating disorder or the depression. And also as in the case of anxiety it can be difficult to know whether the symptoms are being caused by restriction, by withdrawal from the eating disorder behaviors, or an underlying condition. Another common factor: depression doesn't always look like sadness or a Hollywood depiction of this very serious and common mental disorder. Depression can look like anger, apathy, resentment, chronic disappointment in others or society, or social withdrawal.

Depressive symptoms are an expected natural consequence of early malnutrition. This may mean that nutritional recovery alone will bring relief, but rarely immediately. Parents should be aware, however, that the symptoms of depression can temporarily worsen as the body is restored, and it is common for it to take many months for the brain to recover. This period of time is very difficult for the patient and requires careful monitoring and support from family.

Suicide is the leading cause of death in eating disorders. Parents must keep this fact in mind and be prepared to provide around the clock presence and support as needed. Skilled clinicians should be involved, and all suicidal talk or behaviors taken extremely seriously.

Body Dysmorphia

We are all familiar with modern society's focus on appearance and particularly on thinness. But some people suffer actual brain changes which cause "dysmorphia." The person is not exaggerating or over-valuing a physical aspect: the person literally sees the distortion on the body and in the mirror. Eating disorders, by altering brain chemistry, can cause body dysmorphia or make it far worse—often the distortion exaggerates body size or proportions. In some cases, the body dysmorphia is resolved as the patient regains nutritional and medical health.

The standard treatment for pre-existing or continuing body dysmorphic disorder (BDD) is selective serotonin re-uptake inhibitor (SSRI) drugs, which is successful in many cases.

Cutting And Self-Injury

Although it is commonly mistaken for a suicidal impulse, "cutting" is believed by experts to be a self-medicating response to extreme anxiety. It is often found in patients who have had or go on to develop eating disorders, especially bulimia. As a sign of extreme distress, and an indication of a person unable to tolerate their level of anxiety, it should be taken as an indication of extreme feelings. It is never appropriate to get angry or punitive with a person who is compelled to do these behaviors. Parents must take this behavior seriously, seek expert advice, and make sure that treatment for self-injury is coordinated with the eating disorder treatment.

Personality Disorders

Some people have, in addition to an eating disorder, what is called a personality disorder. These disorders make relationships difficult. These disorders are treatable, but are thought of as lifelong conditions that can be managed, not cured. A personality disorder can make eating disorder recovery particularly difficult.

It is very important to provide full family history and a developmental history of your loved one in order to help with a full diagnosis. Many parents find the questions clinicians have to ask very intrusive, even insulting. Since personality disorders are associated with childhood abuse, parents may be rightly indignant to be questioned about these issues. Keep in mind that clinicians must ask these questions and get a full view of your child's history in order to rule out other difficulties. It is prudent, with this very serious and sometimes misunderstood diagnosis, to seek second opinions if a personality disorder is diagnosed. It is also important to keep in mind that many of the symptoms of an eating disorder resemble those of personality disorders, and have a reassessment after full recovery has been achieved and maintained.

Stress

Stress, whether from internal or external origins, complicates eating disorder symptoms and all efforts to recover. It also hampers caregivers in having the energy and resources to provide a safe environment. If your family leads a high-stress lifestyle, or the eating disorder patient's personality has created a schedule which distracts from recovery, many families find that treating eating disorder recovery as one would a grave injury is helpful. Cutting back on expectations and obligations, and letting go of any external calendar deadlines can be beneficial to the whole family. Stress is an emotional and physiological drain, and deserves to be treated seriously during initial recovery and preventing relapse.

Medical Conditions

There are many medical conditions that can complicate or even be mistaken for an eating disorder. Diabetes, thyroid issues, autoimmune disorders, gallstones, achalasia, vitamin deficiencies, Lyme disease, and strep infections are all important for you and your clinical team to assess and treat with the eating disorder in mind.

Chapter 28

Diabetes And Eating Disorders

The daily management of diabetes and the focus on eating and nutrition has the potential to create a preoccupation with food. Sometimes this preoccupation becomes an obsession, building momentum until food is almost viewed as dangerous. Worrying about eating the wrong foods and using terms such as "cheating" are unhealthy perspectives that can contribute to the development of an eating disorder.

Disordered eating or eating disorders are serious illnesses that take their toll both emotionally and physically. For people with diabetes, the price of this condition is particularly high—resulting in uncontrolled blood glucose levels and increasing the risk for diabetes complications.

Diabetes may also contribute to the triggering factors that lead to an eating disorder—namely low self-esteem, depression, anxiety, and loneliness. In many of these cases, the person with diabetes may choose to obsessively control their food and/or weight in efforts to manage their emotions.

Teens, in particular, are vulnerable to eating disorders. A teenager with diabetes may learn that poor glucose control leads to weight loss and that well-controlled glucose levels may contribute to weight gain. The term "diabulimia" has cropped up over the last few years, referencing a frightening trend within the diabetes community. This term refers to the method of weight loss by which a person with diabetes intentionally skips insulin therapy in order to keep their blood sugar elevated to a dangerous level, thus causing them to lose weight. Unfortunately, the long-term effects of uncontrolled blood sugars are often viewed as unimportant in the mind of a person with diabetes who is battling an eating disorder.

About This Chapter: "Signs of an Eating Disorder," reprinted with permission from www.dlife.com. © 2012 LifeMed Media, Inc. All rights reserved. Some text excerpted and adapted from State of Missouri Department of Health and Senior Services, http://health.mo.gov.

There are ways to minimize the catalysts for eating disorders, potentially preventing them entirely.

- Focus on food choices rather than food restrictions. Don't expect perfection in diet compliance.

- Avoid emotional or judgmental labels for foods or eating behaviors. Do not categorize foods as "good or bad," or say that a person is "good or bad" based on how or what they eat.

What is diabetes?

Diabetes is a disorder of metabolism—the way the body uses digested food for growth and energy. Most of the food people eat is broken down into glucose, the form of sugar in the blood. Glucose is the main source of fuel for the body.

After digestion, glucose passes into the bloodstream, where it is used by cells for growth and energy. For glucose to get into cells, insulin must be present. Insulin is a hormone produced by the pancreas, a large gland behind the stomach.

When people eat, the pancreas automatically produces the right amount of insulin to move glucose from blood into the cells. In people with diabetes, however, the pancreas either produces little or no insulin, or the cells do not respond appropriately to the insulin that is produced. Glucose builds up in the blood, overflows into the urine, and passes out of the body in the urine. Thus, the body loses its main source of fuel even though the blood contains large amounts of glucose.

The three main types of diabetes are type 1 diabetes, type 2 diabetes, and gestational diabetes.

- **Type 1 Diabetes:** Type 1 diabetes is an autoimmune disease. The body's immune system attacks and destroys the insulin-producing beta cells in the pancreas. The pancreas then produces little or no insulin. A person who has type 1 diabetes must take insulin daily to live.

- **Type 2 Diabetes:** When type 2 diabetes is diagnosed, the pancreas is usually producing enough insulin, but for unknown reasons the body cannot use the insulin effectively, a condition called insulin resistance. After several years, insulin production decreases. The result is the same as for type 1 diabetes—glucose builds up in the blood and the body cannot make efficient use of its main source of fuel.

- **Gestational Diabetes:** Some women develop gestational diabetes late in pregnancy. Although this form of diabetes usually disappears after the birth of the baby, women who have had gestational diabetes have a 40 to 60 percent chance of developing type 2 diabetes within five to ten years.

Source: Excerpted from "Diabetes Overview," National Institute of Diabetes and Digestive and Kidney Diseases (http://diabetes.niddk.nih.gov), April 4, 2012.

Diabulimia

Diabulimia is an eating disorder in which people with Type 1 diabetes deliberately reduce insulin treatment for the purpose of weight loss. The body goes into a starvation state, resulting in breakdown of muscle and fat into ketone bodies and subsequently ketoacids. The body is unable to process sugars that have been consumed, so the sugars are excreted rather than being used by the body for energy or stored as fat. This typically results in significant weight loss but also places the patient at risk of a life-threatening condition known as diabetic ketoacidosis.

Source: Excerpted from "Eating Disorders Glossary," © 2012 Families Empowered and Supporting Treatment of Eating Disorders (www.feast-ed.org).

- Make exercise a part of your life, not just a method of calorie burning. Becoming involved in life-long recreational sports like hiking or tennis makes exercise more fun and can help remove the exercise obsession as it relates to diabetes management.

- Also, keep talking. Isolating and discussing the stressors in your life may help to alleviate them. Talking with family members, loved ones, or seeking professional counseling is an option. If you or your loved one exhibits the signs of an eating disorder, don't be afraid to talk about it.

What are the signs of an eating disorder, clinically known as disordered eating?

Diabulimia is characterized by a person with diabetes intentionally skipping insulin therapy to keep blood glucose levels elevated, which in turn causes dangerous weight loss. Signs and symptoms may include:

- Excessive exercise
- Intentionally skipped or drastically lowered insulin doses
- Decreased blood glucose monitoring
- Rapid weight loss
- Excessive urination
- Vomiting
- Extreme concern with body weight and shape

Anorexia nervosa is characterized by self-starvation and excessive weight loss. Signs and symptoms may include:

- Refusal to maintain body weight at or above a minimally normal weight for height, body type, age, and activity level

- Intense fear of weight gain or being "fat"

- Feeling "fat" or overweight despite dramatic weight loss

- Loss of menstrual periods

- Extreme concern with body weight and shape

Bulimia is characterized by a secretive cycle of binge eating followed by purging. Bulimia includes eating large amounts of food—more than most people would eat in one meal—in short periods of time, then getting rid of the food and calories through vomiting, laxative abuse, or over-exercising. Signs and symptoms may include:

- Repeated episodes of binging and purging

- Feeling out of control during a binge and eating beyond the point of comfortable fullness

- Purging after a binge (typically by self-induced vomiting, abuse of laxatives, diet pills and/or diuretics, excessive exercise, or fasting)

- Frequent dieting

- Extreme concern with body weight and shape

Eating disorders are serious medical conditions. Combined with diabetes, they can cause illness, long-term complications, and even death. If you suspect that you or your loved one may have an eating disorder, talk to your doctor today about treatment options.

Chapter 29

Depression, Anxiety, And Eating Disorders

Eating Disorders

What are eating disorders?

An eating disorder is an illness that causes serious disturbances to your everyday diet, such as eating extremely small amounts of food or severely overeating. A person with an eating disorder may have started out just eating smaller or larger amounts of food, but at some point, the urge to eat less or more spiraled out of control. Severe distress or concern about body weight or shape may also characterize an eating disorder.

Eating disorders frequently appear during the teen years or young adulthood but may also develop during childhood or later in life. Common eating disorders include anorexia nervosa, bulimia nervosa, and binge-eating disorder.

Eating disorders are real, treatable medical illnesses. They frequently coexist with other illnesses such as depression, substance abuse, or anxiety disorders.

Depression

What is depression?

Everyone occasionally feels blue or sad. But these feelings are usually short-lived and pass within a couple of days. When you have depression, it interferes with daily life and causes pain for you and those who care about you. Depression is a common but serious illness.

About This Chapter: This chapter includes excerpts from the following documents produced by the National Institute of Mental Health (www.nimh.nih.gov): "Eating Disorders," January 10, 2012; "Depression," December 28, 2011; and "Anxiety Disorders," November 2, 2010.

Many people with a depressive illness never seek treatment. But the majority, even those with the most severe depression, can get better with treatment. Medications, psychotherapies, and other methods can effectively treat people with depression.

What are the different forms of depression?

There are several forms of depressive disorders.

Major depressive disorder, or major depression, is characterized by a combination of symptoms that interfere with a person's ability to work, sleep, study, eat, and enjoy once-pleasurable activities. Major depression is disabling and prevents a person from functioning normally. Some people may experience only a single episode within their lifetime, but more often a person may have multiple episodes.

Dysthymic disorder, or dysthymia, is characterized by long-term (two years or longer) symptoms that may not be severe enough to disable a person but can prevent normal functioning or feeling well. People with dysthymia may also experience one or more episodes of major depression during their lifetimes.

Minor depression is characterized by having symptoms for two weeks or longer that do not meet full criteria for major depression. Without treatment, people with minor depression are at high risk for developing major depressive disorder.

Some forms of depression are slightly different, or they may develop under unique circumstances. However, not everyone agrees on how to characterize and define these forms of depression. They include psychotic depression, postpartum depression, and seasonal affective disorder.

Psychotic depression occurs when a person has severe depression plus some form of psychosis, such as having disturbing false beliefs or a break with reality (delusions), or hearing or seeing upsetting things that others cannot hear or see (hallucinations).

Postpartum depression is a form of depression that is much more serious than the baby blues many women experience after giving birth (when hormonal and physical changes and the new responsibility of caring for a newborn can be overwhelming). It is estimated that 10 to 15 percent of women experience postpartum depression after giving birth.

Seasonal affective disorder (SAD) is characterized by the onset of depression during the winter months when there is less natural sunlight. The depression generally lifts during spring and summer. SAD may be effectively treated with light therapy, but nearly half of those with SAD do not get better with light therapy alone. Antidepressant medication and psychotherapy can reduce SAD symptoms, either alone or in combination with light therapy.

Bipolar disorder, also called manic-depressive illness, is not as common as major depression or dysthymia. Bipolar disorder is characterized by cycling mood changes—from extreme highs (mania) to extreme lows (depression).

What are the signs and symptoms of depression?

People with depressive illnesses do not all experience the same symptoms. The severity, frequency, and duration of symptoms vary depending on the individual and his or her particular illness. Signs and symptoms include persistent sad, anxious, or "empty" feelings. They also include feelings of hopelessness or pessimism or feelings of guilt, worthlessness, or helplessness. Other signs and symptoms include irritability, restlessness, loss of interest in activities or hobbies once pleasurable, fatigue and decreased energy, difficulty concentrating or remembering details, difficulty making decisions, insomnia, early-morning wakefulness, excessive sleeping, overeating, appetite loss, and thoughts of suicide or suicide attempts. Aches or pains, headaches, cramps, or digestive problems that do not ease even with treatment can also be signs and symptoms of depression.

What illnesses often co-exist with depression?

Other illnesses may come on before depression, cause it, or be a consequence of it. But depression and other illnesses interact differently in different people.

Anxiety disorders, such as post-traumatic stress disorder (PTSD), obsessive-compulsive disorder, panic disorder, social phobia, and generalized anxiety disorder, often accompany depression. PTSD can occur after a person experiences a terrifying event or ordeal, such as a violent assault, a natural disaster, an accident, terrorism or military combat. People experiencing PTSD are especially prone to having co-existing depression.

Alcohol and other substance abuse or dependence may also co-exist with depression. Research shows that mood disorders and substance abuse commonly occur together.

Depression also may occur with other serious medical illnesses such as heart disease, stroke, cancer, HIV/AIDS, diabetes, and Parkinson disease. People who have depression along with another medical illness tend to have more severe symptoms of both depression and the medical illness, more difficulty adapting to their medical condition, and more medical costs than those who do not have co-existing depression. Treating the depression can also help improve the outcome of treating the co-occurring illness.

What causes depression?

Most likely, depression is caused by a combination of genetic, biological, environmental, and psychological factors.

Depressive illnesses are disorders of the brain. Longstanding theories about depression suggest that important neurotransmitters—chemicals that brain cells use to communicate—are out of balance in depression. But it has been difficult to prove this.

Brain-imaging technologies, such as magnetic resonance imaging (MRI), have shown that the brains of people who have depression look different than those of people without depression. The parts of the brain involved in mood, thinking, sleep, appetite, and behavior appear different. But these images do not reveal why the depression has occurred. They also cannot be used to diagnose depression.

How do children and teens experience depression?

Children who develop depression often continue to have episodes as they enter adulthood. Children who have depression also are more likely to have other more severe illnesses in adulthood.

A child with depression may pretend to be sick, refuse to go to school, cling to a parent, or worry that a parent may die. Older children may sulk, get into trouble at school, be negative and irritable, and feel misunderstood. Because these signs may be viewed as normal mood swings typical of children as they move through developmental stages, it may be difficult to accurately diagnose a young person with depression.

Before puberty, boys and girls are equally likely to develop depression. By age 15, however, girls are twice as likely as boys to have had a major depressive episode.

Depression during the teen years comes at a time of great personal change—when boys and girls are forming an identity apart from their parents, grappling with gender issues and emerging sexuality, and making independent decisions for the first time in their lives. Depression in adolescence frequently co-occurs with other disorders such as anxiety, eating disorders, or substance abuse. It can also lead to increased risk for suicide.

How is depression diagnosed and treated?

Depression, even the most severe cases, can be effectively treated. The earlier that treatment can begin, the more effective it is.

The first step to getting appropriate treatment is to visit a doctor or mental health specialist. Certain medications, and some medical conditions such as viruses or a thyroid disorder, can cause the same symptoms as depression. A doctor can rule out these possibilities by doing a physical exam, interview, and lab tests. If the doctor can find no medical condition that may be causing the depression, the next step is a psychological evaluation.

The doctor may refer you to a mental health professional, who should discuss with you any family history of depression or other mental disorder, and get a complete history of your symptoms. You should discuss when your symptoms started, how long they have lasted, how severe they are, and whether they have occurred before and if so, how they were treated. The mental health professional may also ask if you are using alcohol or drugs, and if you are thinking about death or suicide.

Once diagnosed, a person with depression can be treated in several ways. The most common treatments are medication and psychotherapy.

FDA Warning On Antidepressants

Despite the relative safety and popularity of selective serotonin reuptake inhibitors (SSRIs) and other antidepressants, studies have suggested that they may have unintentional effects on some people, especially adolescents and young adults. In 2004, the Food and Drug Administration (FDA) conducted a thorough review of published and unpublished controlled clinical trials of antidepressants that involved nearly 4,400 children and adolescents. The review revealed that four percent of those taking antidepressants thought about or attempted suicide (although no suicides occurred), compared to two percent of those receiving placebos.

This information prompted the FDA, in 2005, to adopt a "black box" warning label on all antidepressant medications to alert the public about the potential increased risk of suicidal thinking or attempts in children and adolescents taking antidepressants. In 2007, the FDA proposed that makers of all antidepressant medications extend the warning to include young adults up through age 24. A "black box" warning is the most serious type of warning on prescription drug labeling.

The warning emphasizes that patients of all ages taking antidepressants should be closely monitored, especially during the initial weeks of treatment. Possible side effects to look for are worsening depression, suicidal thinking or behavior, or any unusual changes in behavior such as sleeplessness, agitation, or withdrawal from normal social situations. The warning adds that families and caregivers should also be told of the need for close monitoring and that they should report any changes to the doctor. The latest information from the FDA can be found on their website (www.fda.gov).

Results of a comprehensive review of pediatric trials conducted between 1988 and 2006 suggested that the benefits of antidepressant medications likely outweigh their risks to children and adolescents with major depression and anxiety disorders.

Source: NIMH, December 28, 2011.

How can I help myself if I am depressed?

If you have depression, you may feel exhausted, helpless, and hopeless. It may be extremely difficult to take any action to help yourself. But as you begin to recognize your depression and begin treatment, you will start to feel better. Here are some tips to help you get started:

- Do not wait too long to get evaluated or treated. There is research showing the longer one waits, the greater the impairment can be down the road. Try to see a professional as soon as possible.

- Try to be active and exercise. Go to a movie, a ballgame, or another event or activity that you once enjoyed.

- Set realistic goals for yourself.

- Break up large tasks into small ones, set some priorities and do what you can as you can.

- Try to spend time with other people and confide in a trusted friend or relative. Try not to isolate yourself, and let others help you.

- Expect your mood to improve gradually, not immediately. Do not expect to suddenly "snap out of" your depression. Often during treatment for depression, sleep and appetite will begin to improve before your depressed mood lifts.

- Postpone important decisions until you feel better. Discuss decisions with others who know you well and have a more objective view of your situation.

- Remember that positive thinking will replace negative thoughts as your depression responds to treatment.

- Continue to educate yourself about depression.

Anxiety Disorders

What are anxiety disorders?

Anxiety disorders cause people to be filled with fearfulness and uncertainty. Unlike the relatively mild, brief anxiety caused by a stressful event (such as speaking in public or a first date), anxiety disorders last at least six months and can get worse if they are not treated. Anxiety disorders commonly occur along with other mental or physical illnesses, including alcohol or substance abuse, which may mask anxiety symptoms or make them worse. In some cases, these other illnesses need to be treated before a person will respond to treatment for the anxiety disorder.

What if I am or someone I know is in crisis?

If you are thinking about harming yourself, or know someone who is, tell someone who can help immediately.

- Do not leave your friend or relative alone, and do not isolate yourself.
- Call your doctor.
- Call 911 or go to a hospital emergency room to get immediate help, or ask a friend or family member to help you do these things.
- Call the toll-free, 24-hour hotline of the National Suicide Prevention Lifeline at 800-273-TALK (800-273-8255); TTY: 800-799-4TTY (4889) to talk to a trained counselor.

Source: NIMH, December 28, 2011.

Effective therapies for anxiety disorders are available, and research is uncovering new treatments that can help most people with anxiety disorders lead productive, fulfilling lives. If you think you have an anxiety disorder, you should seek information and treatment right away.

There are many different anxiety disorders, including panic disorder, obsessive-compulsive disorder, post-traumatic stress disorder, social phobia (social anxiety disorder), specific phobias, and generalized anxiety disorder. Each anxiety disorder has different symptoms, but all the symptoms cluster around excessive, irrational fear and dread.

What is panic disorder?

Panic disorder is a real illness that can be successfully treated. It is characterized by sudden attacks of terror, usually accompanied by a pounding heart, sweatiness, weakness, faintness, or dizziness. During these attacks, people with panic disorder may flush or feel chilled; their hands may tingle or feel numb; and they may experience nausea, chest pain, or smothering sensations. Panic attacks usually produce a sense of unreality, a fear of impending doom, or a fear of losing control.

A fear of one's own unexplained physical symptoms is also a symptom of panic disorder. People having panic attacks sometimes believe they are having heart attacks, losing their minds, or on the verge of death. They can't predict when or where an attack will occur, and between episodes many worry intensely and dread the next attack.

Panic attacks can occur at any time, even during sleep. An attack usually peaks within 10 minutes, but some symptoms may last much longer.

Panic attacks often begin in late adolescence or early adulthood, but not everyone who experiences panic attacks will develop panic disorder. Many people have just one attack and never have another. The tendency to develop panic attacks appears to be inherited.

People who have full-blown, repeated panic attacks can become very disabled by their condition and should seek treatment before they start to avoid places or situations where panic attacks have occurred. For example, if a panic attack happened in an elevator, someone with panic disorder may develop a fear of elevators that could affect the choice of a job or an apartment, and restrict where that person can seek medical attention or enjoy entertainment.

Some people's lives become so restricted that they avoid normal activities, such as grocery shopping or driving. About one-third becomes housebound or is able to confront a feared situation only when accompanied by a spouse or other trusted person. When the condition progresses this far, it is called agoraphobia, or fear of open spaces.

Early treatment can often prevent agoraphobia, but people with panic disorder may sometimes go from doctor to doctor for years and visit the emergency room repeatedly before someone correctly diagnoses their condition. This is unfortunate, because panic disorder is one of the most treatable of all the anxiety disorders, responding in most cases to certain kinds of medication or certain kinds of cognitive psychotherapy, which help change thinking patterns that lead to fear and anxiety.

Panic disorder is often accompanied by other serious problems, such as depression, drug abuse, or alcoholism. These conditions need to be treated separately.

What is obsessive-compulsive disorder?

People with obsessive-compulsive disorder (OCD) have persistent, upsetting thoughts (obsessions) and use rituals (compulsions) to control the anxiety these thoughts produce. Most of the time, the rituals end up controlling them.

For example, if people are obsessed with germs or dirt, they may develop a compulsion to wash their hands over and over again. If they develop an obsession with intruders, they may lock and relock their doors many times before going to bed. Being afraid of social embarrassment may prompt people with OCD to comb their hair compulsively in front of a mirror—sometimes they get "caught" in the mirror and can't move away from it. Performing such rituals is not pleasurable. At best, it produces temporary relief from the anxiety created by obsessive thoughts.

Other common rituals are a need to repeatedly check things, touch things (especially in a particular sequence), or count things. Some common obsessions include having frequent thoughts of violence and harming loved ones, persistently thinking about performing sexual acts the person dislikes, or having thoughts that are prohibited by religious beliefs. People with OCD may also be preoccupied with order and symmetry, have difficulty throwing things out (so they accumulate), or hoard unneeded items.

Healthy people also have rituals, such as checking to see if the stove is off several times before leaving the house. The difference is that people with OCD perform their rituals even though doing so interferes with daily life and they find the repetition distressing. Although most adults with OCD recognize that what they are doing is senseless, some adults and most children may not realize that their behavior is out of the ordinary.

OCD affects about 2.2 million American adults, and the problem can be accompanied by eating disorders, other anxiety disorders, or depression. It strikes men and women in roughly equal numbers and usually appears in childhood, adolescence, or early adulthood. One-third of adults with OCD develop symptoms as children, and research indicates that OCD might run in families.

OCD usually responds well to treatment with certain medications and/or exposure-based psychotherapy, in which people face situations that cause fear or anxiety and become less sensitive (desensitized) to them.

What is post-traumatic stress disorder?

Post-traumatic stress disorder (PTSD) develops after a terrifying ordeal that involved physical harm or the threat of physical harm. The person who develops PTSD may have been the one who was harmed, the harm may have happened to a loved one, or the person may have witnessed a harmful event that happened to loved ones or strangers.

PTSD was first brought to public attention in relation to war veterans, but it can result from a variety of traumatic incidents, such as mugging, rape, torture, being kidnapped or held captive, child abuse, car accidents, train wrecks, plane crashes, bombings, or natural disasters such as floods or earthquakes.

People with PTSD may startle easily, become emotionally numb (especially in relation to people with whom they used to be close), lose interest in things they used to enjoy, have trouble feeling affectionate, be irritable, become more aggressive, or even become violent. They avoid situations that remind them of the original incident, and anniversaries of the incident are often very difficult. PTSD symptoms seem to be worse if the event that triggered them was deliberately initiated by another person, as in a mugging or a kidnapping.

Most people with PTSD repeatedly relive the trauma in their thoughts during the day and in nightmares when they sleep. These are called flashbacks. Flashbacks may consist of images, sounds, smells, or feelings, and are often triggered by ordinary occurrences, such as a door slamming or a car backfiring on the street. A person having a flashback may lose touch with reality and believe that the traumatic incident is happening all over again.

Not every traumatized person develops full-blown or even minor PTSD. Symptoms usually begin within three months of the incident but occasionally emerge years afterward. They must last more than a month to be considered PTSD. The course of the illness varies. Some people recover within six months, while others have symptoms that last much longer. In some people, the condition becomes chronic.

What is social phobia?

Social phobia, also called social anxiety disorder, is diagnosed when people become overwhelmingly anxious and excessively self-conscious in everyday social situations. People with social phobia have an intense, persistent, and chronic fear of being watched and judged by others and of doing things that will embarrass them. They can worry for days or weeks before a dreaded situation. This fear may become so severe that it interferes with school and other ordinary activities and can make it hard to make and keep friends.

While many people with social phobia realize that their fears about being with people are excessive or unreasonable, they are unable to overcome them. Even if they manage to confront their fears and be around others, they are usually very anxious beforehand, are intensely uncomfortable throughout the encounter, and worry about how they were judged for hours afterward.

Social phobia can be limited to one situation (such as talking to people, eating or drinking, or writing on a blackboard in front of others) or may be so broad (such as in generalized social phobia) that the person experiences anxiety around almost anyone other than the family.

Physical symptoms that often accompany social phobia include blushing, profuse sweating, trembling, nausea, and difficulty talking. When these symptoms occur, people with social phobia feel as though all eyes are focused on them.

Social phobia usually begins in childhood or early adolescence. There is some evidence that genetic factors are involved. Social phobia is often accompanied by other anxiety disorders or depression, and substance abuse may develop if people try to self-medicate their anxiety.

Social phobia can be successfully treated with certain kinds of psychotherapy or medications.

What are specific phobias?

A specific phobia is an intense, irrational fear of something that poses little or no actual danger. Some of the more common specific phobias are centered around closed-in places, heights, escalators, tunnels, highway driving, water, flying, dogs, and injuries involving blood.

Such phobias aren't just extreme fear; they are irrational fear of a particular thing. You may be able to ski the world's tallest mountains with ease but be unable to go above the fifth floor of an office building.

Specific phobias usually appear in childhood or adolescence and tend to persist into adulthood. The causes of specific phobias are not well understood, but there is some evidence that the tendency to develop them may run in families.

If the feared situation or feared object is easy to avoid, people with specific phobias may not seek help; but if avoidance interferes with their careers or their personal lives, it can become disabling and treatment is usually pursued.

Specific phobias respond very well to carefully targeted psychotherapy.

What is generalized anxiety disorder?

People with generalized anxiety disorder (GAD) go through the day filled with exaggerated worry and tension, even though there is little or nothing to provoke it. They anticipate disaster and are overly concerned about health issues, money, family problems, or difficulties at work. Sometimes just the thought of getting through the day produces anxiety.

GAD is diagnosed when a person worries excessively about a variety of everyday problems for at least six months. People with GAD can't seem to get rid of their concerns, even though they usually realize that their anxiety is more intense than the situation warrants. They can't relax, startle easily, and have difficulty concentrating. Often they have trouble falling asleep or staying asleep. Physical symptoms that often accompany the anxiety include fatigue, headaches, muscle tension, muscle aches, difficulty swallowing, trembling, twitching, irritability, sweating, nausea, lightheadedness, having to go to the bathroom frequently, feeling out of breath, and hot flashes.

GAD develops gradually and can begin at any point in the life cycle, although the years of highest risk are between childhood and middle age. There is evidence that genes play a modest role in GAD. Other anxiety disorders, depression, or substance abuse often accompany GAD, which rarely occurs alone. GAD is commonly treated with medication or cognitive-behavioral therapy, but co-occurring conditions must also be treated using the appropriate therapies.

How are anxiety disorders treated?

In general, anxiety disorders are treated with medication, specific types of psychotherapy, or both. Treatment choices depend on the problem and the person's preference. Before treatment begins, a doctor must conduct a careful diagnostic evaluation to determine whether a person's symptoms are caused by an anxiety disorder or a physical problem. If an anxiety disorder is diagnosed, the type of disorder or the combination of disorders that are present must be identified, as well as any coexisting conditions, such as depression or substance abuse. Sometimes alcoholism, depression, or other coexisting conditions have such a strong effect on the individual that treating the anxiety disorder must wait until the coexisting conditions are brought under control.

Chapter 30

Self-Injury Linked To Eating Disorders

An alarming number of adolescents already battling eating disorders are also intentionally cutting themselves, and health-care providers may be failing to diagnose many instances of such self-injury, according to a new study from Stanford University School of Medicine and Lucile Packard Children's Hospital.

The researchers found that 40.8 percent of patients with eating disorders in their study had documented incidents of intentionally harming themselves, most often by cutting and burning. What's more, the study suggests that inadequate clinical screening might mean the count should be much higher.

"These are very high numbers, but they're still conservative estimates," said the study's lead author, Rebecka Peebles, MD, who was an instructor in pediatrics at Stanford when the research was conducted and is joining the faculty at Children's Hospital of Philadelphia.

Peebles noted that clinicians aren't routinely asking about this activity. "We ask 97 percent of children 12 years and up if they smoke cigarettes; we need to get that good with screening for self-injurious behavior," she said.

The study was published online October 8, 2010 in the *Journal of Adolescent Health*. Its senior author is James Lock, MD, PhD, professor of psychiatry and behavioral sciences and of pediatrics. He is also psychiatric director of the Comprehensive Eating Disorders Program at Packard Children's Hospital.

To conduct the study, the researchers examined the intake evaluation records of 1,432 patients, ages 10–21, who were admitted to the hospital's eating disorders program from January 1997 through April 2008. Just over 90 percent of all the patients were female, three-quarters of them white, with a mean age of 15. Among the 40.8 percent identified to be physically harming themselves, the mean age was 16. Many of these patients had a history of binging and purging, and 85.2 percent of the self-injurers were cutting themselves.

The researchers also discovered that slightly fewer than half the charts showed that health-care providers had asked patients if they intentionally injured themselves. If patients aren't asked, they are unlikely to volunteer such information, said Peebles.

Those who were questioned tended to fit previously published profiles of a self-injurer: older, white, female, suffering from bulimia nervosa, or with a history of substance abuse. "The question is, 'Are we missing other kids who are not meeting this profile?'" Peebles said. "This is part of why we wanted to look at this. If you see an innocent-looking 12-year-old boy, you don't even think of asking about self-injurious behavior. We need to get much better about universal screening."

Peebles noted that the profile itself might be flawed. If health-care workers only ask a certain type of patient about a behavior, the profile that emerges will necessarily reflect that bias, she said.

The study did not examine the reasons behind such acts but Peebles said her clinical experience suggested patients "are trying to feel pain."

"Patients describe a feeling of release that comes when they cut or burn themselves," she said. "They'll cut with a razor or a scissor blade. Sometimes we've even had kids who will take the tip of a paper clip and gouge holes. To burn themselves, they'll heat up a metal object and press it to their skin, or they'll use cigarettes."

Physicians and other health-care providers at Packard's Comprehensive Eating Disorders Program now question all new patients about self-injurious behavior. Studies have shown that between 13 and 40 percent of all adolescents engage in some form of self-injury, which is also associated with a higher risk of suicide.

"In clinical practice, kids are fairly open when you engage with them," Peebles said. "They'll come in wearing long sleeves, or hiding the marks on their inner thighs. But then when you ask them, they are usually willing to discuss the behavior."

The study's other author is Jenny Wilson, MD, who was a resident in pediatrics when the study was conducted.

The study was funded in part by the Stanford Child Health Research Program. Information about the Departments of Pediatrics and of Psychiatry and Behavioral Sciences, which also helped to support this study, is available at http://pediatrics.stanford.edu and http://psychiatry.stanford.edu/.

Comments From The Cornell Research Program On Self-Injurious Behavior

Sometimes called "deliberate self-harm," "self-injury," "self-mutilation," "cutting," or "non-suicidal self-injury," self-injury typically refers to a variety of behaviors in which an individual intentionally inflicts harm to his or her body for purposes not socially recognized or sanctioned and without suicidal intent.

Tattoos and body piercing are not typically considered self-injurious unless undertaken with the intention to harm the body.

Those who practice self-injurious behavior also report high levels of perceived loneliness, less dense social networks, less affectionate relationships with their parents, and a history of emotional and/or sexual abuse. They are also more likely to suffer from diminished self-esteem, feelings of invisibility, and shame. Indeed, feeling invisible and inauthentic are common themes among self-injurious students we have interviewed for our studies. Approaches in which adolescents and adults are aided in recognizing and building on existing strengths, in reaching out to and connecting way with others in an authentic and meaningful way, and in participating in activities which allow them to feel meaningfully linked to something larger than themselves may help to shape a more positive view of the self. This may ultimately lessen reliance on potentially damaging coping mechanisms.

As with many risk behaviors, our research shows that peers are most often the first to know or suspect that a friend is using self-injurious practices. As such, peers constitute the "front line" in detection and intervention. We advocate concentrating effort on assisting young people to recognize general symptoms of distress in their peers. Self-injurious behavior could be one of several categories of behaviors and perceptions assessed (mixing both positive and negative indicators avoids a solely deficit-based slant to findings) such as perceived wellbeing, eating disorders, life satisfaction, depression, relationships with adults, suicidality, etc. In addition to educating about how to recognize distress, students could be encouraged to seek assistance and coached on specific strategies for getting help.

Chapter 31

Unresolved Trauma
And Eating Disorders

There is a strong correlation between trauma and eating disorders. A number of studies have shown that people who struggle with eating disorders have a higher incidence of neglect and physical, emotional, and sexual abuse. In particular, binge eating disorder is associated with emotional abuse while sexual abuse has been linked to eating disorders in males.

So what constitutes trauma?

Trauma comes in many forms, including childhood abuse or neglect, growing up in an alcoholic or dysfunctional home, environmental catastrophes such as Hurricane Katrina, a serious accident, loss of a loved one, and violent attacks such as rape and sexual assault. What all of these experiences have in common is that they leave the individual feeling helpless and out of control.

Trauma isn't the same as having post-traumatic stress disorder (PTSD). PTSD is a specific diagnosis with distinct criteria, involving a serious or life-threatening experience that results in nightmares, flashbacks, attempts to avoid situations similar to those that led to the trauma, and a hyperactive startle response, among other symptoms.

How Trauma Contributes To Eating Disorders

An eating disorder may develop in an attempt to cope with the trauma, suppress painful emotions, or to regain a sense of control. Here are a few examples of how trauma manifests in eating disorders:

About This Chapter: "Is Unresolved Trauma Preventing a Full Eating Disorder Recovery?" by Carolyn Coker Ross, MD. © 2012 Psych Central (www.psychcentral.com). All rights reserved. Reprinted with permission.

- **Example 1:** After the death of a parent, a child is sent to live with a grandparent who isn't as loving and kind as her mother. She had pleasant memories around food, cooking, and eating as a family, and used food to comfort herself through the sadness of losing her mom. After bingeing, she feels consumed by guilt and self-loathing and begins purging through self-induced vomiting, use of laxatives or excessive exercise.

- **Example 2:** A young adult woman was raped in college. Because she was powerless to prevent the attack, she began restricting her food intake to feel a sense of control over her body. Losing weight became a way to disappear or to appear childlike so she could be cared for by others or appear less attractive to men. Others who have been sexually abused or traumatized by the men in their lives may overeat, using their weight as a protective mechanism to avoid being hurt again.

Treatment For Trauma And Eating Disorders

Individuals with a history of trauma may not fully recover from an eating disorder, or may experience chronic relapse from their eating disorder, until they address the underlying trauma. As part of an integrative approach to eating disorder treatment, patients may participate in the following interventions.

Somatic Experiencing

Trauma is held in the body and often can't be resolved solely with intellectual processing. Somatic experiencing is a body-awareness technique that was developed by Peter Levine, PhD. With guidance from a therapist, patients explore the sensations in the body as they work to recognize and regulate their feelings of distress.

Eye Movement Desensitization And Reprocessing

In EMDR, the patient focuses on past memories, present triggers, or experiences they anticipate in the future while focusing on an external stimulus (e.g., eye movements, tones, or taps). For example, the patient may be asked to focus on a particular thought or bodily sensation while simultaneously moving their eyes back and forth, following the therapist's fingers as they move across the patient's field of vision for about 20–30 seconds. Each session is guided by a therapist to help the patient develop new insights or associations surrounding their experience of trauma.

Cognitive Behavioral Therapy

Individuals who have experienced trauma often struggle with self-blame or feeling responsible for what happened to them. This maladaptive thought process may follow them into adulthood. Trauma victims may recreate the trauma in some form for themselves or by perpetrating the act of their abuser on others.

Cognitive behavioral therapy helps patients work through anger, shame, guilt, and other emotions by replacing negative thought and behavior patterns with new skills and problem-solving strategies. It is backed by extensive scientific research and is widely used to treat trauma, eating disorders, and a variety of other mental illnesses. In a safe, supportive therapeutic setting, patients are able to openly talk about their traumatic experiences and disordered eating behaviors.

Coping Skills Training

Eating disorders frequently develop as a way to cope with trauma. If trauma occurs at a time in life when the individual lacks the coping mechanisms to process it, they may use food to feel a sense of control.

Rather than judging the coping mechanism as good or bad, the therapist helps the patient identify the purpose the eating disorder has served and recognize that it has begun to cost more than it helps. As an adult, the patient can develop more mature coping strategies and call upon different skills than they could at the time of the traumatic event.

Dialectical behavior therapy helps trauma sufferers build the skills of mindfulness, distress tolerance, emotional regulation, and interpersonal effectiveness to improve body image, manage painful feelings associated with trauma, and guard against relapse. Learning how to trust and express anger in a healthy way are other important recovery tools.

Self-Help Support Groups

Social support is a major determinant of successful coping. A number of 12-step support groups exist for those suffering from an eating disorder, including Eating Disorders Anonymous, Overeaters Anonymous, and Anorexics and Bulimics Anonymous. Many eating disorder treatment programs invite family members to be part of the treatment team and to address their own emotional and psychological issues while their loved one is in treatment.

Nutritional Therapy

Beginning to address trauma can lead to an increase in eating disorder behaviors. By educating patients about nutrition and fueling the body with wholesome foods, patients can practice healthier patterns and boost their energy and mood.

Exercise

When a patient is working to manage their anger, certain forms of exercise may be a tool for healthy release of anger.

Nutraceuticals

Use of nutraceuticals—amino acids, nutrients, and dietary supplements that improve overall health—can decrease distractions from trauma work and reduce some of the physical complaints of eating disorder recovery, such as bloating and constipation. Certain supplements and herbal remedies may also assist with symptoms of depression and co-occurring mood disorders.

Mind-Body Therapies

A number of mind-body therapies can aid in stress management and boost mood and memory. Meditation, acupuncture, yoga, massage, energy healing, self-hypnosis, and breath work are a few examples of therapies that have been helpful in treating eating disorders and trauma.

Remember

The human mind is complex. A traumatic experience in childhood can manifest as an eating disorder years later. Both trauma and eating disorders can have profound, long-term consequences that make recovery challenging. Once the issues have been identified and are being treated simultaneously by a multidisciplinary team of professionals, lasting recovery is possible.

Part Four
Diagnosing And Treating Eating Disorders

Chapter 32

Signs And Symptoms
Of Eating Disorders

There are physical and psychological indicators of eating disorders. Depending on the disorder, some include:

- Preoccupation with food, weight, and body
- Unrelenting fear of gaining weight
- Refusal to eat except for tiny portions
- Dehydration
- Compulsive exercise
- Excessive fine hair on face and body
- Distorted body image
- Abnormal weight loss

- Sensitivity to cold
- Absent menstruation
- Rapid consumption of a large amount of food
- Eating alone or in secret
- Abuse of laxatives, diuretics, diet pills, or emetics
- Depression
- Shame and guilt
- Withdrawal

Mental Functioning

- Feeling dull
- Feeling listless
- Difficulty concentrating or focusing
- Difficulty regulating mood

- Associated mental disorders: depression, anxiety disorders, obsessive-compulsive disorder, substance abuse

Symptoms Specific To Bulimia Nervosa

Symptoms or behavioral signs of bulimia may include:

- Regularly going to the bathroom right after meals
- Suddenly eating large amounts of food or buying large quantities that disappear right away
- Compulsive exercising
- Broken blood vessels in the eyes (from the strain of vomiting)
- Pouch-like appearance to the corners of the mouth due to swollen salivary glands
- Dry mouth
- Tooth cavities, diseased gums, and irreversible enamel erosion from excessive gastric acid produced by vomiting
- Rashes and pimples
- Small cuts and calluses across the tops of finger joints due to self-induced vomiting
- Evidence of discarded packaging for laxatives, diet pills, emetics (drugs that induce vomiting), or diuretics (medications that reduce fluids)

Symptoms Specific To Anorexia Nervosa

The primary symptom of anorexia is major weight loss from excessive and continuous dieting, which may either be restrictive dieting or binge-eating and purging.

Other symptoms of anorexia may include:

- Infrequent or absent menstrual periods
- Compulsive exercising coupled with excessive thinness
- Refusal to eat in front of others
- Ritualistic eating, including cutting food into small pieces
- Hypersensitivity to cold—some women wear several layers of clothing to both keep warm and hide their thinness
- Yellowish skin, especially on the palms of the hands and soles of the feet—from eating too many vitamin A-rich vegetables such as carrots
- Dry skin covered with fine hair
- Thin scalp hair
- Cold or swollen feet and hands
- Stomach problems, including bloating after eating
- Confused or slowed thinking
- Poor memory or judgment

Source: Excerpted from "Eating Disorders: In-Depth Report," © 2012 A.D.A.M., Inc.; reprinted with permission.

Cardiovascular (Heart)

- Slow irregular, pulse
- Low blood pressure
- Dizziness or faintness
- Shortness of breath
- Chest pain
- Decreased potassium levels may result in life-threatening cardiac arrhythmias or arrest
- Electrolyte imbalances may lead to life-threatening cardiac arrhythmias or arrest

Muscular Skeletal (Bones)

- Stunted growth in children
- Stress fractures and broken bones more likely
- Osteoporosis

Mouth

- Enamel erosion
- Loss of teeth
- Gum disease
- "Chipmunk cheeks"—swollen salivary glands from vomiting
- Sore throat because of induced vomiting

Esophagus

- Painful burning in throat or chest
- May vomit blood from small tear(s) in esophagus
- Rupture of the esophagus, may lead to circulatory collapse and death

Endocrine System

- Thyroid abnormalities
- Low energy or fatigue

- Cold intolerance
- Low body temperature
- Hair becomes thin and may fall out
- Development of fine body hair as the body's attempt to keep warm

Stomach

- Stomach may swell following eating or binging (causes discomfort and bloating)
- Gastric rupture due to severe binge eating (gastric rupture has an 80% fatality rate)
- Vomiting causes severe electrolyte imbalance which can lead to sudden cardiac arrest.

Intestines

- Normal movement in intestinal tract often slows down with very restricted eating and severe weight loss
- Frequent constipation
- Chronic irregular bowel movements

Complications Associated With Laxative Abuse

- Kidney complications
- "Cathartic colon," refers to the colon's inability to function normally without the use of large doses of laxatives due to the destruction of the nerves in the colon that control elimination
- Electrolyte imbalance
- Dehydration
- Potassium depletion
- Dependence on laxatives

Complications Associated With Ipecac Abuse

- Toxic to heart (irregular heartbeat, rapid heart rate, cardiac arrest)
- Sudden death

Chapter 33

Eating Disorders Self-Assessment Test

Eating Attitudes Test (EAT-26)

Instructions: This is a screening measure to help you determine whether you might have an eating disorder that needs professional attention. The EAT-26 is not designed to make a diagnosis of an eating disorder or take the place of a professional consultation. Please answer the questions below as accurately, honestly, and completely as possible. There are no right or wrong answers.

Part A

Answer the following questions:

1. Birth date: Month, Day, Year

2. Gender: Male or Female

3. Height: Feet and Inches

4. Current Weight:

5. Highest Weight (excluding pregnancy):

6. Lowest Adult Weight:

7: Ideal Weight:

About This Chapter: This chapter begins with "Eating Attitudes Test (EAT-26)." The EAT-26 has been reproduced with permission. Garner et al. (1982). The Eating Attitudes Test: Psychometric features and clinical correlates. *Psychological Medicine*, 12, 871-878. Text under the heading "Scoring and Interpretation" is excerpted from "Eating Attitudes Test (EAT-26): Scoring and Interpretation," © David M. Garner, Ph.D. Reprinted with permission from www.eat-26.com. All rights reserved. The complete text of this document including references is available at http://www.eat-26.com/Docs/EAT-26IntpretScoring-Test-3-20-10.pdf. Reviewed by David A. Cooke, MD, FACP, August 2012.

Part B

Choose a response for each of the following statements (always; usually; often; sometimes; rarely; never):

1. Am terrified about being overweight.

2. Avoid eating when I am hungry.

3. Find myself preoccupied with food.

4. Have gone on eating binges where I feel that I may not be able to stop.

5. Cut my food into small pieces.

6. Aware of the calorie content of foods that I eat.

7. Particularly avoid food with a high carbohydrate content (that is, bread, rice, potatoes, etc.)

8. Feel that others would prefer if I ate more.

9. Vomit after I have eaten.

10. Feel extremely guilty after eating.

11. Am preoccupied with a desire to be thinner.

12. Think about burning up calories when I exercise.

13. Other people think that I am too thin.

14. Am preoccupied with the thought of having fat on my body.

15. Take longer than others to eat my meals.

16. Avoid foods with sugar in them.

17. Eat diet foods.

18. Feel that food controls my life.

19. Display self-control around food.

20. Give too much time and thought to food.

22. Feel uncomfortable after eating sweets.

23. Engage in dieting behavior.

24. Like my stomach to be empty.

25. Have the impulse to vomit after meals.

26. Enjoy trying new rich foods.

Part C

Behavioral Questions: Answer: Never; once a month or less; two or three times a month; once a week; two to six times a week; or once a day or more.

In the past six months, have you:

A. Gone on eating binges where you feel that you may not be able to stop? (Defined as eating much more than most people would under the same circumstances and feeling that eating is out of control.)

B. Ever made yourself sick (vomited) to control your weight or shape?

C. Ever used laxatives, diet pills, or diuretics (water pills) to control your weight or shape?

D. Exercised more than 60 minutes a day to lose or control your weight?

E. Lost 20 pounds or more in the past six months?

Scoring And Interpretation

The Eating Attitudes Test (EAT-26) is probably the most widely used standardized measure of symptoms and concerns characteristic of eating disorders. The original EAT appeared as a Current Contents Citation Classic in 1993. The 26-item version is highly reliable and valid. The EAT-26 alone does not yield a specific diagnosis of an eating disorder (neither the EAT-26 nor any other screening instrument has been established as highly efficient as the sole means for identifying eating disorders).

Nevertheless, many studies have used the EAT-26 as an economical first step in a two-stage screening process. According to this methodology, individuals who score 20 or more on the test should be interviewed by a qualified professional to determine if they meet the diagnostic criteria for an eating disorder. If you have a low score on the EAT-26 (below 20), you still could have a serious eating problem, so do not let the results deter you from seeking help. The EAT-26 can be used in group or individual settings and is designed to be self-administered or administered by health professionals, school counselors, coaches, camp counselors, and others with an interest in gathering information to determine if an individual should be referred to a specialist for evaluation for an eating disorder.

The EAT-26 has been particularly useful as a screening tool to assess "eating disorder risk" in high school, college, and other special risk samples such as athletes. Screening for eating disorders is based on the assumption that early identification of an eating disorder can lead to earlier treatment, thereby reducing serious physical and psychological complications or even death.

Interpretation

The interpretation of the Eating Attitudes Test (EAT-26) is based on three "referral criteria" that determine if the respondent should seek further evaluation of your risk of having an eating disorder. These are:

1. The total score on the actual EAT test items;
2. Behavioral questions indicating possible eating disorder symptoms or recent significant weight loss;
3. Low body weight compared to age-matched norms.

If the respondent meets one or more of these criteria, they should seek an evaluation by a professional who specializes in the treatment of eating disorders.

Additional Interpretive Information:

EAT-26 Scores: A score at or above 20 on the EAT-26 indicates a high level of concern about dieting, body weight, or problematic eating behaviors. If your score is above 20, you should seek an evaluation by a qualified health professional to determine if your score reflects a problem that warrants clinical attention. However, please keep in mind that high scores do not always reflect over-concern about body weight, body shape, and eating. Screening studies have shown that some people with high scores do not have eating disorders. Regardless of your score, if you are suffering from feelings which are causing you concern or interfering with your daily functioning, you should seek an evaluation from a trained mental health professional.

The EAT-26 items form three subscales: 1) Dieting; 2) Bulimia and Food Preoccupation; and 3) Oral Control. The subscale scores are computed by summing all items assigned to that particular scale:

- Dieting scale items: 1, 6, 7, 10, 11, 12, 14, 16, 17, 22, 23, 24, 26.

- Bulimia and Food Preoccupation scale items: 3, 4, 9, 18, 21, 25.

- Oral Control subscale items: 2, 5, 8, 13, 15, 19, 20.

Because denial can be a problem on self-report screening instruments, low scores should not be taken to mean that either clinically significant eating disorder symptoms or a formal eating disorder is not present. Collateral information from parents, teammates, and coaches is useful information that can correct for denial, limited self-disclosure, and social desirability. High scores on self-report measures do not necessarily mean the respondent has an eating disorder; however, it does denote concerns regarding body weight, body shape, and eating.

Behavioral Questions: If you answered affirmatively to any of the behavioral questions, you should seek an evaluation from a trained mental health professional specializing in the treatment of eating disorders. It is important to consider the frequency, and the context of the behaviors needs to determine the degree of medical risk they represent. For example, both vomiting and using laxatives for weight control confer serious medical dangers in direct relationship to their frequency. However, less frequent use of these behaviors is still a serious reason for concern since these behaviors tend to escalate over time.

Body Mass Index: The EAT-26 includes specific questions on height, weight, and gender that can be used to compute body mass index (BMI) for the purpose of determining if you are "at risk" for an eating disorder because your body weight is extremely underweight according to age-matched population norms. BMI is a formula for estimating body mass that takes both height and weight into account. It is calculated by dividing weight (in kilograms) by height in meters, and then divided again by height in meters (kg/m^2). Alternatively, BMI can be calculated as weight (in pounds) divided by height in inches, then divided again by height in inches and multiplied by 703. We recommend that you seek a professional evaluation for a possible eating disorder if your body weight is "extremely underweight" according to age-matched population norms [see Table 33.1 on page 204].

Although BMI is a convenient and useful weight classification tool, it does have limitations. For example, BMI can overestimate fatness for people who are athletic. Also, some races, ethnic groups, and nationalities have different body fat distributions and body compositions; therefore, the norms used are not appropriate for all groups.

However, if you do have a high score, do not panic. It does not necessarily mean that you have a life-threatening condition and that you will have to immediately seek a form of treatment that may be uncomfortable. If you have a score of 20 or higher, this simply means that you should seek the advice of a qualified mental health professional who has experience with treating eating disorders.

In addition to the EAT-26 questions, identification of those at risk for eating disorders is based on information on the individual's body mass index (BMI) and behavioral symptoms reflective of an eating disorder. Following the methodology described in the Eating Disorder Inventory Referral Form, four behavioral questions are included on this version of the EAT-26 aimed at determining the presence of extreme weight-control behaviors as well as providing an estimate of their frequency. These questions assess self-reported binge eating, self-induced vomiting, use of laxatives, and treatment for an eating disorder over the preceding six months. Although these content areas could be assessed in the same format as other items, this would not provide the type of frequency data required to evaluate the extent of the problem. Body mass index (BMI) is also computed and used to determine if the person is "significantly underweight" compared to age-matched norms. Generally a referral is recommended if a respondent scores "positively" on the EAT-26 items or meets the threshold on one or more of the behavioral criteria.

All self-report measures require open and honest responses in order to provide accurate information. The fact that most people provide honest responses means that the EAT-26 usually provides very useful information about the eating symptoms and concerns that are common in eating disorders.

Interpreting Eating Attitudes Test (EAT-26) Scores

The Eating Attitudes Test (EAT-26) is probably the most widely used test used to assess "eating disorder risk" based on attitudes, feelings, and behaviors related to eating and eating disorder symptoms. It was used as a screening instrument in the 1998 National Eating Disorders Screening program and has been used in many other studies to identify individuals with possible eating disorders. However, the EAT-26 does not provide a diagnosis of an eating disorder. A diagnosis can only be provided by a qualified health care professional.

The version of the Eating Attitudes Test (EAT-26) shown in this chapter has three criteria for determining if you should seek further evaluation of your risk for having an eating disorder. These are:

1. Your score on the actual EAT test items;

2. Low body weight compared to age-matched norms, and

3. Behavioral questions indicating possible eating disorder symptoms or recent significant weight loss.

If you meet one or more of these criteria, you should seek an evaluation by a professional who specializes in the treatment of eating disorders.

1. Your Eating Attitudes Test (EAT-26) Is: _____

A score at or above 20 on the EAT-26 indicates a high level of concern about dieting, body weight, or problematic eating behaviors. Because your score is above 20, you should seek an evaluation by a qualified health professional to determine if your score reflects a problem that warrants clinical attention. However, please keep in mind that high scores do not always reflect over-concern about body weight, body shape, and eating. Screening studies have shown that some people with high scores do not have eating disorders. Regardless of your score, if you are suffering from feelings which are causing you concern or interfering with your daily functioning, you should seek an evaluation from a trained mental health professional.

- Score for questions 1–25:
  - Always: 3
  - Usually: 2
  - Often: 1
  - Sometimes: 0
  - Rarely: 0
  - Never: 0

- Score for question #26:
  - Always: 0
  - Usually: 0
  - Often: 0
  - Sometimes: 1
  - Rarely: 2
  - Never: 3

Add the scores for each item together for a total score.

2. Your Body Mass Index (BMI) Is: _____

If your BMI meets the criterion for "underweight," it is an important risk factor for a serious eating disorder. If your EAT-26 score is 20 or more, then this increases your likelihood of having a serious eating disorder. If your BMI indicates that you are neither "underweight" nor "extremely underweight" compared to age/gender-matched norms, then you could still have a serious eating disorder. It just means that it is unlikely that you have anorexia nervosa. If you believe that your body weight is a problem, then it would be good for you to consult with a qualified health professional for further clarification. [For information about calculating your BMI, see the body mass index section of the box titled "Interpretation."]

3. Behavioral Questions

If you gave any of the following answers, you should seek an evaluation from a trained mental health professional:

In the past six months, have you:

A. Gone on eating binges where you feel that you may not be able to stop? Two or three times a month; once a week; two to six times a week; or once a day or more.

B. Ever made yourself sick (vomited) to control your weight or shape? Once a month or less; two or three times a month; once a week; two to six times a week; or once a day or more.

C. Ever used laxatives, diet pills, or diuretics (water pills) to control your weight or shape? Once a month or less; two or three times a month; once a week; two to six times a week; or once a day or more.

D. Exercised more than 60 minutes a day to lose or control your weight? Once a day or more.

E. Lost 20 pounds or more in the past six months? Yes.

Please remember that the EAT-26 does not provide a diagnosis of an eating disorder. A diagnosis can only be provided by a qualified health provider.

Table 33.1. BMI Considered "Underweight" for Different Ages and Sexes According to Norms

Age	Female (BMI)	Male (BMI)
9	14.0	14.0
10	14.5	14.5
11	14.5	15.0
12	15.0	15.0
13	15.5	16.0
14	16.0	16.5
15	16.5	17.0
16	17.0	17.5
17	17.5	18.0
18	18.0	18.5
19	18.0	19.0
20	18.5	19.5
21+	19.0	20.0

Chapter 34

When You Suspect Someone You Know Has An Eating Disorder

How To Help A Friend With Eating And Body Image Issues

If you are reading this chapter, chances are you are concerned about the eating habits, weight, or body image of someone you care about. We understand that this can be a very difficult and scary time for you. Let us assure you that you are doing a great thing by looking for more information. This list may not tell you everything you need to know about what to do in your specific situation, but it will give you some helpful ideas on what to do to help your friend.

- Learn as much as you can about eating disorders. Read books, articles, and brochures.

- Know the differences between facts and myths about weight, nutrition, and exercise. Knowing the facts will help you reason against any inaccurate ideas that your friend may be using as excuses to maintain their disordered eating patterns.

- Be honest. Talk openly and honestly about your concerns with the person who is struggling with eating or body image problems. Avoiding it or ignoring it won't help.

- Be caring, but be firm. Caring about your friend does not mean being manipulated by them. Your friend must be responsible for their actions and the consequences of those actions. Avoid making rules, promises, or expectations that you cannot or will not uphold. For example, "I promise not to tell anyone." Or, "If you do this one more time I'll never talk to you again."

About This Chapter: This chapter includes "How to Help a Friend with Eating and Body Image Issues" and "What Should I Say?" both reprinted with permission from the National Eating Disorders Association, © 2005. All rights reserved. For more information, visit www.nationaleatingdisorders.org. Reviewed by David A. Cooke, MD, FACP, August 2012.

- Compliment your friend's wonderful personality, successes, or accomplishments. Remind your friend that "true beauty" is not simply skin deep.

- Be a good role model in regard to sensible eating, exercise, and self-acceptance.

- Tell someone. It may seem difficult to know when, if at all, to tell someone else about your concerns. Addressing body image or eating problems in their beginning stages offers your friend the best chance for working through these issues and becoming healthy again. Don't wait until the situation is so severe that your friend's life is in danger. Your friend needs as much support and understanding as possible.

When Someone You Know Has An Eating Disorder

What should I do?

- Know the signs of anorexia and bulimia.
- Learn what community and healthcare resources are available.
- Understand that eating disorders are complex. Recovery is not just a matter of will power.
- Discuss your concerns with the individual.
- Be compassionate; listen.
- Try to understand things from the person's perspective. Understand that persons with eating disorders often make decisions based on their feelings rather than on facts and logic.
- State what you have observed—list evidence of the problem.
- Express your concerns about the person's health and functioning, not just their weight.
- Indicate your conviction that the situation should at least be evaluated by a professional.
- Explain how you can help—with a referral, information, emotional or financial support.
- End the conversation if going nowhere or if the person becomes upset. But if possible, leave the door open for further conversations.
- Have patience: If rejected, try again later, explaining that you are coming back because you think the situation is serious.
- Respond during emergencies: If the person is throwing up several times per day, passing out, complaining of chest pain, or talking about suicide, get help immediately.
- Find support for yourself. Talk to a counselor or healthcare professional; attend a support group for family and friends of those with eating disorders.

Source: Excerpted from "When Someone You Know Has an Eating Disorder," © 2012 Remuda Ranch. All rights reserved. Reprinted with permission. For additional information, visit www.remudaranch.com.

Remember that you cannot force someone to seek help, change their habits, or adjust their attitudes. You will make important progress in honestly sharing your concerns, providing support, and knowing where to go for more information. People struggling with anorexia, bulimia, or binge eating disorder do need professional help. There is help available and there is hope.

What Should I Say?

Tips For Talking To A Friend Who May Be Struggling With An Eating Disorder

If you are worried about your friend's eating behaviors or attitudes, it is important to express your concerns in a loving and supportive way. It is also necessary to discuss your worries early on, rather than waiting until your friend has endured many of the damaging physical and emotional effects of eating disorders. In a private and relaxed setting, talk to your friend in a calm and caring way about the specific things you have seen or felt that have caused you to worry.

What To Say—Step By Step

- Set a time to talk. Set aside a time for a private, respectful meeting with your friend to discuss your concerns openly and honestly in a caring, supportive way. Make sure you will be some place away from other distractions.

- Communicate your concerns. Share your memories of specific times when you felt concerned about your friend's eating or exercise behaviors. Explain that you think these things may indicate that there could be a problem that needs professional attention.

- Ask your friend to explore these concerns with a counselor, doctor, nutritionist, or other health professional who is knowledgeable about eating issues. If you feel comfortable doing so, offer to help your friend make an appointment or accompany your friend on their first visit.

- Avoid conflicts or a battle of the wills with your friend. If your friend refuses to acknowledge that there is a problem, or any reason for you to be concerned, restate your feelings and the reasons for them and leave yourself open and available as a supportive listener.

- Avoid placing shame, blame, or guilt on your friend regarding their actions or attitudes. Do not use accusatory "you" statements like, "You just need to eat." Or, "You are acting irresponsibly." Instead, use "I" statements. For example: "I'm concerned about you because you refuse to eat breakfast or lunch." Or, "It makes me afraid to hear you vomiting."

- Avoid giving simple solutions. For example, "If you'd just stop, then everything would be fine."

- Express your continued support. Remind your friend that you care and want your friend to be healthy and happy.

After talking with your friend, if you are still concerned with their health and safety, find a trusted adult or medical professional to talk to. This is probably a challenging time for both of you. It could be helpful for you, as well as your friend, to discuss your concerns and seek assistance and support from a professional.

When Someone You Know Has An Eating Disorder

What should I NOT do?

- Don't make promises you can't keep; don't promise to keep the person's behavior a secret.
- Don't get over-involved. Know your limits. You are not a substitute for professional care.
- Don't oversimplify. Avoid platitudes like, "Eating disorders are an addiction like alcoholism," or "All you have to do is accept yourself as you are."
- Don't nag about eating or not eating, or spend time talking about food and weight.
- Don't be judgmental; don't say that what the person is doing is "sick", "stupid", or "self-destructive."
- Don't give advice about weight loss, exercise, or appearance.
- Don't say, "I know how you feel." You can demonstrate that you understand by paraphrasing what the person has said.
- Don't feel obliged to agree with the person's perspective or beliefs, even though you are making an effort to understand them.
- Don't bring a group of people to confront the person.

Source: Excerpted from "When Someone You Know Has an Eating Disorder," © 2012 Remuda Ranch. All rights reserved. Reprinted with permission. For additional information, visit www.remudaranch.com.

Chapter 35

Diagnosing Eating Disorders

Anorexia Nervosa

Individuals with anorexia nervosa are unable or unwilling to maintain a body weight that is normal or expected for their age and height. There is no precise boundary dividing "normal" from "too low," but most clinicians use 85% of normal weight as a reasonable guide.

Individuals with anorexia nervosa usually display a pronounced fear of weight gain and a dread of becoming fat even though they are markedly underweight. Concerns about their weight and about how they believe they look have a powerful influence on the individual's self-evaluation. The seriousness of the weight loss and its health implications is usually minimized, if not denied, by the individual.

The diagnosis of anorexia nervosa includes two subtypes of the disorder that describe two behavioral patterns. Individuals with the restricting type maintain their low body weight purely by restricting food intake and, possibly, by exercise. Individuals with the binge-eating/purging type usually restrict their food intake as well, but also regularly engage in binge eating and/or purging behaviors such as self-induced vomiting or the misuse of laxatives, diuretics or enemas.

Available data indicate that the binge-eating/purging type of anorexia nervosa is more frequently associated with other impulsive behaviors, substance use disorders, and mood lability. The longer a person has anorexia nervosa, the more likely they are to binge and purge.

About This Chapter: "Diagnosis of Eating Disorders," © 2012 Academy for Eating Disorders (www.aedweb.org). Reprinted with permission.

Bulimia Nervosa

Individuals with bulimia nervosa regularly engage in discrete periods of overeating, which are followed by attempts to compensate for overeating and to avoid weight gain. There can be considerable variation in the nature of the overeating but the typical episode of overeating involves the consumption of an amount of food that would be considered excessive in normal circumstances. The individual's subjective experience is dominated by a sense of a lack of control over the eating.

Binge eating is followed by attempts to "undo" the consequences of eating too much though behaviors such as self-induced vomiting, misuse of laxatives, enemas, diuretics, severe caloric restriction, or excessive exercising. Profound concerns about weight and shape are also characteristic of individuals with bulimia nervosa. Self-evaluation is centered on the individual's perceptions of her body image.

Diagnosing Bulimia Nervosa

The formal diagnosis of bulimia nervosa requires that the individual not simultaneously meet criteria for anorexia nervosa. In other words, if an individual simultaneously meets criteria for both anorexia nervosa and bulimia nervosa, only the diagnosis of anorexia nervosa, binge-eating/purging type is given.

The bulimia nervosa diagnostic criteria also specify minimum frequency and duration cut-offs for the diagnosis: individuals must binge eat and engage in inappropriate compensatory behavior at least twice weekly for at least three months.

As with anorexia nervosa, there are two subtypes of bulimia nervosa. The purging type describes individuals who regularly compensate for the binge eating with self-induced vomiting or through the use of laxatives, diuretics, or enemas. The non-purging type is used to describe individuals who compensate through excessive exercising or dietary fasting.

Binge Eating Disorder

The term, binge eating disorder, was officially introduced in 1992 to describe individuals who binge eat but do not regularly use inappropriate compensatory weight control behaviors such as fasting or purging to lose weight.

The binge eating may involve rapid consumption of food with a sense of loss of control, uncomfortable fullness after eating, and eating large amounts of food when not hungry. Feelings of shame and embarrassment are prominent.

Course And Outcomes Of Eating Disorders

It is estimated that nearly one-half of patients with anorexia nervosa recover, 33 percent improve somewhat, and 20 percent remain chronically ill. Numerous studies have attempted to identify predictors of the course and recovery of anorexia nervosa, but these findings have been contradictory and unclear.

Similar to anorexia nervosa, approximately 50 percent of bulimic individuals recover, 30 percent improve somewhat, and 20 percent continue to meet full criteria for bulimia nervosa. Long-term followup studies suggest that only 10 percent of bulimic individuals continue to fully meet diagnostic criteria after 10 years of the illness.

Duration of symptoms and level of personality disturbance may predict a more negative outcome in bulimia nervosa. Furthermore, there is some evidence to suggest that cognitive behavioral therapy may speed recovery from the disorder.

Source: "Course and Outcomes of Eating Disorders," © 2012 Academy for Eating Disorders (www.aedweb.org). Reprinted with permission."

Binge Eating And Obesity

Binge eating disorder is often associated with obesity. In the past these individuals were often referred to as compulsive overeaters, emotional overeaters, or food addicts. Available research suggests that approximately one fifth of the people who seek professional treatment for obesity meet the criteria for binge eating disorder.

In the *American Psychiatric Association's Diagnostic and Statistical Manual* (*DSM- IV-TR*), binge eating disorder is not an officially recognized eating disorder, but is included in the category titled Eating Disorder Not Otherwise Specified (EDNOS).

Other Eating Disorders

There are numerous variants of disordered eating in addition to binge eating disorder that do not meet the diagnostic criteria for anorexia nervosa or bulimia nervosa, but nevertheless are eating disorders requiring treatment. Individuals with eating disordered behaviors that resemble anorexia nervosa or bulimia nervosa but whose eating behaviors do not meet one or more essential diagnostic criteria may be diagnosed with EDNOS.

Examples of EDNOS include individuals who regularly purge but do not binge eat, individuals who meet criteria for anorexia nervosa but continue to menstruate, and individuals who meet criteria for bulimia nervosa, but binge eat less than twice weekly.

Chapter 36

Treating Eating Disorders

Patients with eating disorders typically require a treatment team consisting of a primary care physician, dietitian, and a mental health professional knowledgeable about eating disorders. The multidisciplinary membership of the Academy for Eating Disorders reflects the consensus view that treatment must often involve clinicians from different health disciplines including psychologists, psychotherapists, physicians, dietitians, and nurses.

Research on the treatment of eating disorders is exploring how different treatments can be helpful for different types of eating disorders. The American Psychiatric Association has published a set of practice guidelines for the treatment of patients with eating disorders (American Psychiatric Association, *Practice Guidelines for Eating Disorders, American Journal of Psychiatry*, 2000).

There is general agreement that good treatment often requires a spectrum of treatment options. These options can range from basic educational interventions designed to teach nutritional and symptom management techniques to long-term residential treatment (living away from home in treatment centers).

Most individuals with eating disorders are treated on an outpatient basis after a comprehensive evaluation. Individuals with medical complications due to severe weight loss or due to the effects of binge eating and purging may require hospitalization. Other individuals, for whom outpatient therapy has not been effective, may benefit from day-hospital treatment, hospitalization, or residential placement.

About This Chapter: "Treatment," © 2012 Academy for Eating Disorders (www.aedweb.org). Reprinted with permission."

Treatment is usually conducted in the least restrictive setting that can provide adequate safety for the individual. Many patients with eating disorders also have depression, anxiety disorders, drug and/or alcohol use disorders, and other psychiatric problems requiring treatment along with the eating disorder.

Initial Assessment

The initial assessment of individuals with eating disorders involves a thorough review of the patient's history, current symptoms, physical status, weight control measures, and other

Most Teens With Eating Disorders Go Without Treatment

About three percent of U.S. adolescents are affected by an eating disorder, but most do not receive treatment for their specific eating condition, according to a study funded by the National Institute of Mental Health (NIMH) published online ahead of print March 7, 2011, in the *Archives of General Psychiatry*.

Background

Kathleen Merikangas, Ph.D., of NIMH and colleagues analyzed data from the National Co-morbidity Study-Adolescent Supplement (NCS-A), a nationally representative, face-to-face survey of more than 10,000 teens ages 13 to 18. Previously published results found that about 20 percent of youth are affected by a severe mental disorder, and a substantial proportion of these youth do not receive mental health care.

In this new study, the authors tracked the prevalence of eating disorders and the proportion of those youth who received treatment for these disorders.

Results Of The Study

According to the data, 0.3 percent of youth have been affected by anorexia, 0.9 percent by bulimia, and 1.6 percent by binge-eating disorder. The researchers also tracked the rate of some forms of eating disorders not otherwise specified (EDNOS), a catch-all category of symptoms that do not meet full criteria for specific disorders but still impact a person's life. EDNOS is the most common eating disorder diagnosis. Overall, another 0.8 percent had subthreshold anorexia, and another 2.5 percent had symptoms of subthreshold binge-eating disorder.

psychiatric issues or disorders such as depression, anxiety, substance abuse, or personality issues. Consultation with a physician and a registered dietitian is often recommended. The initial assessment is the first step in establishing a diagnosis and treatment plan.

Outpatient Treatment

Outpatient treatment for an eating disorder often involves a coordinated team effort between the patient, a psychotherapist, a physician, and a dietitian (yet, many patients are treated by their pediatrician or physician with or without a mental health professional's involvement).

In addition these results were identified:

- Hispanics reported the highest rates of bulimia, while whites reported the highest rates of anorexia.

- The majority who had an eating disorder also met criteria for at least one other psychiatric disorder, such as depression.

- Each eating disorder was associated with higher levels of suicidal thinking compared to those without an eating disorder.

Significance

The prevalence of these disorders and their association with coexisting disorders, role impairment, and suicidal thinking suggest that eating disorders represent a major public health concern. In addition, the significant rates of subthreshold eating conditions support the notion that eating disorders tend to exist along a spectrum and may be better recognized by doctors if they included a broader range of symptoms. In addition, the findings clearly underscore the need for better access to treatment specifically for eating disorders.

Reference

Swanson SA, Crow SJ, LeGrange D, Swendsen J, Merikangas KR. Prevalence and correlates of eating disorders in adolescents: results from the National Comorbidity Survey Replication Adolescent Supplement. *Archives of General Psychiatry*. Online ahead of print March 7, 2011.

Source: "Most Teens with Eating Disorders Go without Treatment," National Institute of Mental Health (www.nimh.nih .gov), March 7, 2011.

Similarly, many patients are seen and helped by generalist mental health clinicians without specialist involvement. Not all individuals, then, will receive a multidisciplinary approach, but the qualified clinician should have access to all of these resources.

Psychotherapy

There are several different types of outpatient psychotherapies with demonstrated effectiveness in patients with eating disorders. These include cognitive-behavioral therapy, interpersonal psychotherapy, family therapy, and behavioral therapy. Some of these therapies may be relatively short-term (i.e., four-months), but other psychotherapies may last years.

It is very difficult to predict who will respond to short-term treatments versus longer term treatments. Other therapies which some clinicians and patients have found to be useful include feminist therapies, psychodynamic psychotherapies, and various types of group therapy.

Psychopharmacology

Psychiatric medications have a demonstrated role in the treatment of patients with eating disorders. Most of the research to date has involved antidepressant medications such as fluoxetine (for example, Prozac), although some clinicians and patients have found that other types of medications may also be effective.

Nutritional Counseling

Regular contact with a registered dietitian can be an effective source of support and information for patients who are regaining weight or who are trying to normalize their eating behavior. Dietitians may help patients to gain a fundamental understanding of adequate nutrition and may also conduct dietary counseling, which is a more specific process designed to help patients change the nature of their eating behavior.

Medical Treatment

Patients with eating disorders are subject to a variety of physical and medical concerns. Adequate medical monitoring is a cornerstone of effective outpatient treatment. Individuals with anorexia nervosa may be followed quite closely (i.e., weekly or more) because of the significant medical problems that this disorder poses for patients. Individuals with bulimia nervosa should be seen regularly, but may not require the intensive medical monitoring often seen in anorexia nervosa. Individuals with binge eating disorder may need medical treatment for a variety of complications of obesity, such as diabetes and hypertension.

Day Hospital Care

Patients for whom outpatient treatment is ineffective may benefit from the increased structure provided by a day hospital treatment program. Generally, these programs are scheduled from three to eight hours a day and provide several structured eating sessions per day, along with various other therapies, including cognitive behavioral therapy, body image therapies, family therapy, and numerous other interventions. Day hospital care allows the patient to live at home when they are not in treatment and often continue to work or attend school.

Inpatient Treatment

Inpatient treatment provides a structured and contained environment in which the patient with an eating disorder has access to clinical support 24-hours a day. Many programs are now affiliated with a day hospital program so that patients can "step-up" and "step-down" to the appropriate level of care depending on their clinical needs.

Although eating disorder patients can sometimes be treated on general psychiatric units with individuals experiencing other psychiatric disorders, such an approach often poses problems with monitoring and containing eating disorder symptoms. Therefore, most inpatient programs for eating disordered individuals only treat patients with anorexia nervosa, bulimia nervosa, binge eating disorder, or variants of these disorders.

Residential Care

Residential programs provide a longer term treatment option for patients who require longer term treatment. This treatment option generally is reserved for individual who have been hospitalized on several occasions, but have not been able to reach a significant degree of medical or psychological stability.

Chapter 37

Medications And Therapies For Eating Disorders

Standard treatments include medications (prescription drugs), various psychotherapies, nutrition therapy, other nondrug therapies, and supportive or adjunct interventions such as yoga, art, massage, and movement therapy. Some novel treatments are currently under research, such as implantation of a device called a vagus nerve stimulator implanted at the base of the neck. This stimulator is currently in use to treat some forms of depression, and it is under research for treating obesity.

The most commonly used treatments—psychotherapy and medication—are delivered at various levels of inpatient and outpatient care, and in various settings depending on the severity of the illness and the treatment plan that has been developed for a particular patient. Bulimia nervosa and binge eating disorders can often be treated on an outpatient basis, although more severe cases may require inpatient or residential treatment. The levels of care and types of treatment centers are discussed in separate documents in the tool kit [available online from the National Eating Disorders Association at http://www.nationaleatingdisorders.org]. The treatment plan should be developed by a multidisciplinary team in consultation with the patient and family members as deemed appropriate by the patient and his/her team.

Medication

Biochemical abnormalities in the brain and body have been associated with eating disorders. Many types of prescription drugs have been used in treatment of eating disorders; however, only one prescription drug (fluoxetine) actually has a labeled indication for one eating disorder, bulimia nervosa. (This means that the manufacturer requested permission from the U.S. Food and Drug Administration (FDA) to market the drug specifically for treatment of bulimia nervosa and that FDA approved this request based on the evidence the manufacturer provided about the drug's efficacy for bulimia nervosa.) Most prescription drug therapy used for treatment of the disorder is aimed at alleviating major depression, anxiety, or obsessive-compulsive disorder (OCD), which often coexist with an eating disorder. Some prescription drug therapies are intended to make individuals feel full to try to prevent binge eating. Generic and brand names of prescription drugs that have been used to treat eating disorders are listed below. Some of these antidepressants also can exert other effects. Selective serotonin reuptake inhibitors alleviate depression, but may also play a role in making an individual feel full and possibly prevent binge eating in patients with bulimia or binge eating disorder. FDA has issued a warning and labeling to prevent prescription of one particular antidepressant for eating disorders—Wellbutrin, which is available in several brand and generic formulations—because it leads to higher risk of epileptic seizures in these patients.

Medication Names: Generic (Brand)

Antidepressants

Tricyclics

- Amitriptyline (Elavil)
- Clomipramine (Anafranil)
- Desipramine (Norpramin, Pertofrane)
- Imipramine (Janimine, Tofranil)
- Nortriptyline (Aventyl, Pamelor)

Selective Serotonin Reuptake Inhibitors (SSRIs)

- Citalopram (Celexa)
- Escitalopram (Lexapro)
- Fluoxetine (Prozac, Sarafem)
- Fluvoxamine (Luvox)
- Paroxetine (Paxil)
- Sertraline (Zoloft)

Monamine Oxidase Inhibitors

- Brofaromine (Consonar)
- Isocarboxazid (Benazide)
- Moclobemide (Manerix)
- Phenelzine (Nardil)
- Tranylcypromine (Parnate)

Tetracyclics

- Mianserin (Bolvidon)
- Mirtazapine (Remeron)

Modified Cyclic Antidepressants

- Trazodone (Desyrel)

Aminoketone

- Bupropion (Wellbutrin, Zyban): Now contraindicated for treatment of eating disorders because of several reports of drug-related seizures.

Serotonin And Norepinephrine Reuptake Inhibitor

- Duloxetine (Cymbalta)
- Venlafaxine (Effexor)

Opioid Antagonist

- Naltrexone (Nalorex) (Intended to alleviate addictive behaviors such as the addictive drive to eat or binge eat.)

Antiemetic

- Ondansetron (Zofran) (Used to give sensation of satiety and fullness.)

Anticonvulsant

- Topiramate (Topamax) (May help regulate feeding behaviors.)

Other

- Lithium carbonate (Carbolith, Cibalith-S, Duralith, Eskalith, Lithane, Lithizine, Lithobid, Lithonate, Lithotabs) (Used for patients who also have bipolar disorder, but may be contraindicated for patients with substantial purging.)

Psychological Therapy

Several types of psychotherapy are used in individual and group settings and with families. Patients must be medically stable to be able to participate meaningfully in any type of psychological therapy. Thus, a patient who has required hospitalization for refeeding and to stabilize his/her medical condition will ordinarily not be able to participate in therapy until after he/she has recovered sufficiently to enable cognitive function to return to normal.

A given psychologist or psychiatrist may use several different approaches tailored to the situation. The types of psychotherapy used are listed here and defined below. Cognitive behavior therapy (CBT) and behavior therapy (BT) have been used for many years as first-line treatment, and they are the most-used types of psychotherapy for bulimia. CBT involves three overlapping phases. The first phase focuses on helping people to resist the urge to engage in the cycle of behavior by educating them about the dangers. The second phase introduces procedures to reduce dietary restraint and increase eating regularity. The last phase involves teaching people relapse-prevention strategies to help prepare them for possible setbacks. A course of individual CBT for bulimia nervosa usually involves 16 to 20 hour-long sessions over a period of four to five months. BT uses principles of learning to increase the frequency of desired behavior and decrease the frequency of problem behavior. When used to treat bulimia nervosa, BT focuses on teaching relaxation techniques and coping strategies that individuals can use instead of binge eating and purging or excessive exercise or fasting.

Self-help groups are listed here because they may be the only option available to people who have no insurance. However, self-help groups can also have negative effects on a person with an eating disorder if they are not well-moderated by a trained professional.

For information about what types of treatments are recommended for particular situations and types of patients, please refer to the document, "The evidence on what treatment works" [available from the National Eating Disorders Association online at http://www.nationaleatingdisorders.org/uploads/file/toolkits/NEDA-TKP-B02-TreatmentEvidence.pdf].

Psychological Therapies

Individual Psychotherapy

- Behavior therapy
- Exposure with response prevention
- Hypnobehavior therapy
- Cognitive therapy
- Cognitive analytic therapy
- Cognitive behavior therapy (all forms)
- Cognitive remediation therapies
- Scheme-based cognitive therapy
- Self-guided cognitive behavioral therapy

- Dialectical behavior therapy
- Guided imagery
- Psychodynamic therapy
- Self psychology
- Psychoanalysis
- Interpersonal psychotherapy
- Motivational enhancement therapy
- Psychoeducation
- Supportive therapy

Family Therapy

- Involving family members in psychotherapy sessions with and without the patient

Group Psychotherapy

- Cognitive behavioral therapy
- Psychodynamic
- Psychoeducational
- Interpersonal

Self-Help Groups

- ANAD (Anorexia Nervosa and Associated Disorders)
- 12-step approaches
- Eating Disorders Anonymous
- Web-based on-line programs

Other Adjunctive And Alternative Treatments

Creative Arts Therapies

- Art Therapy
- Movement Therapy
- Psychodrama

Nutritional Counseling

- Individual, group, family, and mealtime-support therapy

Other Therapies

Although little research exists to support the use of the following interventions, individual patients have sometimes found some of these approaches to be useful, particularly as adjuncts to conventional treatments. However, these approaches should not be used in place of evidence-based treatments where the latter are available.

- Biofeedback
- Coaching
- Emailing for support or coaching
- Eye movement desensitization
- Exercise
- Journaling
- Mandometer
- Massage
- Meditation
- Relaxation training
- Yoga

Treatments Defined

Antidepressants: Prescription drugs used for treatment of eating disorders and aimed at alleviating major depression, anxiety, or obsessive-compulsive disorder, which often coexist with an eating disorder.

Behavior Therapy (BT): A type of psychotherapy that uses principles of learning to increase the frequency of desired behaviors and/or decrease the frequency of problem behaviors. Subtypes of BT include dialectical behavior therapy (DBT), exposure and response prevention (ERP), and hypnobehavioral therapy.

Cognitive Therapy (CT): A type of psychotherapeutic treatment that attempts to change a patient's feelings and behaviors by changing the way the patient thinks about or perceives his/her significant life experiences. Subtypes include cognitive analytic therapy and cognitive orientation therapy.

Cognitive Analytic Therapy (CAT): A type of cognitive therapy that focuses its attention on discovering how a patient's problems have evolved and how the procedures the patient has devised to cope with them may be ineffective or even harmful. CAT is designed to enable people to gain an understanding of how the difficulties they experience may be made worse by their habitual coping mechanisms. Problems are understood in the light of a person's personal history and life experiences. The focus is on recognizing how these coping procedures originated and how they can be adapted.

Cognitive Behavior Therapy (CBT): CBT is a goal-oriented, short-term treatment that addresses the psychological, familial, and societal factors associated with eating disorders. Therapy is centered on the principle that there are both behavioral and attitudinal disturbances regarding eating, weight, and shape.

Cognitive Orientation Therapy (COT): A type of cognitive therapy that uses a systematic procedure to understand the meaning of a patient's behavior by exploring certain themes such as aggression and avoidance. The procedure for modifying behavior then focuses on systematically changing the patient's beliefs related to the themes, not beliefs that refer directly to eating behavior.

Cognitive Remediation Therapy (CRT): Since patients with anorexia nervosa (AN) have a tendency to get trapped in detail rather than seeing the big picture, and have difficulty shifting thinking among perspectives, this newly investigated brief psychotherapeutic approach targets these specific thinking styles and their role in the development and maintenance of an eating disorder. Currently, it's usually conducted side by side with other forms of psychotherapies.

Dialectical Behavior Therapy (DBT): A type of behavioral therapy that views emotional deregulation as the core problem in eating disorders. It involves teaching people new skills to regulate negative emotions and replace dysfunctional behavior. (See also Behavioral Therapy.)

Equine/Animal-Assisted Therapy: A treatment program in which people interact with horses and become aware of their own emotional states through the reactions of the horse to their behavior.

Exercise Therapy: An individualized exercise plan that is written by a doctor or rehabilitation specialist, such as a clinical exercise physiologist, physical therapist, or nurse. The plan takes into account an individual's current medical condition and provides advice for what type of exercise to perform, how hard to exercise, how long, and how many times per week.

Exposure With Response Prevention (ERP): A type of behavior therapy strategy that is based on the theory that purging serves to decrease the anxiety associated with eating. Purging is therefore negatively reinforced via anxiety reduction. The goal of ERP is to modify the association between anxiety and purging by preventing purging following eating until the anxiety associated with eating subsides.(See also Behavioral Therapy.)

Expressive Therapy: A nondrug, nonpsychotherapy form of treatment that uses the performing and/or visual arts to help people express their thoughts and emotions. Whether through dance, movement, art, drama, drawing, painting, etc., expressive therapy provides an opportunity for communication that might otherwise remain repressed.

Eye Movement Desensitization And Reprocessing (EMDR): A nondrug and nonpsychotherapy form of treatment in which a therapist waves his or her fingers back and forth in front of the patient's eyes, and the patient tracks the movements while also focusing on a traumatic event. It is thought that the act of tracking while concentrating allows a different level of processing to occur in the brain so that the patient can review the event more calmly or more completely than before.

Family Therapy: A form of psychotherapy that involves members of an immediate or extended family. Some forms of family therapy are based on behavioral or psychodynamic principles; the most common form is based on family systems theory. This approach regards the family as the unit of treatment and emphasizes factors such as relationships and communication patterns. With eating disorders, the focus is on the eating disorder and how the disorder affects family relationships. Family therapies may also be educational and behavioral in approach.

Hypnobehavioral Therapy: A type of behavioral therapy that uses a combination of behavioral techniques such as self-monitoring to change maladaptive eating disorders and hypnotic techniques intended to reinforce and encourage behavior change.

Interpersonal Therapy (IPT): IPT (also called interpersonal psychotherapy) is designed to help people with eating disorders identify and address their interpersonal problems, specifically those involving grief, interpersonal role conflicts, role transitions, and interpersonal deficits. In this therapy, no emphasis is placed directly on modifying eating habits. Instead, the expectation is that the therapy enables people to change as their interpersonal functioning improves. IPT usually involves 16 to 20 hour-long, one-on-one treatment sessions over a period of four to five months.

Light Therapy (also called phototherapy): Treatment that involves regular use of a certain spectrum of lights in a light panel or light screen that bathes the person in that light. Light therapy is also used to treat conditions such as seasonal affective disorder (seasonal depression).

Mandometer Therapy: Treatment program for eating disorders based on the idea that psychiatric symptoms of people with eating disorders emerge as a result of poor nutrition and are not a cause of the eating disorder. A Mandometer is a computer that measures food intake and is used to determine a course of therapy.

Massage Therapy: A generic term for any of a number of various types of therapeutic touch in which the practitioner massages, applies pressure to, or manipulates muscles, certain points on the body, or other soft tissues to improve health and well-being. Massage therapy is thought to relieve anxiety and depression in patients with eating disorders.

Maudsley Method: A family-centered treatment program with three distinct phases. During the first phase parents are placed in charge of the child's eating patterns in hopes to break the cycle of not eating, or of binge eating and purging. The second phase begins once the child's refeeding and eating is under control with a goal of returning independent eating to the child. The goal of the third and final phase is to address the broader concerns of the child's development.

Mealtime Support Therapy: Treatment program developed to help patients with eating disorders eat healthfully and with less emotional upset.

Motivational Enhancement Therapy (MET): A treatment based on a model of change, with focus on the stages of change. Stages of change represent constellations of intentions and behaviors through which individuals pass as they move from having a problem to doing something to resolve it. The stages of change move from "pre-contemplation," in which individuals show no intention of changing, to the "action" stage, in which they are actively engaged in overcoming their problem. Transition from one stage to the next is sequential, but not linear. The aim of MET is to help individuals move from earlier stages into the action stage using cognitive and emotional strategies.

Movement/Dance Therapy: The psychotherapeutic use of movement as a process that furthers the emotional, cognitive, social, and physical integration of the individual, according to the American Dance Therapy Association.

Nutritional Therapy: Therapy that provides patients with information on the effects of eating disorders, techniques to avoid binge eating, and advice about making meals and eating. For example, the goals of nutrition therapy for individuals with bulimia nervosa are to help individuals maintain blood sugar levels, help individuals maintain a diet that provides them with enough nutrients, and help restore overall physical health.

Opioid Antagonists: A type of drug therapy that interferes with the brain's opioid receptors and is sometimes used to treat eating disorders.

Pharmacotherapy: Treatment of a disease or condition using clinician-prescribed drugs.

Progressive Muscle Relaxation: A deep relaxation technique based on the simple practice of tensing or tightening one muscle group at a time followed by a relaxation phase with release of the tension. This technique has been purported to reduce symptoms associated with night eating syndrome.

Psychoanalysis: An intensive, nondirective form of psychodynamic therapy in which the focus of treatment is exploration of a person's mind and habitual thought patterns. It is insight oriented, meaning that the goal of treatment is for the patient to increase understanding of the sources of his/her inner conflicts and emotional problems.

Psychodrama: A method of psychotherapy in which patients enact the relevant events in their lives instead of simply talking about them.

Psychodynamic Therapy: Psychodynamic theory views the human personality as developing from interactions between conscious and unconscious mental processes. The purpose of all forms of psychodynamic treatment is to bring unconscious thoughts, emotions, and memories into full consciousness so that the patient can gain more control over his/her life.

Psychodynamic Group Therapy: Psychodynamic groups are based on the same principles as individual psychodynamic therapy and aim to help people with past difficulties, relationships, and trauma, as well as current problems. The groups are typically composed of eight members plus one or two therapists.

Psychotherapy: The treatment of mental and emotional disorders through the use of psychological techniques designed to encourage communication of conflicts and insight into problems, with the goal being symptom relief, changes in behavior leading to improved social and vocational functioning, and personality growth.

Psychoeducational Therapy: A treatment intended to teach people about their problem, how to treat it, and how to recognize signs of relapse so that they can get necessary treatment before their difficulty worsens or recurs. Family psychoeducation includes teaching coping strategies and problem-solving skills to families, friends, and/or caregivers to help them deal more effectively with the individual.

Self-Guided Cognitive Behavior Therapy: A modified form of cognitive behavior therapy in which a treatment manual is provided for people to proceed with treatment on their own or with support from a nonprofessional. Guided self-help usually implies that the support person may or may not have some professional training, but is usually not a specialist in eating disorders. The important characteristics of the self-help approach are the use of a highly structured and detailed manual-based CBT, with guidance as to the appropriateness of self-help, and advice on where to seek additional help.

Self Psychology: A type of psychoanalysis that views anorexia and bulimia as specific cases of pathology of the self. According to this viewpoint, people with eating disorders cannot rely on human beings to fulfill their self-object needs (e.g., regulation of self-esteem, calming, soothing, vitalizing). Instead, they rely on food (its consumption or avoidance) to fulfill these needs. Self psychological therapy involves helping people with eating disorders give up their pathologic preference for food as a self-object and begin to rely on human beings as self-objects, beginning with their therapist.

Supportive Therapy: Psychotherapy that focuses on the management and resolution of current difficulties and life decisions using the patient's strengths and available resources.

Telephone Therapy: A type of psychotherapy provided over the telephone by a trained professional.

Chapter 38

Improving Your Body Image And Self-Esteem

Body Image And Self-Esteem

I'm fat. I'm too skinny. I'd be happy if I were taller, shorter, had curly hair, straight hair, a smaller nose, bigger muscles, longer legs.

Do any of these statements sound familiar? Are you used to putting yourself down? If so, you're not alone. As a teen, you're going through a ton of changes in your body. And as your body changes, so does your image of yourself. Lots of people have trouble adjusting, and this can affect their self-esteem.

Why Are Self-Esteem And Body Image Important?

Self-esteem is all about how much people value themselves, the pride they feel in themselves, and how worthwhile they feel. Self-esteem is important because feeling good about yourself can affect how you act. A person who has high self-esteem will make friends easily, is more in control of his or her behavior, and will enjoy life more.

Body image is how someone feels about his or her own physical appearance.

For many people, especially those in their early teens, body image can be closely linked to self-esteem. That's because as kids develop into teens, they care more about how others see them.

About This Chapter: This chapter includes "Body Image and Self-Esteem," May 2009, and "How Can I Improve My Self-Esteem?" March 2009, reprinted with permission from www.kidshealth.org. This information was provided by KidsHealth®, one of the largest resources online for medically reviewed health information written for parents, kids, and teens. For more articles like this, visit www.KidsHealth.org, or www.TeensHealth.org. Copyright © 1995-2012 The Nemours Foundation. All rights reserved.

What Influences A Person's Self-Esteem?

Puberty

Some teens struggle with their self-esteem when they begin puberty because the body goes through many changes. These changes, combined with a natural desire to feel accepted, mean it can be tempting for people to compare themselves with others. They may compare themselves with the people around them or with actors and celebs they see on TV, in movies, or in magazines.

But it's impossible to measure ourselves against others because the changes that come with puberty are different for everyone. Some people start developing early; others are late bloomers. Some get a temporary layer of fat to prepare for a growth spurt, others fill out permanently, and others feel like they stay skinny no matter how much they eat. It all depends on how our genes have programmed our bodies to act.

The changes that come with puberty can affect how both girls and guys feel about themselves. Some girls may feel uncomfortable or embarrassed about their maturing bodies. Others may wish that they were developing faster. Girls may feel pressure to be thin but guys may feel like they don't look big or muscular enough.

Outside Influences

It's not just development that affects self-esteem, though. Many other factors (like media images of skinny girls and bulked-up guys) can affect a person's body image too.

Family life can sometimes influence self-esteem. Some parents spend more time criticizing their kids and the way they look than praising them, which can reduce kids' ability to develop good self-esteem.

People also may experience negative comments and hurtful teasing about the way they look from classmates and peers. Sometimes racial and ethnic prejudice is the source of such comments. Although these often come from ignorance, sometimes they can affect someone's body image and self-esteem.

Healthy Self-Esteem

If you have a positive body image, you probably like and accept yourself the way you are. This healthy attitude allows you to explore other aspects of growing up, such as developing good friendships, growing more independent from your parents, and challenging yourself physically and mentally. Developing these parts of yourself can help boost your self-esteem.

A positive, optimistic attitude can help people develop strong self-esteem—for example, saying, "Hey, I'm human" instead of "Wow, I'm such a loser" when you've made a mistake, or not blaming others when things don't go as expected.

Knowing what makes you happy and how to meet your goals can help you feel capable, strong, and in control of your life. A positive attitude and a healthy lifestyle (such as exercising and eating right) are a great combination for building good self-esteem.

Tips For Improving Your Body Image

Some people think they need to change how they look or act to feel good about themselves. But actually all you need to do is change the way you see your body and how you think about yourself.

The first thing to do is recognize that your body is your own, no matter what shape, size, or color it comes in. If you're very worried about your weight or size, check with your doctor to verify that things are okay. But it's no one's business but your own what your body is like—ultimately, you have to be happy with yourself.

Next, identify which aspects of your appearance you can realistically change and which you can't. Everyone (even the most perfect-seeming celeb) has things about themselves that they can't change and need to accept—like their height, for example, or their shoe size.

If there are things about yourself that you want to change and can (such as how fit you are), do this by making goals for yourself. For example, if you want to get fit, make a plan to exercise every day and eat nutritious foods. Then keep track of your progress until you reach your goal. Meeting a challenge you set for yourself is a great way to boost self-esteem.

When you hear negative comments coming from within yourself, tell yourself to stop. Try building your self-esteem by giving yourself three compliments every day. While you're at it, every evening list three things in your day that really gave you pleasure. It can be anything from the way the sun felt on your face, the sound of your favorite band, or the way someone laughed at your jokes. By focusing on the good things you do and the positive aspects of your life, you can change how you feel about yourself.

Resilience

People who believe in themselves are better able to recognize mistakes, learn from them, and bounce back from disappointment. This skill is called resilience.

Source: Nemours Foundation, May 2009.

Where Can I Go If I Need Help?

Sometimes low self-esteem and body image problems are too much to handle alone. A few teens may become depressed, lose interest in activities or friends—and even hurt themselves or resort to alcohol or drug abuse.

If you're feeling this way, it can help to talk to a parent, coach, religious leader, guidance counselor, therapist, or an adult friend. A trusted adult—someone who supports you and doesn't bring you down—can help you put your body image in perspective and give you positive feedback about your body, your skills, and your abilities.

If you can't turn to anyone you know, call a teen crisis hotline (check the yellow pages under social services or search online). The most important thing is to get help if you feel like your body image and self-esteem are affecting your life.

How Can I Improve My Self-Esteem?

Steve's mind wanders as he does his homework. "I'm never going to do well on this history test," he thinks. "My dad's right, I'm just like him—I'll never amount to much." Distracted, he looks down and thinks how skinny his legs are. "Ugh," he says to himself. "I bet the football coach won't even let me try out when he sees what a wimp I am."

Julio is studying for the same history test as Steve, and he's also not too fond of the subject. But that's where the similarity ends. Julio has a completely different outlook. He's more likely to think, "OK, history again, what a pain. Thank goodness I'm acing the subject I really love—math." And when Julio thinks about the way he looks, it's also a lot more positive. Although he is shorter and skinnier than Steve, Julio is less likely to blame or criticize his body and more likely to think, "I may be skinny, but I can really run. I'd be a good addition to the football team."

Self-Esteem Defined

We all have a mental picture of who we are, how we look, what we're good at, and what our weaknesses might be. We develop this picture over time, starting when we're very young kids. The term self-image is used to refer to a person's mental picture of himself or herself. A lot of our self-image is based on interactions we have with other people and our life experiences. This mental picture (our self-image) contributes to our self-esteem.

Self-esteem is all about how much we feel valued, loved, accepted, and thought well of by others—and how much we value, love, and accept ourselves. People with healthy self-esteem are able to feel good about themselves, appreciate their own worth, and take pride in their abilities, skills, and accomplishments. People with low self-esteem may feel as if no one will like them or accept them or that they can't do well in anything.

We all experience problems with self-esteem at certain times in our lives—especially during our teens when we're figuring out who we are and where we fit in the world. The good news is that, because everyone's self-image changes over time, self-esteem is not fixed for life. So if you feel that your self-esteem isn't all it could be, you can improve it.

Self-Esteem Problems

Before a person can overcome self-esteem problems and build healthy self-esteem, it helps to know what might cause those problems in the first place. Two things in particular—how others see or treat us and how we see ourselves—can have a big impact on our self-esteem.

Parents, teachers, and other authority figures influence the ideas we develop about ourselves—particularly when we are little kids. If parents spend more time criticizing than praising a child, it can be harder for a kid to develop good self-esteem. Because teens are still forming their own values and beliefs, it's easy to build self-image around what a parent, coach, or other person says.

Obviously, self-esteem can be damaged when someone whose acceptance is important (like a parent or teacher) constantly puts you down. But criticism doesn't have to come from other people. Like Steve in the story above, some teens also have an "inner critic," a voice inside that seems to find fault with everything they do. And, like Steve, people sometimes unintentionally model their inner voice after a critical parent or someone else whose opinion is important to them.

Over time, listening to a negative inner voice can harm a person's self-esteem just as much as if the criticism were coming from another person. Some people get so used to their inner critic being there that they don't even notice when they're putting themselves down.

Unrealistic expectations can also affect a person's self-esteem. People have an image of who they want to be (or who they think they should be). Everyone's image of the ideal person is different. For example, some people admire athletic skills and others admire academic abilities. People who see themselves as having the qualities they admire—such as the ability to make friends easily—usually have high self-esteem.

People who don't see themselves as having the qualities they admire may develop low self-esteem. Unfortunately, people who have low self-esteem often do have the qualities they admire. They just can't see that they do because their self-image is trained that way.

Why Is Self-Esteem Important?

How we feel about ourselves can influence how we live our lives. People who feel that they are likable and lovable (in other words people with good self-esteem) have better relationships. They're more likely to ask for help and support from friends and family when they need it. People who believe they can accomplish goals and solve problems are more likely to do well in school. Having good self-esteem allows you to accept yourself and live life to the fullest.

Retrain Your Inner Critic

Because it comes from inside you, you can take back control over that inner voice that puts you down or tells you not to bother trying something because you're sure to fail. Decide that your inner voice will only give you constructive feedback from now on.

Source: Nemours Foundation, March 2009.

Steps To Improving Self-Esteem

If you want to improve your self-esteem, here are some steps to start empowering yourself:

- **Try To Stop Thinking Negative Thoughts About Yourself:** If you're used to focusing on your shortcomings, start thinking about positive aspects of yourself that outweigh them. When you catch yourself being too critical, counter it by saying something positive about yourself. Each day, write down three things about yourself that make you happy.

- **Aim For Accomplishments Rather Than Perfection:** Some people become paralyzed by perfection. Instead of holding yourself back with thoughts like, "I won't audition for the play until I lose 10 pounds," think about what you're good at and what you enjoy, and go for it.

Beware The Perfectionist

Are you expecting the impossible? It's good to aim high, but your goals for yourself should be within reach. So go ahead and dream about being a star athlete—but set your sights on improving your game in specific ways.

Source: Nemours Foundation, March 2009.

- **View Mistakes As Learning Opportunities:** Accept that you will make mistakes because everyone does. Mistakes are part of learning. Remind yourself that a person's talents are constantly developing, and everyone excels at different things—it's what makes people interesting.

- **Try New Things:** Experiment with different activities that will help you get in touch with your talents. Then take pride in new skills you develop.

- **Recognize What You Can Change And What You Can't:** If you realize that you're unhappy with something about yourself that you can change, then start today. If it's something you can't change (like your height), then start to work toward loving yourself the way you are.

- **Set Goals:** Think about what you'd like to accomplish, then make a plan for how to do it. Stick with your plan and keep track of your progress.

- **Take Pride In Your Opinions And Ideas:** Don't be afraid to voice them.

- **Make A Contribution:** Tutor a classmate who's having trouble, help clean up your neighborhood, participate in a walkathon for a good cause, or volunteer your time in some other way. Feeling like you're making a difference and that your help is valued can do wonders to improve self-esteem.

- **Exercise:** You'll relieve stress, and be healthier and happier.

- **Have Fun:** Ever found yourself thinking stuff like "I'd have more friends if I were thinner"? Enjoy spending time with the people you care about and doing the things you love. Relax and have a good time—and avoid putting your life on hold.

It's never too late to build healthy, positive self-esteem. In some cases where the emotional hurt is deep or long lasting, it can take the help of a mental health professional, like a counselor or therapist. These experts can act as a guide, helping people learn to love themselves and realize what's unique and special about them.

Self-esteem plays a role in almost everything you do. People with high self-esteem do better in school and find it easier to make friends. They tend to have better relationships with peers and adults, feel happier, find it easier to deal with mistakes, disappointments, and failures, and are more likely to stick with something until they succeed. It takes some work to develop good self-esteem, but once you do it's a skill you'll have for life.

Chapter 39

Re-Establishing Normal Eating

Not only is it important to deal with the underlying issues causing the eating disorder, it is also important to work towards developing a healthy eating pattern. Many people are afraid to start eating normally for fear that once they start eating, they won't be able to stop. This won't happen. Beginning to eat normally takes time and it should be done slowly so that you don't start to panic and lose control. Your ultimate goal will be to learn to eat three non-dieting meals and 2–3 snacks per day. Carbohydrates such as cereals, pasta, rice, bread, fruit, and vegetables should make up 50–60% of your total daily intake. Fat is also an essential nutrient and should make up about 25% of your total daily intake. Proteins such as eggs, red meats, dairy products, and poultry should make up about 10–15% of your total daily intake. A qualified nutritionist can help you to gradually develop a healthy eating pattern. Below is a list of suggestions that might help when trying to return to normal eating.

- If you are anorexic, try eating 6–8 small meals per day. Small meals will be easier to eat than three normal meals. Small meals will not leave you feeling quite so bloated and full. It is important to remember that in the beginning, you will experience bloating that can be uncomfortable. Many think this is a sign they are becoming fat, but it is natural for this to happen. It is only temporary and can last from 6–8 weeks. Instead of thinking of the bloating as you becoming fat, remind yourself that it is a part of the refeeding process and it is a sign that your body is healing.

- If you are bulimic or a compulsive eater, try eating three non-dieting meals and three snacks each day. Try to eat them at the same time each day. You may find it beneficial to follow a meal plan in the beginning so that you will know what you will be eating in advance. Do not allow yourself to eat more than planned. Eating more could lead to feelings of "I've blown it" and may cause you to binge or purge.

- In the beginning try to avoid foods that tend to trigger a binge or cause you to much feelings of guilt after eating. Later on you can reintroduce those foods into your meals.

- If anorexic, you may wish to begin the refeeding process with foods that will be easier to digest (i.e., applesauce, mashed potatoes, macaroni and cheese, oatmeal, etc.). Once the body starts to get used to having food, you can then begin to introduce more solid foods.

- Throw out your scale. Scales can prevent you from your reaching your goal of healthy eating. Also, it is important to remember that you are not a number and that number on the scale can never change the wonderful person you are inside.

- After eating, try and distract yourself with an activity you enjoy or if you feel very uncomfortable, try deep breathing exercises.

- Stop counting calories. Counting calories will prevent you from eating normally. Concentrate on learning about what normal eating is. Sometimes watching others eat can help to show us what normal eating really is.

- Start living one day at a time and one meal at a time.

- Sometimes it helps to think of food as medicine. You may not want to take it, but it is necessary for you to eat it, in order to recover. You can also think of food as fuel. Your body needs that fuel in order to be able to function properly.

- Remember that the voice in your head is lying to you. You need to do the opposite of what it tells you. If it tells you not to eat, go against it and eat. By doing this, you will be able to start taking back the control the eating disorder has. Many people believe that if they don't eat, they are the ones in control. The reality is, if you do not allow yourself to eat, the eating disorder is the one controlling you.

- If you exercise excessively, try to slowly cut back.

- In the beginning practice "mechanical eating." This means to eat your meals at predetermined times, whether you are hungry or not. The physiological mechanisms that signal hunger and fullness may not be functioning properly. In time, these signals will return, allowing you to know when you are hungry and when you are full.

- Remind yourself constantly that NO food will make you fat, as long as it is eaten in moderation.

- Stop buying "diet" foods. Buy foods that you would like to eat, do not buy them because they are low in calories.

Normal eating does take time and it should be done slowly so that you do not become too overwhelmed. It does take a lot of hard work in the beginning, but in time it will become a normal part of your day.

Refeeding (Also Called Renutrition)

Evidence-based treatment providers consider refeeding the essential first step in modern treatment of anorexia nervosa. Food is seen as primary medicine, both for the body and the brain. In hospital inpatient or residential settings, refeeding is often carried out through systematic use of behavior motivation techniques. If a patient is unable to cooperate with refeeding efforts, nasogastric feeding or even intravenous feeding may be prescribed. Inpatient refeeding is usually ramped up gradually to prevent refeeding syndrome. In Maudsley/family-based treatment, the overall goal of weight restoration is similar. Here, families work to replicate basic structures that would be typical of inpatient settings in their homes. Parents are called upon to manage and enforce eating until full weight restoration is achieved. A variation of refeeding protocol is the Mandometer method, where patients use a biofeedback device to relearn the "habit" of eating.

Refeeding syndrome is a serious, potentially fatal, complication of nutritional restoration. Major causes include low phosphorus blood levels following intake of foods high in calories or glucose. Phosphorous depletion causes abnormalities in the cardiorespiratory system, which left untreated can be fatal. Symptoms also develop in response to changes in potassium and magnesium levels. Rapid changes in intake can place excessive strain on the impaired heart which is then unable to maintain adequate circulation. Symptoms include: development of edema, increased liver function tests, hypophosphatemia, cardiac failure, central nervous system depression. Medical and dietary guidelines used to prevent refeeding syndrome include graded refeeding.

Graded refeeding refers to gradual increases in caloric intake during refeeding from very low weight, with aim to avoid complications such as refeeding syndrome. Graded refeeding is often used as protocol for newly arrived patients in the hospital.

Source: Excerpted from "Eating Disorders Glossary," © 2012 Families Empowered and Supporting Treatment of Eating Disorders (www.feast-ed.org).

Chapter 40

Eating Disorders Relapse And Relapse Prevention

Dealing With An Eating Disorder Relapse

Although complete recovery from eating disorders is possible, many experience slips and relapses during the recovery process. A slip is a once or twice, perhaps occasional, return to maladaptive behavior. A relapse is a complete and longer-lasting return to the behavior or worse. In a relapse, someone with an eating disorder would be back where she was before she entered recovery.

The best way to deal with relapse is prevention. Those in recovery need to identify risky situations in advance. A suitable analogy is black ice. When a driver encounters black ice, she skids out of control. Yet, if the driver knows where the black ice is, she can take precautions by going slower, driving more deliberately, or taking another route. For women and adolescents recovering from eating disorders, black ice is anything likely to trigger the eating disorder. Triggers are highly individualized. Often, but not always, they are the same situations and experiences that caused the eating disorder in the first place. Identifying these risky situations in advance allows the person to strategize how she will cope with the thoughts and emotions associated with her trigger situations.

Even with rigorous planning, slips may occur. If so, it is important for the individual to understand why the slip happened. Using a behavior chain analysis, she can identify the links in the chain—the events and her reactions—that led to the unhealthy behavior.

She can process what happened step by step, understanding what transpired in her mind and emotions at each step. With this information, she may not need her eating disorder when encountering the same situation in the future, because she can break the chain with different, pre-planned choices.

If relapse occurs, the individual can:

- Be hopeful and choose recovery again.

- Acknowledge her behavior is destructive and will damage her life now and in the future if she chooses to continue.

- Seek help from a healthcare professional.

- List the pros and cons of returning to the eating disorder. This list can re-establish the value of recovery.

- Talk to someone rather than choosing the eating disorder for support.

- Think about her accomplishments and what she will lose with a relapse.

- Identify goals and activities that relapse will prevent.

- Set small goals that can lead back to recovery, and congratulate herself for every success.

- Acknowledge that although her eating disorder has advantages, she already knows of healthier and less dangerous ways to obtain these same advantages.

- Remember her personal rights—the right to say "no", to express her feelings and opinions, to ask to have her needs met.

- Start a journal to help her identify feelings, internal messages, and triggers leading to the relapse.

- Let go of faultfinding, blame, guilt, and shame. Focus on the present and what she can change today.

- Ask her Higher Power for guidance.

Parents and spouses can also help during relapses by speaking to their loved one with truth and love. The dialogue takes place in a nonthreatening environment. Confrontation must always be preceded by listening, understanding, and validation. Validation comes through words such as "I love you and am really proud of you," or "I know how difficult this is for you." Confrontation without validation is perceived as an attack and the person will retaliate or withdraw.

When addressing the relapse, cite actual behavioral examples to prevent denial. Present the facts using supportive statements, such as "Help me understand what's going on," or "Obviously this fills a need; how can I help?" Encourage the person to seek renewed treatment.

In case of self harm or imminent death, take action—up to and including legal action—to ensure the person receives the help she needs.

Eating Disorder Relapse Prevention: Support Is Key

We know it is possible to experience complete recovery from an eating disorder because we have seen it again and again. However, with that said, we also recognize it's not unusual for a woman or girl to have multiple slips during the process. A "slip" is a return to unhealthy behaviors that does not last more than a few hours or days. A relapse, on the other hand, is a return to eating disorder behaviors that places the person back where they were prior to entering recovery—where many eating disorder behaviors are being practiced day after day. No one wants a relapse to occur; no one wants to go back to square one. This is why relapse prevention is so important.

Relapse

Relapse occurs commonly during recovery process, with studies showing relapse rates for anorexia nervosa and bulimia nervosa in the range of 35–60%. Relapse is defined as returning to a level of disordered eating after a period of full or partial remission from those behaviors. In particular: failure to maintain body weight range; cessation of menstrual periods; resumption of purging or restrictive behavior; and resumption of maladaptive attitudes regarding diet and food.

Studies indicate the highest risk for relapse is 6–7 months following partial symptom remission, and that if a full year can be reached relapse chances are reduced. Relapse may be often confused with less severe lapses or setbacks. But because it is impossible to tell the difference when such periods begin, it is vital for parents to be ready for immediate action if signs of a relapse appear.

A relapse prevention plan is a pre-planned strategy designed to quickly interrupt an eating disorder relapse.

Source: Excerpted from "Eating Disorders Glossary," © 2012 Families Empowered and Supporting Treatment of Eating Disorders (www.feast-ed.org).

Support is key when entering into any recovery process. For those recovering from an eating disorder, three types of support are essential: family, peer, and professional. Family support is quite important, especially if the recovering individual is still living with the family. Because eating disorders are complex, family-embedded, and often extremely difficult to understand, family therapy can often help. In terms of friends, peer support must be "recovery friendly." By this we mean that the patient's friends should not be highly invested in dieting, weight management, or appearance concerns. The third type of support—professional—is often the most important of all. At the very least, an individual should have an outpatient therapist and a dietitian for support, guidance, and accountability. In addition, if on medication, a psychiatrist should also be part of the team.

Anyone entering recovery must identify their eating disorder triggers. These are the situations and experiences that provoked the eating disorder in the first place. Triggers are highly individualized, meaning that what might trigger one woman may not affect another. It is important not only to identify these triggers, but also to decide in advance with one's treatment team how to deal with each of them using effective coping methods.

If a slip does occur, eating disorder patients can take positive steps to understand the "whys" behind it and what can be done differently in the future to change the outcome. It's called a behavior chain analysis, in which she identifies the links in the chain—the events and her reactions to them—that led to the unhealthy behavior. By examining what happened step by step, then making a new plan for the future, she may not need to rely on her eating disorder the next time she encounters the same situation. Again, professional support in this process greatly increases the chances of success.

Recovery from any addiction is not easy, and an eating disorder is no different. But it can be done. Remember... plan your life around your recovery, not your recovery around your life.

Part Five
Maintaining Healthy Eating And Fitness Habits

Chapter 41

Identifying The Right Weight For Your Height

"What's the right weight for my height?" is one of the most common questions girls and guys have.

It seems like a simple question. But, for teens, it's not always an easy one to answer. Why not? People have different body types, so there's no single number that's the right weight for everyone. Even among people who are the same height and age, some are more muscular or more developed than others. That's because not all teens have the same body type or develop at the same time.

It is possible to find out if you are in a healthy weight range for your height, though—it just takes a little effort. Read on to discover how this works. You'll also be able to go online and put your measurements into the KidsHealth calculator and get an idea of how you're doing.

Growth And Puberty

Not everyone grows and develops on the same schedule, but teens do go through a period of faster growth. During puberty, the body begins making hormones that spark physical changes like faster muscle growth (particularly in guys) and spurts in height and weight gain in both guys and girls.

Once these changes start, they continue for several years. The average person can expect to grow as much as 10 inches (25 centimeters) during puberty before he or she reaches full adult height.

About This Chapter: "What's the Right Weight for My Height?" March 2011, reprinted with permission from www.kidshealth.org. This information was provided by KidsHealth®, one of the largest resources online for medically reviewed health information written for parents, kids, and teens. For more articles like this, visit www.KidsHealth.org, or www.TeensHealth.org. Copyright © 1995-2012 The Nemours Foundation. All rights reserved.

Why You Need More Than A Scale

People overweight for their height can have major differences in body composition (the amounts of muscle, fat, and bone they have). An athlete might have a high body mass index (BMI) because of extra muscle, so may not be overweight. But a less fit person of the same height and weight may be considered overweight because of too much body fat.

Most guys and girls gain weight more rapidly during this time as the amounts of muscle, fat, and bone in their bodies changes. All that new weight gain can be perfectly fine—as long as body fat, muscle, and bone are in the right proportion.

Because some kids start developing as early as age eight and some not until age 14 or so, it can be normal for two people who are the same height and age to have very different weights.

It can feel quite strange adjusting to suddenly feeling heavier or taller. So it's perfectly normal to feel self-conscious about weight during adolescence—a lot of people do.

Figuring Out Fat Using BMI

Experts have developed a way to help figure out if a person is in the healthy weight range for his or her height. It's called the body mass index, or BMI. BMI is a formula that doctors use to estimate how much body fat a person has based on his or her weight and height.

The BMI formula uses height and weight measurements to calculate a BMI number. This number is then plotted on a chart, which tells a person whether he or she is underweight, average weight, overweight, or obese.

Figuring out the body mass index is a little more complicated for teens than it is for adults (that puberty thing again). BMI charts for teens use percentile lines to help individuals compare their BMIs with those of a very large group of people the same age and gender. There are different BMI charts for guys and girls under the age of 20.

A person's BMI number is plotted on the chart for their age and gender. A teen whose BMI is at the 50th percentile is close to the average of the age group and is considered in the healthy weight range (greater than or equal to the 5th percentile but less than 84th percentile). A BMI greater than or equal to 85th but less than the 95th percentile is in the overweight range. A teen with a BMI equal to or greater than the 95th percentile is in the obese range. A teen with a BMI below the 5th percentile is considered underweight.

BMI Calculator

To figure out your BMI, use the tool available online on the KidsHealth website (go to http://kidshealth.org/teen/food_fitness/dieting/weight_height.html#). Before you start, you'll need an accurate height and weight measurement. Bathroom scales and tape measures aren't always precise. So the best way to get accurate measurements is by being weighed and measured at your doctor's office or school.

What Does BMI Tell Us?

Although you can calculate BMI on your own, it's a good idea to ask your doctor, school nurse, or fitness counselor to help you figure out what it means. That's because a doctor can do more than just use BMI to assess a person's current weight. He or she can take into account where a girl or guy is during puberty and use BMI results from past years to track whether that person may be at risk for becoming overweight. Spotting this risk early on can be helpful because the person can then make changes in diet and exercise to help avert developing a weight problem.

People think of weight as a looks issue, but weight problems be more serious than someone's appearance. People who are overweight as teens increase their risk of developing health problems, such as diabetes and high blood pressure.

Being overweight as a teen also makes a person more likely to be overweight as an adult. And adults who are overweight may develop other serious health conditions, such as heart disease.

Although BMI can be a good indicator of a person's body fat, it doesn't always tell the full story. People can have a high BMI because they have a large frame or a lot of muscle (like a bodybuilder or athlete) instead of excess fat. Likewise, a small person with a small frame may have a normal BMI but could still have too much body fat. These are other good reasons to talk about your BMI with your doctor.

Some teens, especially those who go through puberty on a later time schedule, may feel too skinny. The good news is that their growth, development, and weight gain almost always catch up to other people their age later on.

How Can I Be Sure I'm Not Overweight Or Underweight?

If you think you've gained too much weight or are too skinny, a doctor should help you decide whether it's normal for you or whether you really have a weight problem. Your doctor has measured your height and weight over time and knows whether you're growing normally.

If concerned about your height, weight, or BMI, your doctor may ask questions about your health, physical activity, and eating habits. Your doctor may also ask about your family background to find out if you've inherited traits that might make you taller, shorter, or a late bloomer (someone who develops later than other people the same age). The doctor can then put all this information together to decide whether you might have a weight or growth problem.

If your doctor thinks your weight isn't in a healthy range, you will probably get specific dietary and exercise recommendations based on your individual needs. Following a doctor's or dietitian's plan that's designed especially for you will work way better than following fad diets. For teens, fad diets or severely cutting back on calories can actually slow down growth and sexual development, and the weight loss usually doesn't last.

What if you're worried about being too skinny? Most teens who weigh less than other teens their age are just fine. They may be going through puberty on a different schedule than some of their peers, and their bodies may be growing and changing at a different rate. Most underweight teens catch up in weight as they finish puberty during their later teen years and there's rarely a need to try to gain weight.

In a few cases, teens can be underweight because of a health problem that needs treatment. If you feel tired or ill a lot, or if you have symptoms like a cough, stomachache, diarrhea, or other problems that have lasted for more than a week or two, be sure to let your parents or your doctor know. Some teens are underweight because of eating disorders, like anorexia or bulimia, that require attention.

Getting Into Your Genes

Heredity plays a role in body shape and what a person weighs. People from different races, ethnic groups, and nationalities tend to have different body fat distribution (meaning they accumulate fat in different parts of their bodies) or body composition (amounts of bone and muscle versus fat).

But genes are not destiny. (That may be a relief if you're looking at Aunt Mildred and wondering if you'll end up with her physique!) No matter whose genes you inherit, you can have a healthy body and keep your weight at a level that's normal for you by eating right and being active.

Genes aren't the only things that family members may share. It's also true that unhealthy eating habits can be passed down, too. The eating and exercise habits of people in the same household probably have an even greater effect than genes on a person's risk of becoming overweight. If your family eats a lot of high-fat foods or snacks or doesn't get much exercise, you may tend to do the same. The good news is these habits can be changed for the better. Even simple forms of exercise, such as walking, have huge benefits on a person's health.

It can be tough dealing with the physical changes our bodies go through during puberty. But at this time, more than any other, it's not a specific number on the scale that's important. It's keeping your body healthy—inside and out.

Chapter 42

What Should You Really Eat?

Let's Eat For The Health Of It

Build A Healthy Plate

Before you eat, think about what goes on your plate or in your cup or bowl. Foods like vegetables, fruits, whole grains, low-fat dairy products, and lean protein foods contain the nutrients you need without too many calories. Try some of these options:

- Make half your plate fruits and vegetables.
- Switch to skim or 1% milk.
- Make at least half your grains whole.
- Vary your protein food choices.
- Keep your food safe to eat—learn more at www.FoodSafety.gov.

Cut Back On Solid Fats, Added Sugars, And Salt

Many people eat foods with too much solid fats, added sugars, and salt (sodium). Added sugars and fats load foods with extra calories you don't need. Too much sodium may increase your blood pressure.

About This Chapter: This chapter includes excerpts from the following documents produced by the U.S. Department of Agriculture (USDA) in June 2011 and available online at ChooseMyPlate.gov: "Let's Eat for the Health of It!" "Build a Healthy Meal: 10 Tips for Healthy Meals," "Why Is It Important to Eat Fruit?" "Why Is It Important to Eat Vegetables?" "Why Is It Important to Eat Grains, Especially Whole Grains?" "Why Is It Important to Make Lean or Low-Fat Choices from the Protein Foods Group?" and "Dairy: Health Benefits and Nutrients." The chapter concludes with a summary from "How to Eat for Health," Office on Women's Health (www.womenshealth.gov), June 17, 2008.

- Choose foods and drinks with little or no added sugars.

- Look out for salt (sodium) in foods you buy—it all adds up.

- Eat fewer foods that are high in solid fats.

The Right Amount Of Calories

Everyone has a personal calorie limit. Staying within yours can help you get to or maintain a healthy weight. People who are successful at managing their weight have found ways to keep track of how much they eat in a day, even if they don't count every calorie.

Ten Tips For A Healthy Meal

A healthy meal starts with more vegetables and fruits and smaller portions of protein and grains. Think about how you can adjust the proportions of your plate to get more of what you need without too many calories. And, don't forget dairy—make it the beverage with your meal or add fat-free or low-fat dairy products.

1. Make half your plate veggies and fruits. Vegetables and fruits are full of nutrients and may help to promote good health. Choose red, orange, and dark-green vegetables such as tomatoes, sweet potatoes, and broccoli.

2. Add lean protein. Choose protein foods, such as lean beef and pork, or chicken, turkey, beans, or tofu. Twice a week make seafood the protein on your plate.

3. Include whole grains. Aim to make at least half your gains whole grains. Look for the words "100% whole grain" or "100% whole wheat" on the food label. Whole grains provide more nutrients, like fiber, than refined grains.

4. Don't forget the dairy. Pair your meal with a cup of fat-free or low-fat milk. They provide the same amount of calcium and other essential nutrients as whole milk, but less fat and calories. Don't drink milk? Try soymilk (soy beverage) as your beverage or include fat-free or low-fat yogurt in your meal.

5. Avoid extra fat. Using heavy gravies or sauces will add fat and calories to otherwise healthy choices. For example, steamed broccoli is great, but avoid topping it with cheese sauce. Try other options, like a sprinkling of low-fat parmesan cheese or a squeeze of lemon.

6. Take your time. Savor your food. Eat slowly, enjoy the taste and textures, and pay attention to how you feel. Be mindful. Eating very quickly may cause you to eat too much.

7. Use a smaller plate. Use a smaller plate at meals to help with portion control. That way you can finish your entire plate and feel satisfied without overeating.

8. Take control of your food. Eat at home more often so you know exactly what you are eating. If you eat out, check and compare the nutrition information. Choose healthier options such as baked instead of fried.

9. Try new foods. Keep it interesting by picking out new foods you've never tried before, like mango, lentils, or kale. You may find a new favorite. Trade fun and tasty recipes with friends or find them online.

10. Satisfy your sweet tooth in a healthy way. Indulge in a naturally sweet dessert dish—fruit. Serve a fresh fruit cocktail or a fruit parfait made with yogurt. For a hot dessert, bake apples and top with cinnamon.

Food Groups

Why is it important to eat fruits and vegetables?

Eating fruits and vegetables provides health benefits—people who eat more fruits and vegetables as part of an overall healthy diet are likely to have a reduced risk of some chronic diseases. Fruits and vegetables provide nutrients vital for health and maintenance of your body.

Health Benefits

- Eating a diet rich in vegetables and fruits as part of an overall healthy diet may reduce risk for heart disease, including heart attack and stroke.

Everyday Foods Vs. Treats

Teens need to eat a good mix of foods each day. These everyday foods are fruits, vegetables, low-fat or fat-free milk or dairy foods (like low-fat yogurt and cheese), whole grain foods (like oatmeal, wholegrain breads, and brown rice) and lean meats, poultry, fish, beans and tofu.

Some foods and drinks are treats to have only from time to time. They may have a lot of extra things you don't need, like extra calories, added sugar, salt, trans fatty acids, saturated fat, or cholesterol. Examples include candy, onion rings, cookies, french fries, chips, and sugar-sweetened sodas.

Source: Excerpted from "BodyWorks For Teens," Office on Women's Health (www.womenshealth.gov), 2008.

- Eating a diet rich in some vegetables and fruits as part of an overall healthy diet may protect against certain types of cancers.

- Diets rich in foods containing fiber, such as some vegetables and fruits, may reduce the risk of heart disease, obesity, and type 2 diabetes.

- Eating vegetables and fruits rich in potassium as part of an overall healthy diet may lower blood pressure, and may also reduce the risk of developing kidney stones and help to decrease bone loss.

- Eating foods such as fruits and vegetables that are lower in calories per cup instead of some other higher-calorie food may be useful in helping to lower calorie intake.

Nutrients

- Most fruits are naturally low in fat, sodium, and calories. None have cholesterol. Most vegetables are naturally low in fat and calories. None have cholesterol. (Sauces or seasonings may add fat, calories, or cholesterol.)

Power Foods

Vitamin A: Good vision, healthy skin and hair, helps you grow

Some Food Sources: Fortified instant cereals (cereals that have vitamin A added to them); cantaloupe; dark green leafy vegetables like spinach, collards, and kale; carrots, sweet potatoes, pumpkin, and winter squash

Vitamin C: Healthy bones, skin, blood cells, gums, and teeth

Some Food Sources: Strawberries, grapefruits, oranges, melons, mangos, tomatoes, broccoli, red sweet peppers, cauliflower, and sweet potatoes

Vitamin E: Protects body cells

Some Food Sources: Nuts (almonds, hazelnuts, peanuts), sunflower seeds, pine nuts, and vegetable oils

Calcium: Strong bones and teeth

Some Food Sources: Low-fat or fat-free milk, yogurt, and cheese; calcium-fortified cereals, juices, soy beverages, and tofu; canned sardines, salmon, and trout

Folate (Folic Acid): Helps your body make red blood cells

Some Food Sources: Cooked or dry beans, peas, peanuts, oranges, orange juice, dark green leafy vegetables (like spinach), and enriched grain products

- Fruits are sources of many essential nutrients that are under-consumed, including potassium, dietary fiber, vitamin C, and folate (folic acid). Vegetables are also important sources of many nutrients, including potassium, dietary fiber, folate (folic acid), vitamin A, and vitamin C.

- Diets rich in potassium may help to maintain healthy blood pressure. Fruit sources of potassium include bananas, prunes and prune juice, dried peaches and apricots, cantaloupe, honeydew melon, and orange juice. Vegetable sources of potassium include sweet potatoes, white potatoes, white beans, tomato products (paste, sauce, and juice), beet greens, soybeans, lima beans, spinach, lentils, and kidney beans.

- Dietary fiber from fruits and vegetables, as part of an overall healthy diet, helps reduce blood cholesterol levels and may lower risk of heart disease. Fiber is important for proper bowel function. It helps reduce constipation and diverticulosis. Fiber-containing foods such as fruits and vegetables help provide a feeling of fullness with fewer calories. Whole or cut-up fruits are sources of dietary fiber; fruit juices contain little or no fiber.

Fiber: May help reduce risk for coronary heart disease; helps you feel full and have regular bowel movements

Some Food Sources: Cooked dry beans, ready-to-eat 100% bran cereals, sweet potatoes and baked potatoes with skin, and pears and apples with skin

Magnesium: Helps contract and relax muscles

Some Food Sources: Ready-to-eat 100% brain cereals, spinach, almonds, cashews, pine nuts, halibut (fish), and haddock

Iron: Helps red blood cells carry oxygen to different parts of the body to help produce energy; lack of iron in red blood cells (called anemia) can make you feel weak and tired

Some Food Sources: Lean beef, lamb, clams, oysters, shrimp, canned sardines, spinach, cooked dry beans (white, navy, and kidney), lentils, roasted pumpkin and squash seeds, and iron-fortified cereals

Potassium: Helps muscles work; reduces risk of high blood pressure and stroke

Some Food Sources: Baked white or sweet potatoes, tomato products, squash (pumpkin, butternut, and acorn); bananas and plantains; dried peaches, prunes, and apricots; oranges and orange juice, cantaloupe and honeydew melon; and low-fat or fat-free yogurt

Source: Excerpted from "BodyWorks For Teens," Office on Women's Health (www.womenshealth.gov), 2008.

- Vitamin A keeps eyes and skin healthy and helps to protect against infections.

- Vitamin C is important for growth and repair of all body tissues, helps heal cuts and wounds, and keeps teeth and gums healthy. Vitamin C also aids in iron absorption.

- Folate (folic acid) helps the body form red blood cells. Women of childbearing age who may become pregnant should consume adequate folate from foods, and in addition 400 mcg of synthetic folic acid from fortified foods or supplements. This reduces the risk of neural tube defects, spina bifida, and anencephaly during fetal development.

Why is it important to eat grains, especially whole grains?

Eating grains, especially whole grains, provides health benefits. People who eat whole grains as part of a healthy diet have a reduced risk of some chronic diseases. Grains provide many nutrients that are vital for the health and maintenance of our bodies.

Health Benefits

- Consuming whole grains as part of a healthy diet may reduce the risk of heart disease.

- Consuming foods containing fiber, such as whole grains, as part of a healthy diet, may reduce constipation.

- Eating whole grains may help with weight management.

- Eating grain products fortified with folate before and during pregnancy helps prevent neural tube defects during fetal development.

Nutrients

- Grains are important sources of many nutrients, including dietary fiber, several B vitamins (thiamin, riboflavin, niacin, and folate), and minerals (iron, magnesium, and selenium).

- Dietary fiber from whole grains or other foods, may help reduce blood cholesterol levels and may lower risk of heart disease, obesity, and type 2 diabetes. Fiber is important for proper bowel function. It helps reduce constipation and diverticulosis. Fiber-containing foods such as whole grains help provide a feeling of fullness with fewer calories.

- The B vitamins thiamin, riboflavin, and niacin play a key role in metabolism—they help the body release energy from protein, fat, and carbohydrates. B vitamins are also essential for a healthy nervous system. Many refined grains are enriched with these B vitamins.

- Folate (folic acid), another B vitamin, helps the body form red blood cells. Women of childbearing age who may become pregnant should consume adequate folate from foods, and in addition 400 mcg of synthetic folic acid from fortified foods or supplements. This reduces the risk of neural tube defects, spina bifida, and anencephaly during fetal development.

- Iron is used to carry oxygen in the blood. Many teenage girls and women in their childbearing years have iron-deficiency anemia. They should eat foods high in heme-iron (meats) or eat other iron containing foods along with foods rich in vitamin C, which can improve absorption of non-heme iron. Whole and enriched refined grain products are major sources of non-heme iron in American diets.

- Whole grains are sources of magnesium and selenium. Magnesium is a mineral used in building bones and releasing energy from muscles. Selenium protects cells from oxidation. It is also important for a healthy immune system.

Why is it important to eat protein foods and make lean or low-fat choices?

Foods in the meat, poultry, fish, eggs, nuts, and seed group provide nutrients that are vital for health and maintenance of your body. However, choosing foods from this group that are high in saturated fat and cholesterol may have health implications.

Health Benefits

- Meat, poultry, fish, dry beans and peas, eggs, nuts, and seeds supply many nutrients. These include protein, B vitamins (niacin, thiamin, riboflavin, and B6), vitamin E, iron, zinc, and magnesium.

- Proteins function as building blocks for bones, muscles, cartilage, skin, and blood. They are also building blocks for enzymes, hormones, and vitamins. Proteins are one of three nutrients that provide calories (the others are fat and carbohydrates).

- B vitamins found in this food group serve a variety of functions in the body. They help the body release energy, play a vital role in the function of the nervous system, aid in the formation of red blood cells, and help build tissues.

- Iron is used to carry oxygen in the blood. Many teenage girls and women in their child-bearing years have iron-deficiency anemia. They should eat foods high in heme-iron (meats) or eat other non-heme iron containing foods along with a food rich in vitamin C, which can improve absorption of non-heme iron.

- Magnesium is used in building bones and in releasing energy from muscles.

- Zinc is necessary for biochemical reactions and helps the immune system function properly.

- EPA (eicosapentaenoic acid) and DHA (docosahexaenoic acid) are omega-3 fatty acids found in varying amounts in seafood. Eating eight ounces per week of seafood may help reduce the risk for heart disease.

Nutrients

- Diets that are high in saturated fats raise "bad" cholesterol levels in the blood. The "bad" cholesterol is called LDL (low-density lipoprotein) cholesterol. High LDL cholesterol, in turn, increases the risk for coronary heart disease. Some food choices in this group are high in saturated fat. These include fatty cuts of beef, pork, and lamb; regular (75% to 85% lean) ground beef; regular sausages, hot dogs, and bacon; some luncheon meats such as regular bologna and salami; and some poultry such as duck. To help keep blood cholesterol levels healthy, limit the amount of these foods you eat.

- Diets that are high in cholesterol can raise LDL cholesterol levels in the blood. Cholesterol is only found in foods from animal sources. Some foods from this group are high in cholesterol. These include egg yolks (egg whites are cholesterol-free) and organ meats such as liver and giblets. To help keep blood cholesterol levels healthy, limit the amount of these foods you eat.

- A high intake of fats makes it difficult to avoid consuming more calories than are needed.

Why is it important to eat eight ounces of seafood per week?

Seafood contains a range of nutrients, notably the omega-3 fatty acids, EPA and DHA. Eating about eight ounces per week of a variety of seafood contributes to the prevention of heart disease. Smaller amounts of seafood are recommended for young children.

Seafood varieties that are commonly consumed in the United States that are higher in EPA and DHA and lower in mercury include salmon, anchovies, herring, sardines, Pacific oysters, trout, and Atlantic and Pacific mackerel (not king mackerel, which is high in mercury). The health benefits from consuming seafood outweigh the health risk associated with mercury, a heavy metal found in seafood in varying levels.

What are the benefits of eating nuts and seeds?

Eating peanuts and certain tree nuts (for example, walnuts, almonds, and pistachios) may reduce the risk of heart disease when consumed as part of a diet that is nutritionally adequate and within calorie needs. Because nuts and seeds are high in calories, eat them in small portions and use them to replace other protein foods, like some meat or poultry, rather than adding them to what you already eat. In addition, choose unsalted nuts and seeds to help reduce sodium intakes.

Why is it important to consume dairy products and make low-fat choices?

Consuming dairy products provides health benefits—especially improved bone health. Foods in the dairy group provide nutrients that are vital for health and maintenance of your body. These nutrients include calcium, potassium, vitamin D, and protein.

Choosing foods from the dairy group that are high in saturated fats and cholesterol, however, can have health implications. Diets high in saturated fats raise "bad" cholesterol levels in the blood. The "bad" cholesterol is called LDL (low-density lipoprotein) cholesterol. High LDL cholesterol, in turn, increases the risk for coronary heart disease. Many cheeses, whole milk, and products made from them are high in saturated fat. To help keep blood cholesterol levels healthy, limit the amount of these foods you eat. In addition, a high intake of fats makes it difficult to avoid consuming more calories than are needed.

Health Benefits

- Intake of dairy products is linked to improved bone health, and may reduce the risk of osteoporosis.
- The intake of dairy products is especially important to bone health during childhood and adolescence, when bone mass is being built.
- Intake of dairy products is also associated with a reduced risk of cardiovascular disease and type 2 diabetes, and with lower blood pressure in adults.

Nutrients

- Calcium is used for building bones and teeth and in maintaining bone mass. Dairy products are the primary source of calcium in American diets. Diets that provide three cups or the equivalent of dairy products per day can improve bone mass.
- Diets rich in potassium may help to maintain healthy blood pressure. Dairy products, especially yogurt, fluid milk, and soymilk (soy beverage), provide potassium.
- Vitamin D functions in the body to maintain proper levels of calcium and phosphorous, thereby helping to build and maintain bones. Milk and soymilk (soy beverage) that are fortified with vitamin D are good sources of this nutrient. Other sources include vitamin D–fortified yogurt and vitamin D–fortified ready-to-eat breakfast cereals.

- Milk products that are consumed in their low-fat or fat-free forms provide little or no solid fat.

Why is it important to consume oils?

Oils are not a food group, but they do provide essential nutrients and are therefore included in USDA recommendations for what to eat. Note that only small amounts of oils are recommended.

Most of the fats you eat should be polyunsaturated (PUFA) or monounsaturated (MUFA) fats. Oils are the major source of MUFAs and PUFAs in the diet. PUFAs contain some fatty acids that are necessary for health—called "essential fatty acids." Because oils contain these essential fatty acids, there is an allowance for oils in the food guide.

The MUFAs and PUFAs found in fish, nuts, and vegetable oils do not raise LDL ("bad") cholesterol levels in the blood. In addition to the essential fatty acids they contain, oils are the major source of vitamin E in typical American diets.

While consuming some oil is needed for health, oils still contain calories. In fact, oils and solid fats both contain about 120 calories per tablespoon. Therefore, the amount of oil consumed needs to be limited to balance total calorie intake. The Nutrition Facts label provides information to help you make smart choices.

Dieting Is Not The Answer

- Don't skip meals because missing meals often leads to overeating at later meals.

- Don't starve yourself because it's not likely you'll keep weight off in the long term. Also you'll miss out on important nutrients your body needs for growth.

- Don't leave out a whole food group or eat just a few foods. You need to balance different food groups to make sure you get all the nutrients you need.

- Don't make yourself vomit because vomiting can keep your body from absorbing the nutrients you need for good health. In particular, your body can't take in electrolytes, which affect the functioning of your heart.

Source: Excerpted from "BodyWorks For Teens," Office on Women's Health (www.womenshealth.gov), 2008.

Summary: How To Eat For Health

You've probably seen many articles in the media telling you what to eat and not eat. All this information can be confusing. You may be left wondering how much of different types of foods you should eat to stay healthy.

To help you choose foods wisely, the U.S. Departments of Health and Human Services and Agriculture have developed several tools:

- Healthy eating plans with interactive websites that help you choose foods based on your height, weight, and other information (visit http://www.choosemyplate.gov and http://www.womenshealth.gov/fitness-nutrition/how-to-eat-for-health/mypyramid.cfm)

- The Nutrition Facts label on food packages (for details, visit http://www.womenshealth.gov/fitness-nutrition/how-to-eat-for-health/food-labels.cfm#nutritionFacts)

- A Nutrient Database for foods that don't come in packages (available at http://www.womenshealth.gov/fitness-nutrition/how-to-eat-for-health/food-labels.cfm#noLabel)

Eating in a healthy manner isn't hard at all. To help prevent heart disease, stroke, and perhaps other diseases, you should eat mainly these types of foods:

- Fruits and vegetables

- Grains (at least half of your grains should be whole grains, such as whole wheat, oatmeal, and brown rice)

- Fat-free or low-fat versions of milk, cheese, yogurt, and other milk products

- Fish, skinless poultry, lean red meats, dry beans, eggs, and nuts

- Polyunsaturated and monounsaturated fats

Also, you should limit the amount of foods you eat that contain saturated fat, trans fat, cholesterol, sodium, and added sugars.

Following a healthy eating plan doesn't mean that you can't indulge every now and then. If what you eat is generally low in fat (especially saturated and trans fat) and sugars and you are getting enough vitamins and minerals, you may indulge in a rich dessert or serving of fried food every once in a while. If, on the other hand, you eat a lot of high-calorie foods, you are likely to get all the calories you need quickly without getting enough vital nutrients.

Chapter 43

Eat The Right Amount Of Calories For You

Get Started Eating The Right Amount Of Calories

Everyone has a personal calorie limit. Staying within yours can help you get to or maintain a healthy weight. Reaching a healthier weight is a balancing act. The secret is learning how to balance your "energy in" and "energy out" over the long run. "Energy in" is the calories from foods and beverages you have each day. "Energy out" is the calories you burn for basic body functions and physical activity.

To learn about your personal daily calorie limit, you can obtain a customized daily food plan from the U.S. Department of Agriculture (USDA). Visit http://www.choosemyplate.gov/myplate/index.aspx, enter your age, sex, height, weight, and activity level in the Daily Food Plan entry box.

Keep your calorie limit in mind when deciding what to eat and drink. For example, if your calorie limit is 1,800 calories per day, think about how those calories can be split up among meals, snacks, and beverages over the course of a day. It doesn't have to be the same each day.

Compare food and beverage options and think about how they fit within your calorie limit. For example, a snack with 200 calories may be a better option than another with 500 calories. Use your daily calorie limit to help you decide which foods and drinks to choose.

About This Chapter: This chapter begins with text from "Eat the Right Amount of Calories for You," U. S. Department of Agriculture (USDA), 2011. It also contains text from "Sample Menus for a 2000 Calorie Food Pattern," USDA, 2010; "Focus on Foods You Need," USDA, 2011; "What Are Empty Calories?" USDA, 2011; "Calories: How Many Can I Have?" USDA, 2011; and "Eat Fewer Empty Calories," USDA, 2011. For more information on nutrition and dietary guidelines, visit www.choosemyplate.gov.

A Balancing Act: Where is your energy balance?

Maintaining Weight: Your weight will stay the same when the calories you eat and drink equal the calories you burn.

Losing Weight: You will lose weight when the calories you eat and drink are less than the calories you burn.

Gaining Weight: You will gain weight when the calories you eat and drink are greater than the calories you burn.

Source: "Eat the Right Amount of Calories for You," USDA, 2011.

For a healthier you, use the Nutrition Facts label to make smart food choices quickly and easily. Check the label of similar products for calories and nutrients, and choose the food that's best for you. Be sure to look at the serving size and how many servings you are actually consuming, as well. If you eat twice the serving size, you double the calories. When eating out, calorie information may be available on menus, in a pamphlet, or online. You can also find calorie information about a specific food using the online Food-a-pedia, available at https://www.choosemyplate.gov/SuperTracker/foodapedia.aspx.

Stumbling Blocks

Concerned about being able to eat the right amount of calories? Here are some common stumbling blocks and ideas to help you overcome these barriers:

Don't Understand Calories: *Calorie* is just the term used to describe the amount of energy a food or drink provides when you eat it. Carbohydrates, fat, and protein all provide energy—and this energy is measured in calories. Think of calories as a measurement unit—like inches, pounds, or gallons. You need energy from foods and drinks to fuel your body—for everything from breathing to physical activity.

It's important to consider more than just calories when making food choices. Your Daily Food Plan is designed to provide the nutrients you need while staying within your calorie limits. Use your Daily Food Plan to determine how much you should eat from each of the five food groups: Fruits, vegetables, grains, protein, and dairy.

Don't Have Time To Count Calories: People who are successful at managing their weight have found ways to keep track of how much they eat in a day, even if they don't count every calorie. Most people eat the same general types of food on a regular basis. Take some time up front to compare calorie labels, and over time, you will learn which options are the better choices.

No Idea How Many Calories To Eat: Your calorie needs depend on a number of factors including: your height, weight, and physical activity level. You can get your personal daily calorie limit with your Daily Food Plan. The calories in your Daily Food Plan are averages. For best results, track your body weight over time.

Sample Menus For A 2000 Calorie Food Pattern

Use this seven-day menu as a motivational tool to help put a healthy eating pattern into practice and to identify creative new ideas for healthy meals. Averaged over a week, this menu provides the recommended amounts of key nutrients and foods from each food group. The menus feature a large number of different foods to inspire ideas for adding variety to food choices. They are not intended to be followed day-by-day as a specific prescription for what to eat.

Average amounts for weekly menu:

Food group	Daily average over 1 week
GRAINS	6.2 oz eq
Whole grains	3.8
Refined grains	2.4
VEGETABLES	2.6 cups
Vegetable subgroups (amount per week)	
Dark green	1.6 cups per week
Red/Orange	5.6
Starchy	5.1
Beans and Peas	1.6
Other Vegetables	4.1
FRUITS	2.1 cups
DAIRY	3.1 cups
PROTEIN FOODS	5.7 oz eq
Seafood	8.8 oz per week
OILS	29 grams
CALORIES FROM ADDED FATS AND SUGARS	245 calories

Figure 43.1. Sample Menus for a 2000 Calorie Food Pattern, Food Groups Average Amounts

Nutrient	Daily average over 1 week
Calories	1975
Protein	96 g
Protein	19% kcal
Carbohydrate	275 g
Carbohydrate	56% kcal
Total fat	59 g
Total fat	27% kcal
Saturated fat	13.2 g
Saturated fat	6.0% kcal
Monounsaturated fat	25 g
Polyunsaturated fat	16 g
Linoleic Acid	13 g
Alpha-linolenic Acid	1.8 g
Cholesterol	201 mg
Total dietary fiber	30 g
Potassium	4701 mg
Sodium	1810 mg
Calcium	1436 mg
Magnesium	468 mg
Copper	2.0 mg
Iron	18 mg
Phosphorus	1885 mg
Zinc	14 mg
Thiamin	1.6 mg
Riboflavin	2.5 mg
Niacin Equivalents	24 mg
Vitamin B6	2.4 mg
Vitamin B12	12.3 mcg
Vitamin C	146 mg
Vitamin E	11.8 mg (AT)
Vitamin D	9.1 mcg
Vitamin A	1090 mcg (RAE)
Dietary Folate Equivalents	530 mcg
Choline	386 mg

Figure 43.2. Sample Menus for a 2000 Calorie Food Pattern, Average Nutrient Amounts

Spices and herbs can be used to taste. Try spices such as chili powder, cinnamon, cumin, curry powder, ginger, nutmeg, mustard, garlic powder, onion powder, or pepper. Try fresh or dried herbs such as basil, parsley, cilantro, chives, dill, mint, oregano, rosemary, thyme, or tarragon. Also try salt-free spice or herb blends.

Day 1

Breakfast

Creamy oatmeal (cooked in milk):

> ½ cup uncooked oatmeal
>
> 1 cup fat-free milk
>
> 2 Tablespoons raisins
>
> 2 teaspoons brown sugar

Beverage: 1 cup orange juice

Lunch

Taco salad:

> 2 ounces tortilla chips
>
> 2 ounces cooked ground turkey
>
> 2 teaspoons corn/canola oil (to cook turkey)
>
> ¼ cup kidney beans*
>
> ½ ounce low-fat cheddar cheese
>
> ½ cup chopped lettuce
>
> ½ cup avocado
>
> 1 teaspoon lime juice (on avocado)
>
> 2 Tablespoons salsa

Beverage:
1 cup water, coffee, or tea**

Dinner

Spinach lasagna roll-ups:

1 cup lasagna noodles (2 oz. dry)

½ cup cooked spinach

½ cup ricotta cheese

1 ounce part–skim mozzarella cheese

½ cup tomato sauce*

1 ounce whole wheat roll

1 teaspoon tub margarine

Beverage: 1 cup fat-free milk

Snacks

2 Tablespoons raisins

1 ounce unsalted almonds

Day 2

Breakfast

Breakfast burrito:

1 flour tortilla (8" diameter)

1 scrambled egg

⅓ cup black beans*

2 Tablespoons salsa

½ large grapefruit

Beverage:

1 cup water, coffee, or tea**

Lunch

Roast beef sandwich:

1 small whole grain hoagie bun

2 ounces lean roast beef

1 slice part–skim mozzarella cheese

2 slices tomato

¼ cup mushrooms

1 teaspoon corn/canola oil (to cook mushrooms)

1 teaspoon mustard

Baked potato wedges:

1 cup potato wedges

1 tsp corn/canola oil (to cook potato)

1 Tablespoon ketchup

Beverage: 1 cup fat-free milk

Dinner

Baked salmon on beet greens:

4 ounce salmon filet

1 tsp olive oil

2 teaspoons lemon juice

⅓ cup cooked beet greens

(sauteed in 2 teaspoons

corn/canola oil)

Quinoa with almonds:

½ cup quinoa

½ ounce slivered almonds

Beverage: 1 cup fat-free milk

Snacks

1 cup cantaloupe balls

269

Day 3

Breakfast

Cold cereal:

> *1 cup ready-to-eat oat cereal*
>
> *1 medium banana*
>
> *½ cup fat-free milk*

1 slice whole wheat toast

> *1 teaspoon tub margarine*

Beverage: 1 cup prune juice

Lunch

Tuna salad sandwich:

> *2 slices rye bread*
>
> *2 ounces tuna*
>
> *1 Tablespoon mayonnaise*
>
> *1 Tablespoon chopped celery*
>
> *½ cup shredded lettuce*

1 medium peach

Beverage: 1 cup fat-free milk

Dinner

Roasted chicken:

> *3 ounces cooked chicken breast*

1 large sweet potato, roasted

½ cup succotash (limas and corn)

> *1 teaspoon tub margarine*

1 ounce whole wheat roll

> *1 teaspoon tub margarine*

Beverage:

1 cup water, coffee, or tea**

Snacks

¼ cup dried apricots

1 cup flavored yogurt (chocolate)

Day 4

Breakfast

1 whole wheat English muffin

> *1 Tablespoon all-fruit preserves*

1 hard-cooked egg

Beverage:

1 cup water, coffee, or tea**

Lunch

White bean-vegetable soup:

> *1¼ cup chunky vegetable soup with pasta*
>
> *½ cup white beans**

6 saltine crackers*

½ cup celery sticks

Beverage: 1 cup fat-free milk

Dinner

Rigatoni with meat sauce:

> *1 cup rigatoni pasta (2 oz. dry)*
>
> *2 ounces cooked ground beef (95% lean)*
>
> *2 teaspoon corn/canola oil (to cook beef)*
>
> *½ cup tomato sauce**
>
> *3 Tablespoons grated parmesan cheese*

Spinach salad:

> *1 cup raw spinach leaves*
>
> *½ cup tangerine sections*
>
> *½ ounce chopped walnuts*
>
> *4 teaspoons oil and vinegar dressing*

Beverage:

1 cup water, coffee, or tea**

Snacks

1 cup nonfat fruit yogurt

Day 5

Breakfast

Cold cereal:

    1 cup shredded wheat

    ½ cup sliced banana

    ½ cup fat-free milk

1 slice whole wheat toast

    2 teaspoon all-fruit preserves

Beverage:

1 cup fat-free chocolate milk

Lunch

Turkey sandwich

    1 whole wheat pita bread (2 oz)

    3 ounces roasted turkey, sliced

    2 slices tomato

    ¼ cup shredded lettuce

    1 teaspoon mustard

    1 Tablespoon mayonnaise

½ cup grapes

Beverage: 1 cup tomato juice*

Dinner

Steak and potatoes:

    4 ounces broiled beef steak

    ⅔ cup mashed potatoes made with

    milk and 2 teaspoons tub margarine

½ cup cooked green beans

    1 teaspoon tub margarine

    1 teaspoon honey

1 ounce whole wheat roll

    1 teaspoon tub margarine

Frozen yogurt and berries:

    ½ cup frozen yogurt (chocolate)

    ¼ cup sliced strawberries

Beverage: 1 cup fat-free milk

Snacks

1 cup frozen yogurt (chocolate)

Day 6

Breakfast

French toast:

    2 slices whole wheat bread

    3 Tablespoons fat-free milk and

    ⅔ egg (in French toast)

    2 teaspoon tub margarine

    1 Tablespoon pancake syrup

½ large grapefruit

Beverage: 1 cup fat-free milk

Lunch

3-bean vegetarian chili on baked potato:

> *¼ cup each cooked kidney beans,* navy beans,* and black beans**
>
> *½ cup tomato sauce**
>
> *¼ cup chopped onion*
>
> *2 Tablespoon chopped jalapeno peppers*
>
> *1 teaspoon corn/canola oil (to cook onion and peppers)*
>
> *¼ cup cheese sauce*
>
> *1 large baked potato*

½ cup cantaloupe

Beverage:

1 cup water, coffee, or tea**

Dinner

Hawaiian pizza

> *2 slices cheese pizza, thin crust*
>
> *1 ounce lean ham*
>
> *¼ cup pineapple*
>
> *¼ cup mushrooms*
>
> *1 teaspoon safflower oil (to cook mushrooms)*

Green salad:

> *1 cup mixed salad greens*
>
> *4 teaspoon oil and vinegar dressing*

Beverage: 1 cup fat-free milk

Snacks

3 Tablespoons hummus

5 whole wheat crackers*

Day 7

Breakfast

Buckwheat pancakes with berries:

> *2 large (7") pancakes*
>
> *1 Tablespoon pancake syrup*
>
> *¼ cup sliced strawberries*

Beverage: 1 cup orange juice

Lunch

New England clam chowder:

> *3 ounces canned clams*
>
> *½ small potato*
>
> *2 Tablespoons chopped onion*
>
> *2 Tablespoons chopped celery*
>
> *6 Tablespoons evaporated milk*
>
> *¼ cup fat-free milk*

> *1 slice bacon*
>
> *1 Tablespoon white flour*

10 whole wheat crackers*

1 medium orange

Beverage: 1 cup fat-free milk

Dinner

Tofu-vegetable stir-fry:

> *4 ounces firm tofu*
>
> *½ cup chopped Chinese cabbage*
>
> *¼ cup sliced bamboo shoots*
>
> *2 Tablespoons chopped sweet red peppers*
>
> *2 Tablespoons chopped green peppers*
>
> *1 Tablespoon corn/canola oil (to cook stir-fry)*

1 cup cooked brown rice (2 ounces raw)

Honeydew yogurt cup:

¾ cup honeydew melon

½ cup plain fat-free yogurt

Beverage:

1 cup water, coffee, or tea**

Snacks

1 large banana spread with 2 Tablespoons peanut butter*

1 cup nonfat fruit yogurt

Notes

*Foods that are reduced sodium, low sodium, or no-salt added products. These foods can also be prepared from scratch with no added salt. All other foods are regular commercial products, which contain variable levels of sodium. Average sodium level of the seven-day menu assumes that no salt is added in cooking or at the table.

**Unless indicated, all beverages are unsweetened and without added cream or whitener.

Italicized foods are part of the dish or food that precedes it.

Focus On Foods You Need

Building a healthier plate can help you meet your nutrient needs and maintain your weight. Foods like vegetables, fruits, whole grains, low-fat dairy products, and lean protein foods contain the nutrients you need.

When making food choices, use your Daily Food Plan. Focus on the five food groups. Most of what you eat and drink each day should fit within one or more of the five food groups. Smart choices are the foods with low amounts of solid fats or added sugars: such as, fat-free (skim) milk instead of whole milk, unsweetened applesauce instead of sweetened applesauce, and 95% lean ground beef instead of regular (75% lean) ground beef. Also think about how the food was prepared. For example, choose skinless baked chicken instead of fried chicken and choose fresh fruit instead of a fruit pastry.

Does it matter how much carbohydrate, protein, and fat you eat? Carbohydrate, protein, and fat are components of foods and drinks that provide calories. You should not select a diet that avoids or severely limits carbohydrates, protein, or fat. Similarly, you should not select a diet that avoids any of the five food groups. There are choices within each food group that provide the nutrients you need.

Get Started Focusing On Foods You Need

- Start with breakfast. Eat a breakfast that helps you meet your food group needs.

- Have healthy snacks available at home and bring healthy snacks to eat when on-the-go, such as carrot and celery sticks with peanut butter or whole grain crackers and low-fat cheese.

- When preparing meals, include vegetables, fruits, whole grains, fat-free or low-fat dairy products, and lean protein foods.

- Follow the advice to make half your plate fruits and vegetables.

Stumbling Blocks

Concerned about focusing on the foods you need? Here are some common stumbling blocks and ideas to help you overcome these barriers:

Don't Like Many Vegetables Or Fruit: Explore the wide range of different vegetables that are available and choose some you're willing to try. If you're not fond of cooked vegetables, experiment with salads and raw vegetables. Or, try mixed dishes that include vegetables, like stir-fries, chili con carne, vegetable soups, or pasta with marinara sauce. When eating out, choose a vegetable (other than french fries) as a side dish. For fruits, try adding fruit to salads, making fruit smoothies, or snacking on dried fruit. You can find more suggestions online from the "10 Tips Nutrition Education Series" available at http://www.choosemyplate.gov/healthy-eating-tips/ten-tips.html.

Don't/Can't Drink Milk: You don't need to drink milk, but you do need the nutrients it provides. You can get these nutrients from yogurt, from fortified soymilk (soy beverage), or from low-fat cheese. Milk or other foods from the Dairy Group can also be incorporated into lots of foods and drinks including lattes, puddings, and soups. Try some new ways to include milk or other foods from the Dairy Group in your meals and snacks.

Fruits And Vegetables Are Too Expensive: It is possible to fit vegetables and fruits into any budget. Buy fresh fruits and vegetables that are in season; they are easy to get, have more flavor, and are usually less expensive. You can also try canned or frozen. For canned items, choose fruit canned in 100% fruit juice and vegetables with "low sodium" or "no salt added" on the label. And don't forget to check the local newspaper, online, and at the store for sales, coupons, and specials that will cut food costs.

Empty Calories

Currently, many of the foods and beverages Americans eat and drink contain empty calories—calories from solid fats and/or added sugars. Solid fats and added sugars add calories to the food but few or no nutrients. For this reason, the calories from solid fats and added sugars in a food are often called empty calories. Learning more about solid fats and added sugars can help you make better food and drink choices.

Solid fats are fats that are solid at room temperature, like butter, beef fat, and shortening. Some solid fats are found naturally in foods. They can also be added when foods are processed by food companies or when they are prepared.

Added sugars are sugars and syrups that are added when foods or beverages are processed or prepared.

Solid fats and added sugars can make a food or beverage more appealing, but they also can add a lot of calories. The foods and beverages that provide the most empty calories for Americans are:

- Cakes, cookies, pastries, and donuts (contain both solid fat and added sugars)

- Sodas, energy drinks, sports drinks, and fruit drinks (contain added sugars)

- Cheese (contains solid fat)

- Pizza (contains solid fat)

- Ice cream (contains both solid fat and added sugars)

- Sausages, hot dogs, bacon, and ribs (contain solid fat)

These foods and beverages are the major sources of empty calories, but many of them can be found in forms with less or no solid fat or added sugars. For example, low-fat cheese and low-fat hot dogs can be purchased. You can choose water, milk, or sugar-free soda instead of drinks with sugar. Check that the calories in these products are less than in the regular product.

In some foods, like most candies and sodas, all the calories are empty calories. These foods are often called "empty calorie foods." However, empty calories from solid fats and added sugars can also be found in some other foods that contain important nutrients. Table 43.1 illustrates some examples of foods that provide nutrients, in forms with and without empty calories. Making better choices, like unsweetened applesauce or extra lean ground beef, can help keep your intake of added sugars and solid fats low.

How Many Empty Calories Can I Have?

The limit for empty calories is based on estimated calorie needs by age/gender group. Physical activity increases calorie needs, so those who are more physically active need more total calories and have a larger limit for empty calories. Table 43.2 gives a general guide.

Table 43.1. Foods With Nutrients In Forms With And Without Empty Calories

Food with some empty calories	Food with few or no empty calories
Sweetened applesauce (contains added sugars)	Unsweetened applesauce
Regular ground beef (75% lean) (contains solid fats)	Extra lean ground beef (95% or more lean)
Fried chicken (contains solid fats from frying and skin)	Baked chicken breast without skin
Sugar-sweetened cereals (contain added sugars)	Unsweetened cereals
Whole milk (contains solid fats)	Fat-free milk

Table 43.2. Estimated Allowance Of Empty Calories For People Who Are Not Physically Active

Age and gender	Total daily calorie needs*	Daily limit for empty calories
Children 2–3 yrs	1000 cals	135**
Children 4–8 yrs	1200–1400 cals	120
Girls 9–13 yrs	1600 cals	120
Boys 9–13 yrs	1800 cals	160
Girls 14–18 yrs	1800 cals	160
Boys 14–18 yrs	2200 cals	265
Females 19–30 yrs	2000 cals	260
Males 19–30 yrs	2400 cals	330
Females 31–50 yrs	1800 cals	160
Males 31–50 yrs	2200 cals	265
Females 51+ yrs	1600 cals	120
Males 51+ yrs	2000 cals	260

* These amounts are appropriate for individuals who get less than 30 minutes of moderate physical activity most days. Those who are more active need more total calories, and have a higher limit for empty calories.

** The limit for empty calories is higher for children two and three years old than it is for some older children, because younger children have lower nutrient needs and smaller recommended intakes from the basic food groups.

If You Need To Eat Fewer Empty Calories

Regardless of your weight status, empty calories should not be a major part of the diet. For most people, no more than 15% of calories should come from solid fats and added sugars.

Get Started Eating Fewer Empty Calories

Here are three ways to cut back on empty calories:

- Choose foods and drinks with little or no added sugars or solid fats. For example, drink water instead of sugary drinks. There are about ten packets of sugar in a 12-ounce can of soda, while water has no added sugars. Select lean cuts of meats or poultry and fat-free or low-fat milk and cheese. Fatty meats, poultry skin, and whole milk or regular cheese have more solid fats.

- Select products that contain added sugars and solid fats less often. For example, eat sugary desserts only once in a while. Most days, select fruit for dessert instead of a sugary option. Make major sources of solid fats—such as cakes, cookies, ice cream, pizza, regular cheese, sausages, and hot dogs—occasional choices, not everyday foods.

- When you have foods and drinks with added sugars and solid fats, choose a small portion. For example, instead of eating three scoops of ice cream, order one scoop.

Stumbling Blocks

Concerned about eating fewer empty calories? Here are some common "stumbling blocks" and ideas to help you overcome these barriers:

Empty Calories Not On Food Labels: While empty calories are not listed on the food label, you can use the label to see if there are solid fats and added sugars in the food. Check the Nutrition Facts label to choose foods with little or no saturated fat and no trans fat to choose foods with less solid fat. Use the ingredients list to help identify added sugars in the food.

Total Calories Vs. Empty Calories: Foods that are high in empty calories tend to be high in total calories too. It is the total amount of calories consumed each day that can affect weight. If you currently eat too many empty calories, eating fewer is a great way to help you eat fewer total calories.

Cravings For Something Sweet: Replace foods high in empty calories with better choices. For example, try a yogurt parfait with low-fat or fat-free yogurt and sliced fruit or frozen grapes for a sweet treat. You can still get the sweet you want without the excess calories.

Chapter 44

Use Food Labels To Help You Make Healthier Choices

Consumers often compare prices of food items in the grocery store to choose the best value for their money. But comparing items using the food label can help them choose the best value for their health.

The food label identifies a variety of information about a product, such as the ingredients, net weight, and nutrition facts.

"The food label is one of the most valuable tools consumers have," says Barbara Schneeman, Ph.D., Director of the Food and Drug Administration's (FDA's) Office of Nutrition, Labeling and Dietary Supplements. "The food label gives consumers the power to compare foods quickly and easily so they can judge for themselves which products best fit their dietary needs."

For example, someone with high blood pressure who needs to watch salt (sodium) intake may be faced with five different types of tomato soup on the shelf, says Schneeman. You can quickly and easily compare the sodium content of each product by looking at the part of the label that lists nutrition information (Nutrition Facts Label) to choose the one with the lowest sodium content.

FDA regulations require nutrition information to appear on most foods, and any claims on food products must be truthful and not misleading. In addition, "low sodium," "reduced fat," and "high fiber" must meet strict government definitions. FDA has defined other terms used to describe the content of a nutrient, such as "low," "reduced," "high," "free," "lean," "extra lean," "good source," "less," "light," and "more." So a consumer who wants to reduce sodium intake can be assured that the manufacturer of a product claiming to be "low sodium" or "reduced in sodium" has met these definitions.

About This Chapter: Excerpted from "Food Label Helps Consumers Make Healthier Choices," U.S. Food and Drug Administration (www.fda.gov), December 8, 2011.

But you don't have to memorize the definitions. Just look at the Nutrition Facts Label to compare the claims of different products with similar serving sizes.

What Is In Food?

Food provides your body with all of the materials it needs to grow, and to be healthy and active. These are some of the building blocks in food.

- Carbohydrates are the body's main source of fuel. Starchy foods like breads, spaghetti, rice, potatoes, corn and cereals are made up mostly of carbohydrates. Sugary foods like candy, jam, and syrups also are carbohydrates. Some carbohydrates, called fiber or roughage, are hard to digest. They help move waste through the digestive system.

- Fats include butter, margarine, lard, shortening, and cooking oil. Cheese, cream, chocolate, some meats and many desserts have a lot of fat. Fats are very concentrated sources of energy, so only a little is needed.

- Proteins are important for growth and repair of the body. Protein-rich foods include eggs, milk products, meat, dried beans, chicken, turkey, and fish. The body also can use protein as fuel for movement and growth.

- Minerals are found in small amounts in foods. They are needed for many of the body's functions. For example, calcium is used to build bones and teeth, and also is important for muscles and the nervous system. Iron becomes part of red blood cells.

- Vitamins are other chemicals found naturally in food. They are needed in very small amounts by the body.

- Did you know that water also is a major part of almost all food?

Source: Excerpted from "From the Label to the Table," National Institute of Environmental Health Sciences, undated; available at kids.niehs.nih.gov, accessed January 30, 2012.

Nutrient Highs And Lows

Most nutrients must be declared on the Nutrition Facts Label as "percent Daily Value" (%DV), which tells the percent of the recommended daily intake in a serving of that product and helps the consumer create a balanced diet. The %DV allows you to see at a glance if a product has a high or low amount of a nutrient. The rule of thumb is 20% DV or more is high and 5% DV or less is low.

Health experts recommend keeping your intake of saturated fat, trans fat, and cholesterol as low as possible because these nutrients may increase your risk for heart disease. This is where the %DV on the Nutrition Facts Label can be helpful, says Schneeman. There is no %DV for trans fat, but you can use the label to find out whether the saturated fat and cholesterol are high or low, she says. When comparing products, look at the total amount of saturated fat plus trans fat to find the one lowest in both of these types of fat.

For beneficial nutrients, like fiber or calcium, you can use the %DV to choose products that contain higher amounts. Research has shown that eating a diet rich in fiber may lower your chances of getting heart disease and some types of cancer. And eating foods containing calcium may help lower your risk of getting the bone-weakening disease, osteoporosis.

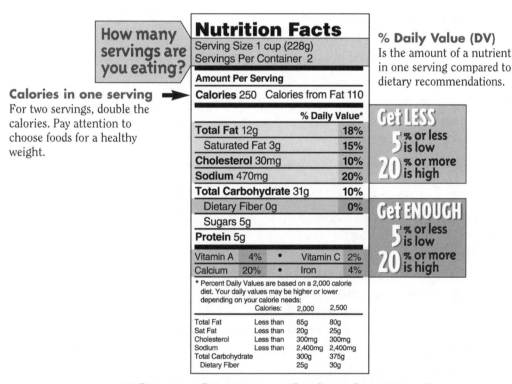

What's the Best Choice for You?

Use the 5%-20% Guide to Daily Values to choose foods.

Figure 44.1. Read It Before You Eat It. Nutrition Facts on food labels tell you the calories (or food energy) and nutrients in one serving of food inside the package. Look for the nutrition information in the store, near fresh fruit, vegetables, meat, poultry, or fish, too. Check the calories in one serving. For two servings, double the calories. Pay attention to choose foods for a healthy weight. (Source: "Healthful Eating...Food Labels Help!" U.S. Department of Agriculture, 2008.)

Confusing Claims

The terms "natural," "healthy," and "organic" often cause confusion. "Consumers seem to think that 'natural' and 'organic' imply 'healthy'," says Schneeman. "But these terms have different meanings from a regulatory point of view."

According to FDA policy, "natural" means the product does not contain synthetic or artificial ingredients. "Healthy," which is defined by regulation, means the product must meet certain criteria that limit the amounts of fat, saturated fat, cholesterol, and sodium, and require specific minimum amounts of vitamins, minerals, or other beneficial nutrients.

Food labeled "organic" must meet the standards set by the Department of Agriculture (USDA). Organic food differs from conventionally produced food in the way it is grown or produced. But USDA makes no claims that organically produced food is safer or more nutritious than conventionally produced food.

For example, says Schneeman, "A premium ice cream could be 'natural' or 'organic' and still be high in fat or saturated fat, so would not meet the criteria for 'healthy'."

Nutrition Facts—The Labels On Food Products

Beginning in 1994, the US government began requiring manufacturers to put information about nutritional value on food labels. You can use this information to make better choices about what you eat—watch for the following information:

- Pay close attention to serving sizes.
- Products labeled "light" or "lite" must have a third fewer calories or half the fat of the foods to which they are compared. "Light" also can mean that salt has been reduced by half.
- Look for foods with lower levels of saturated fats.
- The sodium level tells you how much salt is in food.
- Look for products that have more fiber and less sugar.
- Vitamins and minerals help your body function properly.
- Calcium is important for bones and teeth.
- Use the "percentage of daily values" section of the label as a guide for daily planning.
- The amount of calories a person needs each day depends on many factors, including exercise.

Source: Excerpted from "From the Label to the Table," National Institute of Environmental Health Sciences, undated; available at kids.niehs.nih.gov, accessed January 30, 2012.

Chapter 45

Healthy Eating For Vegetarians

Vegetarian diets can meet all the recommendations for nutrients. The key is to consume a variety of foods and the right amount of foods to meet your calorie needs. Follow the food group recommendations for your age, sex, and activity level to get the right amount of food and the variety of foods needed for nutrient adequacy. Nutrients that vegetarians may need to focus on include protein, iron, calcium, zinc, and vitamin B12.

Nutrients To Focus On For Vegetarians

- Protein has many important functions in the body and is essential for growth and maintenance. Protein needs can easily be met by eating a variety of plant-based foods. Combining different protein sources in the same meal is not necessary. Sources of protein for vegetarians and vegans include beans, nuts, nut butters, peas, and soy products (tofu, tempeh, veggie burgers). Milk products and eggs are also good protein sources for lacto-ovo vegetarians.

- Iron functions primarily as a carrier of oxygen in the blood. Iron sources for vegetarians and vegans include iron-fortified breakfast cereals, spinach, kidney beans, black-eyed peas, lentils, turnip greens, molasses, whole wheat breads, peas, and some dried fruits (dried apricots, prunes, raisins).

- Calcium is used for building bones and teeth and in maintaining bone strength. Sources of calcium for vegetarians and vegans include calcium-fortified soymilk, calcium-fortified breakfast cereals and orange juice, tofu made with calcium sulfate, and some

About This Chapter: From "Tips for Vegetarians," U.S. Department of Agriculture (www.choosemyplate.gov), 2011.

dark-green leafy vegetables (collard greens, turnip greens, bok choy, mustard greens). The amount of calcium that can be absorbed from these foods varies. Consuming enough plant foods to meet calcium needs may be unrealistic for many. Milk products are excellent calcium sources for lacto vegetarians. Calcium supplements are another potential source.

- Zinc is necessary for many biochemical reactions and also helps the immune system function properly. Sources of zinc for vegetarians and vegans include many types of beans (white beans, kidney beans, and chickpeas), zinc-fortified breakfast cereals, wheat germ, and pumpkin seeds. Milk products are a zinc source for lacto vegetarians.

- Vitamin B12 is found in animal products and some fortified foods. Sources of vitamin B12 for vegetarians include milk products, eggs, and foods that have been fortified with vitamin B12. These include breakfast cereals, soymilk, veggie burgers, and nutritional yeast.

Ten Suggestions For Healthy Vegetarian Eating Patterns

A vegetarian eating pattern can be a healthy option. The key is to consume a variety of foods and the right amount of foods to meet your calorie and nutrient needs.

1. **Think About Protein:** Your protein needs can easily be met by eating a variety of plant foods. Sources of protein for vegetarians include beans and peas, nuts, and soy products (such as tofu, tempeh). Lacto-ovo vegetarians also get protein from eggs and dairy foods.

2. **Bone Up On Sources Of Calcium:** Calcium is used for building bones and teeth. Some vegetarians consume dairy products, which are excellent sources of calcium. Other sources of calcium for vegetarians include calcium-fortified soymilk (soy beverage), tofu made with calcium sulfate, calcium-fortified breakfast cereals and orange juice, and some dark-green leafy vegetables (collard, turnip, and mustard greens; and bok choy).

3. **Make Simple Changes:** Many popular main dishes are or can be vegetarian—such as pasta primavera, pasta with marinara or pesto sauce, veggie pizza, vegetable lasagna, tofu-vegetable stir-fry, and bean burritos.

4. **Enjoy A Cookout:** For barbecues, try veggie or soy burgers, soy hot dogs, marinated tofu or tempeh, and fruit kabobs. Grilled veggies are great, too.

5. **Include Beans And Peas:** Because of their high nutrient content, consuming beans and peas is recommended for everyone, vegetarians and non-vegetarians alike. Enjoy some vegetarian chili, three-bean salad, or split pea soup. Make a hummus filled pita sandwich.

Tips For Vegetarians

- Build meals around protein sources that are naturally low in fat, such as beans, lentils, and rice. Don't overload meals with high-fat cheeses to replace the meat.

- Calcium-fortified soymilk provides calcium in amounts similar to milk. It is usually low in fat and does not contain cholesterol.

- Many foods that typically contain meat or poultry can be made vegetarian. This can increase vegetable intake and cut saturated fat and cholesterol intake. Consider the following:

  - Pasta primavera or pasta with marinara or pesto sauce
  - Veggie pizza
  - Vegetable lasagna

  - Tofu-vegetable stir-fry
  - Vegetable lo mein
  - Vegetable kabobs
  - Bean burritos or tacos

---

6. **Try Different Veggie Versions:** A variety of vegetarian products look—and may taste—like their non-vegetarian counterparts but are usually lower in saturated fat and contain no cholesterol. For breakfast, try soy-based sausage patties or links. For dinner, rather than hamburgers, try bean burgers or falafel (chickpea patties).

7. **Make Some Small Changes At Restaurants:** Most restaurants can make vegetarian modifications to menu items by substituting meatless sauces or nonmeat items, such as tofu and beans for meat, and adding vegetables or pasta in place of meat. Ask about available vegetarian options.

8. **Nuts Make Great Snacks:** Choose unsalted nuts as a snack and use them in salads or main dishes. Add almonds, walnuts, or pecans instead of cheese or meat to a green salad.

9. **Get Your Vitamin B12:** Vitamin B12 is naturally found only in animal products. Vegetarians should choose fortified foods such as cereals or soy products, or take a vitamin B12 supplement if they do not consume any animal products. Check the Nutrition Facts label for vitamin B12 in fortified products.

10. **Find A Vegetarian Pattern For You:** Go to www.dietaryguidelines.gov and check appendices 8 and 9 of the Dietary Guidelines for Americans, 2010 for vegetarian adaptations of the USDA food patterns at 12 calorie levels.

Source: From "Healthy Eating For Vegetarians: 10 Tips for Vegetarians," U.S. Department of Agriculture, June 2011.

- A variety of vegetarian products look (and may taste) like their non-vegetarian counterparts, but are usually lower in saturated fat and contain no cholesterol.

  - For breakfast, try soy-based sausage patties or links.

  - Rather than hamburgers, try veggie burgers. A variety of kinds are available, made with soy beans, vegetables, and/or rice.

  - Add vegetarian meat substitutes to soups and stews to boost protein without adding saturated fat or cholesterol. These include tempeh (cultured soybeans with a chewy texture), tofu, or wheat gluten (seitan).

  - For barbecues, try veggie burgers, soy hot dogs, marinated tofu or tempeh, and veggie kabobs.

  - Make bean burgers, lentil burgers, or pita halves with falafel (spicy ground chick pea patties).

  - Some restaurants offer soy options (texturized vegetable protein) as a substitute for meat, and soy cheese as a substitute for regular cheese.

- Most restaurants can accommodate vegetarian modifications to menu items by substituting meatless sauces, omitting meat from stir-fries, and adding vegetables or pasta in place of meat. These substitutions are more likely to be available at restaurants that make food to order.

- Many Asian and Indian restaurants offer a varied selection of vegetarian dishes.

Chapter 46

Healthy Eating For Athletes

What diet is best for athletes?

It's important that an athlete's diet provides the right amount of energy, the 50-plus nutrients the body needs and adequate water. No single food or supplement can do this. A variety of foods are needed every day. But, just as there is more than one way to achieve a goal, there is more than one way to follow a nutritious diet.

Do the nutritional needs of athletes differ from non-athletes?

Competitive athletes, sedentary individuals, and people who exercise for health and fitness all need the same nutrients. However, because of the intensity of their sport or training program, some athletes have higher calorie and fluid requirements. Eating a variety of foods to meet increased calorie needs helps to ensure that the athlete's diet contains appropriate amounts of carbohydrate, protein, vitamins, and minerals.

Are there certain dietary guidelines athletes should follow?

Health and nutrition professionals recommend that 55–60% of the calories in our diet come from carbohydrate, no more than 30% from fat and the remaining 10–15% from protein. While the exact percentages may vary slightly for some athletes based on their sport or training program, these guidelines will promote health and serve as the basis for a diet that will maximize performance.

About This Chapter: "Questions Most Frequently Asked about Sports Nutrition," President's Council on Fitness, Sports, and Nutrition (www.fitness.gov), 2012.

How many calories do I need a day?

This depends on your age, body size, sport, and training program. For example, a 250-pound weight lifter needs more calories than a 98-pound gymnast. Exercise or training may increase calorie needs by as much as 1,000 to 1,500 calories a day. The best way to determine if you're getting too few or too many calories is to monitor your weight. Keeping within your ideal competitive weight range means that you are getting the right amount of calories.

Which is better for replacing fluids—water or sports drinks?

Depending on how muscular you are, 55–70% of your body weight is water. Being "hydrated" means maintaining your body's fluid level. When you sweat, you lose water which must be replaced if you want to perform your best. You need to drink fluids before, during, and after all workouts and events.

Whether you drink water or a sports drink is a matter of choice. However, if your workout or event lasts for more than 90 minutes, you may benefit from the carbohydrates provided by sports drinks. A sports drink that contains 15–18 grams of carbohydrate in every eight ounces of fluid should be used. Drinks with a higher carbohydrate content will delay the absorption of water and may cause dehydration, cramps, nausea, or diarrhea. There are a variety of sports drinks on the market. Be sure to experiment with sports drinks during practice instead of trying them for the first time the day of an event.

What are electrolytes?

Electrolytes are nutrients that affect fluid balance in the body and are necessary for our nerves and muscles to function. Sodium and potassium are the two electrolytes most often added to sports drinks. Generally, electrolyte replacement is not needed during short bursts

A Weighty Matter

- Your calorie needs depend on your age, body size, sport, and training program.
- The best way to make sure you are not getting too many or too few calories is to check your weight from time to time.
- If you're keeping within your ideal weight range, you're probably getting the right amount of calories.

Source: Excerpted from "Fast Facts about Sports Nutrition," President's Council on Fitness, Sports, and Nutrition (www.fitness.gov), 2012.

of exercise since sweat is approximately 99% water and less than 1% electrolytes. Water, in combination with a well-balanced diet, will restore normal fluid and electrolyte levels in the body. However, replacing electrolytes may be beneficial during continuous activity of longer than two hours, especially in a hot environment.

Water, Water Everywhere

- You can survive for a month without food, but only a few days without water.
- Water is the most important nutrient for active people.
- When you sweat, you lose water, which must be replaced. Drink fluids before, during, and after workouts.
- Water is a fine choice for most workouts. However; during continuous workouts of greater than 90 minutes, your body may benefit from a sports drink.
- Sports drinks have two very important ingredients—electrolytes and carbohydrates
- Sports drinks replace electrolytes lost through sweat during workouts lasting several hours.
- Carbohydrates in sports drinks provide extra energy. The most effective sports drinks contain 15 to 18 grams of carbohydrate in every eight ounces of fluid.

Source: Excerpted from "Fast Facts about Sports Nutrition," President's Council on Fitness, Sports, and Nutrition (www .fitness.gov), 2012.

What do muscles use for energy during exercise?

Most activities use a combination of fat and carbohydrate as energy sources. How hard and how long you work out, your level of fitness and your diet will affect the type of fuel your body uses. For short-term, high-intensity activities like sprinting, athletes rely mostly on carbohydrate for energy. During low-intensity exercises like walking, the body uses more fat for energy.

What are carbohydrates?

Carbohydrates are sugars and starches found in foods like breads, cereals, fruits, vegetables, pasta, milk, honey, syrups, and table sugar. Carbohydrates are the preferred source of energy for your body. Regardless of origin, your body breaks down carbohydrates into glucose that your blood carries to cells to be used for energy. Carbohydrates provide four calories per gram, while fat provides nine calories per gram. Your body cannot differentiate between glucose that comes from starches or sugars. Glucose from either source provides energy for working muscles.

Is it true that athletes should eat a lot of carbohydrates?

When you are training or competing, your muscles need energy to perform. One source of energy for working muscles is glycogen which is made from carbohydrates and stored in your muscles. Every time you work out, you use some of your glycogen. If you don't consume enough carbohydrates, your glycogen stores become depleted, which can result in fatigue. Both sugars and starches are effective in replenishing glycogen stores.

When and what should I eat before I compete?

Performance depends largely on the foods consumed during the days and weeks leading up to an event. If you regularly eat a varied, carbohydrate-rich diet you are in good standing and probably have ample glycogen stores to fuel activity. The purpose of the pre-competition meal is to prevent hunger and to provide the water and additional energy the athlete will need during competition.

Most athletes eat two to four hours before their event. However, some athletes perform their best if they eat a small amount 30 minutes before competing, while others eat nothing for six hours beforehand.

For many athletes, carbohydrate-rich foods serve as the basis of the meal. However, there is no magic pre-event diet. Simply choose foods and beverages that you enjoy and that don't bother your stomach. Experiment during the weeks before an event to see which foods work best for you.

Will eating sugary foods before an event hurt my performance?

In the past, athletes were warned that eating sugary foods before exercise could hurt performance by causing a drop in blood glucose levels. Recent studies, however, have shown that consuming sugar up to 30 minutes before an event does not diminish performance. In fact, evidence suggests that a sugar-containing pre-competition beverage or snack may improve performance during endurance workouts and events.

What is carbohydrate loading?

Carbohydrate loading is a technique used to increase the amount of glycogen in muscles. For five to seven days before an event, the athlete eats 10–12 grams of carbohydrate per kilogram body weight and gradually reduces the intensity of the workouts. (To find out how much you weigh in kilograms, simply divide your weight in pounds by 2.2.) The day before the event, the athlete rests and eats the same high-carbohydrate diet. Although carbohydrate loading may be beneficial for athletes participating in endurance sports which require 90 minutes or more of non-stop effort, most athletes needn't worry about carbohydrate loading. Simply eating a diet that derives more than half of its calories from carbohydrates will do.

Rev Up Your Engine With Carbohydrates

- Carbohydrates are your body's main source of energy.
- Carbohydrates are sugars and starches, and they are found in foods such as breads, cereals, fruits, vegetables, pasta, milk, honey, syrups and table sugar.
- Sugars and starches are broken down by your body into glucose, which is used by your muscles for energy.
- For health and peak performance, more than half your daily calories should come from carbohydrates.
- Sugars and starches have four calories per gram, while fat has nine calories per gram. In other words, carbohydrates have less than half the calories of fat.

If you regularly eat a carbohydrate-rich diet you probably have enough carbohydrate stored to fuel activity. Even so, be sure to eat a pre-competition meal for fluid and additional energy. What you eat as well as when you eat your pre-competition meal will be entirely individual.

Source: Excerpted from "Fast Facts about Sports Nutrition," President's Council on Fitness, Sports, and Nutrition (www .fitness.gov), 2012.

As an athlete, do I need to take extra vitamins and minerals?

Athletes need to eat about 1,800 calories a day to get the vitamins and minerals they need for good health and optimal performance. Since most athletes eat more than this amount, vitamin and mineral supplements are needed only in special situations. Athletes who follow vegetarian diets or who avoid an entire group of foods (for example, never drink milk) may need a supplement to make up for the vitamins and minerals not being supplied by food. A multivitamin-mineral pill that supplies 100% of the Recommended Dietary Allowance (RDA) will provide the nutrients needed. An athlete who frequently cuts back on calories, especially below the 1,800 calorie level, is not only at risk for inadequate vitamin and mineral intake, but also may not be getting enough carbohydrate. Since vitamins and minerals do not provide energy, they cannot replace the energy provided by carbohydrates.

Will extra protein help build muscle mass?

Many athletes, especially those on strength-training programs or who participate in power sports, are told that eating a ton of protein or taking protein supplements will help them gain muscle weight. However, the true secret to building muscle is training hard and consuming enough calories. While some extra protein is needed to build muscle, most American diets provide more than enough protein. Between 1.0 and 1.5 grams of protein per kilogram body weight per day is sufficient if your calorie intake is adequate and you're eating a variety of foods. For a 150-pound athlete, that represents 68–102 grams of protein a day.

Score With Vitamins And Minerals

Eating a varied diet will give you all the vitamins and minerals you need for health and peak performance. Exceptions include active people who follow strict vegetarian diets, avoid an entire group of foods, or eat less than 1800 calories a day. If you fall into any of these categories, a multivitamin and mineral pill may provide the vitamins and minerals missing in your diet. Taking large doses of vitamins and minerals will not help your performance and may be bad for your health. Vitamins and minerals do not supply the body with energy and, therefore are not a substitute for carbohydrates.

Source: Excerpted from "Fast Facts about Sports Nutrition," President's Council on Fitness, Sports, and Nutrition (www .fitness.gov), 2012.

Why is iron so important?

Hemoglobin, which contains iron, is the part of red blood cells that carries oxygen from the lungs to all parts of the body, including muscles. Since your muscles need oxygen to produce energy, if you have low iron levels in your blood, you may tire quickly. Symptoms of iron deficiency include fatigue, irritability, dizziness, headaches, and lack of appetite. Many times, however; there are no symptoms at all. A blood test is the best way to find out if your iron level is low. It is recommended that athletes have their hemoglobin levels checked once a year.

The RDA for iron is 15 milligrams a day for women and 10 milligrams a day for men. Red meat is the richest source of iron, but fish and poultry also are good sources. Fortified breakfast cereals, beans and green leafy vegetables also contain iron. Our bodies absorb the iron found in animal products best.

Should I take an iron supplement?

Taking iron supplements will not improve performance unless an athlete is truly iron deficient. Too much iron can cause constipation, diarrhea, and nausea and may interfere with the absorption of other nutrients such as copper and zinc. Therefore, iron supplements should not be taken without proper medical supervision.

Flexing Your Options To Build Bigger Muscles

- It is a myth that eating lots of protein and/or taking protein supplements and exercising vigorously will definitely turn you into a big, muscular person.

- Building muscle depends on your genes, how hard you train, and whether you get enough calories.

- The average American diet has more than enough protein for muscle building. Extra protein is eliminated from the body or stored as fat.

Source: Excerpted from "Fast Facts about Sports Nutrition," President's Council on Fitness, Sports, and Nutrition (www .fitness.gov), 2012.

Why is calcium so important?

Calcium is needed for strong bones and proper muscle function. Dairy foods are the best source of calcium. However, studies show that many female athletes who are trying to lose weight cut back on dairy products. Female athletes who don't get enough calcium may be at risk for stress fractures and, when they're older, osteoporosis. Young women between the ages of 11 and 24 need about 1,200 milligrams of calcium a day. After age 25, the recommended intake is 800 milligrams. Low-fat dairy products are a rich source of calcium and also are low in fat and calories.

Popeye And All That Spinach

- Iron supplies working muscles with oxygen.

- If your iron level is low, you may tire easily and not have enough stamina for activity.

- The best sources of iron are animal products, but plant foods such as fortified breads, cereals, beans and green leafy vegetables also contain iron.

- Iron supplements may have side effects, so take them only if your doctor tells you to.

Source: Excerpted from "Fast Facts about Sports Nutrition," President's Council on Fitness, Sports, and Nutrition (www .fitness.gov), 2012.

No Bones About It, You Need Calcium Everyday

- Many people do not get enough of the calcium needed for strong bones and proper muscle function.

- Lack of calcium can contribute to stress fractures and the bone disease, osteoporosis.

- The best sources of calcium are dairy products, but many other foods such as salmon with bones, sardines, collard greens, and okra also contain calcium. Additionally, some brands of bread, tofu, and orange juice are fortified with calcium.

Source: Excerpted from "Fast Facts about Sports Nutrition," President's Council on Fitness, Sports, and Nutrition (www .fitness.gov), 2012.

Chapter 47

Healthy Eating And Weight Management

A Healthy Weight Is Important

Reaching and maintaining a healthy weight is good for your overall health and will help you prevent and control many diseases and conditions. Maintaining a healthy weight has many benefits, including feeling good about yourself and having more energy to enjoy life.

A person's weight is the result of many things—height, genes, metabolism, behavior, and environment. Maintaining a healthy weight requires keeping a balance, a balance of energy. You must balance the calories you get from food and beverages with the calories you use to keep your body going and being physically active.

- The same amount of energy IN and energy OUT over time = weight stays the same

- More IN than OUT over time = weight gain

- More OUT than IN over time = weight loss

Your energy IN and OUT don't have to balance exactly every day. It's the balance over time that will help you to maintain a healthy weight in the long run.

Identifying Your Risk

First, gather some information—check your body mass index (BMI). Your (BMI) is a good indicator of your risk for a variety of diseases since it gives an accurate estimate of your total body fat. There are three ways to check your BMI.

About This Chapter: Excerpted and adapted from "Aim for a Healthy Weight," National Heart, Lung, and Blood Institute (www.nhlbi.nih.gov), NIH Publication No. 05-5213, August 2005. Revised by David A. Cooke, MD, FACP, August 2012.

One way is to use the chart shown in Figure 47.1 to find your weight and height and then go above that column to find your BMI.

A second way is to use the BMI calculator on the National Heart Lung and Blood Institute (NHLBI) website at http://www.nhlbisupport.com/bmi.

A third way to check your BMI is to calculate it: Divide your weight in pounds by your height in inches, divide by your height in inches again, and then multiply the total by 703. The answer is your BMI. The BMI ranges for underweight, normal weight, overweight, and obesity are as follows:

- Underweight: Less than 18.5

- Normal: 18.5–24.9

- Overweight: 25.0–29.9

- Obesity: 30.0 or more

- Extreme Obesity: 40.0 or more

While BMI is valid for most men and women, it does have some limitations. It may overestimate body fat in athletes and others who have a muscular build. It may underestimate body fat in older persons and others who have lost muscle mass.

A Healthy Eating Plan

Calories

If your doctor wants you to lose weight, you may need to consider your energy balance. To lose weight, most people need to cut down on the number of calories (units of energy) they get from food and beverages and increase their physical activity. For a weight loss of one to two pounds per week, daily intake should be reduced by 500 to 1,000 calories. In general eating plans containing 1,000–1,200 calories will help most women to lose weight safely. Eating plans between 1,200 calories and 1,600 calories each day are suitable for men and may also be appropriate for women who weigh 165 pounds or more or who exercise regularly. If you are hungry on either diet, you may want to boost your calories by 100 to 200 per day.

Foods That Make Up A Healthy Eating Plan

A healthy eating plan is one that gives your body the nutrients it needs every day while staying within your daily calorie level.

Body Mass Index Table

Height (inches) / BMI	Normal						Overweight					Obese										Extreme Obesity															
BMI	19	20	21	22	23	24	25	26	27	28	29	30	31	32	33	34	35	36	37	38	39	40	41	42	43	44	45	46	47	48	49	50	51	52	53	54
	Body Weight (pounds)																																			
58	91	96	100	105	110	115	119	124	129	134	138	143	148	153	158	162	167	172	177	181	186	191	196	201	205	210	215	220	224	229	234	239	244	248	253	258
59	94	99	104	109	114	119	124	128	133	138	143	148	153	158	163	168	173	178	183	188	193	198	203	208	212	217	222	227	232	237	242	247	252	257	262	267
60	97	102	107	112	118	123	128	133	138	143	148	153	158	163	168	174	179	184	189	194	199	204	209	215	220	225	230	235	240	245	250	255	261	266	271	276
61	100	106	111	116	122	127	132	137	143	148	153	158	164	169	174	180	185	190	195	201	206	211	217	222	227	232	238	243	248	254	259	264	269	275	280	285
62	104	109	115	120	126	131	136	142	147	153	158	164	169	175	180	186	191	196	202	207	213	218	224	229	235	240	246	251	256	262	267	273	278	284	289	295
63	107	113	118	124	130	135	141	146	152	158	163	169	175	180	186	191	197	203	208	214	220	225	231	237	242	248	254	259	265	270	278	282	287	293	299	304
64	110	116	122	128	134	140	145	151	157	163	169	174	180	186	192	197	204	209	215	221	227	232	238	244	250	256	262	267	273	279	285	291	296	302	308	314
65	114	120	126	132	138	144	150	156	162	168	174	180	186	192	198	204	210	216	222	228	234	240	246	252	258	264	270	276	282	288	294	300	306	312	318	324
66	118	124	130	136	142	148	155	161	167	173	179	186	192	198	204	210	216	223	229	235	241	247	253	260	266	272	278	284	291	297	303	309	315	322	328	334
67	121	127	134	140	146	153	159	166	172	178	185	191	198	204	211	217	223	230	236	242	249	255	261	268	274	280	287	293	299	306	312	319	325	331	338	344
68	125	131	138	144	151	158	164	171	177	184	190	197	203	210	216	223	230	236	243	249	256	262	269	276	282	289	295	302	308	315	322	328	335	341	348	354
69	128	135	142	149	155	162	169	176	182	189	196	203	209	216	223	230	236	243	250	257	263	270	277	284	291	297	304	311	318	324	331	338	345	351	358	365
70	132	139	146	153	160	167	174	181	188	195	202	209	216	222	229	236	243	250	257	264	271	278	285	292	299	306	313	320	327	334	341	348	355	362	369	376
71	136	143	150	157	165	172	179	186	193	200	208	215	222	229	236	243	250	257	265	272	279	286	293	301	308	315	322	329	338	343	351	358	365	372	379	386
72	140	147	154	162	169	177	184	191	199	206	213	221	228	235	242	250	258	265	272	279	287	294	302	309	316	324	331	338	346	353	361	368	375	383	390	397
73	144	151	159	166	174	182	189	197	204	212	219	227	235	242	250	257	265	272	280	288	295	302	310	318	325	333	340	348	355	363	371	378	386	393	401	408
74	148	155	163	171	179	186	194	202	210	218	225	233	241	249	256	264	272	280	287	295	303	311	319	326	334	342	350	358	365	373	381	389	396	404	412	420
75	152	160	168	176	184	192	200	208	216	224	232	240	248	256	264	272	279	287	295	303	311	319	327	335	343	351	359	367	375	383	391	399	407	415	423	431
76	156	164	172	180	189	197	205	213	221	230	238	246	254	263	271	279	287	295	304	312	320	328	336	344	353	361	369	377	385	394	402	410	418	426	435	443

Source: Adapted from Clinical Guidelines on the Identification, Evaluation, and Treatment of Overweight and Obesity In Adults: The Evidence Report.

Figure 47.1. Body Mass Index (BMI). Find your height in inches in the left-hand column. Read across to your weight, then look at the top to determine your BMI.

Foods that can be eaten more often include those that are lower in calories, total fat, saturated and trans fat, cholesterol, and sodium (salt). Examples of these foods include fat-free and low-fat dairy products; lean meat, fish, and poultry; high-fiber foods such as whole grains, breads, and cereals; fruits; and vegetables. Canola or olive oils and soft margarines made from these oils are heart healthy and can be used in moderate amounts. Unsalted nuts can also be built into a healthy diet as long as you watch the amount.

Foods higher in fats are typically higher in calories. Foods that should be limited include those with higher amounts of saturated and trans fats and cholesterol. These particular fats raise blood cholesterol levels, which increases the risk for heart disease. Saturated fat is found mainly in fresh and processed meats; high-fat dairy products (like cheese, whole milk, cream, butter, and ice cream), lard, and in the coconut and palm oils found in many processed foods. Trans fat is found in foods with partially hydrogenated oils such as many hard margarines and shortening, commercially fried foods, and some bakery goods. Cholesterol is found in eggs, organ meats, and dairy fats.

It's also important to limit foods and beverages with added sugars such as many desserts, canned fruit packed in syrup, fruit drinks, and sweetened beverages (nondiet drinks). Foods and beverages with added sugars will add calories to your diet without giving you needed nutrients.

Food Groups

A healthy eating plan includes foods from all the basic food groups. It is low in saturated fats, trans fat, cholesterol, salt (sodium), and added sugars. It contains enough calories for good health but not too many. A healthy eating plan also emphasizes fruits, vegetables, whole grains, fat-free or low-fat milk and milk products, lean meats, poultry, fish, beans, eggs, and nuts. It also allows for reasonable portion sizes.

Grains: Grains such as wheat, rice, oats, cornmeal, and barley are naturally low in fat and provide vitamins, minerals, and carbohydrates—all important for good health. Examples of grain products are breads, pasta, breakfast cereals, grits, tortillas, couscous, and crackers. Whole grain foods such as whole wheat bread, brown rice, and oatmeal also have fiber that helps protect you against certain diseases and keeps your body regular. Fiber can also help you feel full with fewer calories.

Vegetables: Most vegetables are naturally low in calories, fat, and cholesterol, and are filling. They are also important sources of many nutrients, including potassium, fiber, folate (folic acid), vitamin A, vitamin E, and vitamin C. People who eat more vegetables as part of an overall healthy diet are likely to have a lower risk of some chronic diseases such as heart disease and diabetes. Any vegetable or 100 percent-vegetable juice counts as a member of the vegetable group. Vegetables may be raw or cooked; fresh, frozen, canned, or dried/dehydrated; and may be whole, cut up, or mashed. To get the most health benefits, vary the types of vegetables you eat. Eat more dark green and orange vegetables.

A Healthy Eating Plan

- Emphasizes fruits, vegetables, whole grains, and fat-free or low-fat milk and milk products
- Includes lean meats, poultry, fish, beans, eggs, and nuts
- Is low in saturated fats, trans fat, cholesterol, salt (sodium), and added sugars
- Controls portion sizes

Source: National Heart Lung and Blood Institute, 2005; reviewed 2012.

Fruits: Most fruits are naturally low in fat, sodium, and calories. None have cholesterol. Fruits are important sources of many nutrients, including potassium, fiber, vitamin C, and folate (folic acid). Whole or cut up fruits also contain fiber which can provide a feeling of fullness with fewer calories. People who eat more fruits as part of an overall healthy diet are likely to have a reduced risk of some chronic diseases such as heart disease and diabetes. Any fruit or 100 percent fruit juice counts as part of the fruit group. Fruits may be fresh, canned, frozen, or dried, and may be whole, cut up, or pureed. To get the most health benefits, eat a variety of fruits and go easy on fruit juices to avoid getting too many calories.

Milk: Milk and milk products such as yogurt and cheese provide nutrients that are vital for the health and maintenance of your body. These nutrients include calcium, potassium, vitamin D, and protein. People who have a diet rich in milk and milk products can lower their risk of low bone mass (osteoporosis) and maintain healthy bones throughout the life cycle. Whole milk dairy foods contain unhealthy saturated fats, so it's a good idea to choose low-fat or fat-free milk products such as milk, cheese, and yogurt. If you can't tolerate milk, try lactose-free milk products.

Meat And Beans: All foods made from meat, poultry, fish, dry beans or peas, eggs, nuts, and seeds are considered part of this group. The foods in this group give you many nutrients, including protein; B vitamins (niacin, thiamin, riboflavin, and B6); vitamin E; and minerals such as iron, zinc, and magnesium. Meats, especially high-fat processed meats such as bologna, contain saturated fats and cholesterol, so it's a good idea to limit these, or to try lower fat varieties. Also choose poultry, fish, beans, and peas more often. Nuts and seeds can be included for variety since they contain healthy fats, however, limit the amount to avoid getting too many calories. Bake, broil, or grill your meats.

Oils (Fats): Unsaturated oils are necessary for good health in small amounts. Oils and solid fats both contain about 120 calories per tablespoon so the amount of oil you use needs to be limited to balance your total calorie intake. It's especially important to limit saturated fat, which is found in whole dairy foods, many meats, butter, and lard, and raises blood cholesterol levels and thus the risk for heart disease. Most of your fat should be from fish, nuts, and vegetable oils. Limit solid fats like butter, stick margarine, shortening, and lard.

Low Calorie, Lower Fat Alternatives

These low calorie alternatives provide new ideas for old favorites. When making a food choice, remember to consider vitamins and minerals. Some foods provide most of their calories from sugar and fat but give you few, if any, vitamins and minerals. This guide is not meant to be an exhaustive list. Reading food labels to find out just how many calories are in the specific products you decide to buy.

When Weight Gain Is The Goal

Most of the nutritional advice you see is written for people who are trying lose weight or avoid weight gain. However, for people with very low body weight, weight gain is necessary. How do you accomplish this, when all the "healthy eating" advice seems geared towards weight loss?

Actually, most healthy eating advice also applies to people who are trying to gain weight. In this situation, it is important that calories taken in exceed calories being burned, but as with weight loss, this should be done in moderation. For weight gain, consuming 500–1000 calories per day more than you burn is probably a reasonable initial target.

As with weight loss diets, getting your calories from fresh fruits and vegetables is healthier than from processed foods and simple sugars. Plant sources of protein, such as beans, legumes, and tofu, are also better in general than red meats.

Weight gain usually requires eating more calorie-dense foods, and this tends to mean more fat. This is not necessarily a bad thing. Fats are an important part of any diet, and the types of fat you eat can make a big difference towards your health. Fats from plant sources such as vegetables and nuts are preferred over animal fats. Similarly, meats such as fish and poultry are better choices than red meats, but can still provide you with the calories you need for nourishment. Many kinds of reduced fat dairy products such as cheeses and milk are available, and may represent a good compromise between full fat and fat free varieties.

Source: David A. Cooke, MD, FACP, 2012.

Dairy Products

- Evaporated whole milk, replace with evaporated fat-free (skim) or reduced fat (2%) milk

- Whole milk, replace with low-fat (1%), reduced fat (2%), or fat-free (skim) milk

- Ice cream, replace with sorbet, sherbet, low-fat or fat-free frozen yogurt, or ice milk (check label for calorie content)

- Whipping cream, replace with imitation whipped cream (made with fat-free [skim] milk) or low-fat vanilla yogurt

- Sour cream, replace with plain low-fat yogurt

- Cream cheese, replace with Neufchatel or "light" cream cheese or fat-free cream cheese

- Cheese (cheddar, American, Swiss, jack), replace with reduced calorie cheese, low calorie processed cheeses, etc.; fat-free cheese

- Regular (4%) cottage cheese, replace with low-fat (1%) or reduced fat (2%) cottage cheese

- Whole milk mozzarella cheese, replace with part skim milk, low moisture mozzarella cheese

- Whole milk ricotta cheese, replace with part skim milk ricotta cheese

- Coffee cream (half and half) or nondairy creamer (liquid, powder), replace with low-fat (1%) or reduced fat (2%) milk or fat-free dry milk powder

Cereals, Grains, And Pasta

- Ramen noodles, replace with rice or noodles (spaghetti, macaroni, etc.)

- Pasta with white sauce (Alfredo), replace with pasta with red sauce (marinara)

- Pasta with cheese sauce, replace with pasta with vegetables (primavera)

- Granola, replace with bran flakes, crispy rice, etc.; cooked grits or oatmeal; whole grains (for example, couscous, barley, bulgur, etc.); reduced fat granola

Meat, Fish, And Poultry

- Cold cuts or lunch meats, replace with low-fat cold cuts (95% to 97% fat-free lunch meats, (bologna, salami, liverwurst, etc.) low-fat pressed meats)

- Hot dogs (regular), replace with lower fat hot dogs

- Bacon or sausage, replace with Canadian bacon or lean ham

- Regular ground beef, replace with extra lean ground beef such as ground round or ground turkey (read labels)

- Chicken or turkey with skin, duck or goose, replace with chicken or turkey without skin (white meat)

- Oil-packed tuna, replace with water-packed tuna (rinse to reduce sodium content)

- Beef (chuck, rib, brisket), replace with beef (round, loin) trimmed of external fat (choose select grades)

- Pork (spareribs, untrimmed loin), replace with pork tenderloin or trimmed, lean smoked ham

- Frozen breaded fish or fried fish, replace with fish or shellfish, unbreaded (fresh, frozen, canned in water—homemade or commercial)

- Whole eggs, replace with egg whites or egg substitutes

- Frozen TV dinners containing more than 13 grams of fat per serving, replace with frozen TV dinners containing less than 13 grams of fat per serving and lower in sodium

- Chorizo sausage, replace with turkey sausage, drained well (read label); vegetarian sausage (made with tofu)

Baked Goods

- Croissants, brioches, etc., replace with hard french rolls or soft "brown 'n serve" rolls

- Donuts, sweet rolls, muffins, scones, or pastries, replace with English muffins, bagels, reduced fat or fat-free muffins or scones

- Party crackers, replace with low-fat crackers (choose lower in sodium); saltine or soda crackers (choose lower in sodium)

- Cake (pound, chocolate, yellow), replace with cake (angel food, white, gingerbread)

- Cookies, replace with reduced fat or fat-free cookies (graham crackers, ginger snaps, fig bars) (compare calorie level)

Snacks And Sweets

- Nuts, replace with popcorn (air-popped or light microwave), fruits, vegetables

- Ice cream, for example, cones or bars, replace with frozen yogurt, frozen fruit, or chocolate pudding bars

- Custards or puddings (made with whole milk), replace with puddings (made with skim milk)

Fats, Oils, And Salad Dressings

- Regular margarine or butter, replace with light-spread margarines, diet margarine, or whipped butter, tub or squeeze bottle

- Regular mayonnaise, replace with light or diet mayonnaise or mustard

- Regular salad dressings, replace with reduced calorie or fat-free salad dressings, lemon juice, or plain, herb-flavored, or wine vinegar

- Butter or margarine on toast or bread, replace with jelly, jam, or honey on bread or toast

- Oils, shortening, or lard, replace with nonstick cooking spray for stir-frying or sauteing; as a substitute for oil or butter, use applesauce or prune puree in baked goods

Miscellaneous

- Canned cream soups, replace with canned broth-based soups

- Canned beans and franks, replace with canned baked beans in tomato sauce

- Gravy (homemade with fat and/or milk), replace with gravy mixes made with water or homemade with the fat skimmed off and fat-free milk included

- Fudge sauce, replace with chocolate syrup

- Avocado on sandwiches, replace with cucumber slices or lettuce leaves

- Guacamole dip or refried beans with lard, replace with salsa

Food Preparation Tips

Cooking low calorie, low-fat dishes may not take a long time, but best intentions can be lost with the addition of butter or other added fats at the table. It is important to learn how certain ingredients can add unwanted calories and fat to low-fat dishes—making them no longer lower in calories and lower in fat. The following list provides examples of lower fat cooking methods and tips on how to serve your low-fat dishes.

Low-Fat Cooking Methods

These cooking methods tend to be lower in fat:

- Bake

- Broil

- Microwave

- Roast—for vegetables and/or chicken without skin

- Steam

- Lightly stir-fry or sauté in cooking spray, small amounts of vegetable oil, or reduced sodium broth

- Grill seafood, chicken, or vegetables

How To Save Calories And Fat

Look at the following examples for how to save calories and fat when preparing and serving foods. You might be surprised at how easy it is.

- Two tablespoons of butter on a baked potato adds an extra 200 calories and 22 grams of fat. However, ¼ cup salsa adds only 18 calories and no fat.

- Two tablespoons of regular clear Italian salad dressing will add an extra 136 calories and 14 grams of fat. Reduced fat Italian dressing adds only 30 calories and 2 grams of fat.

Try These Low-Fat Flavorings

- Herbs—oregano, basil, cilantro, thyme, parsley, sage, or rosemary

- Spices—cinnamon, nutmeg, pepper, or paprika

- Reduced fat or fat-free salad dressing

- Mustard

- Ketchup

- Fat-free mayonnaise

- Fat-free or reduced fat sour cream

- Fat-free or reduced fat yogurt

- Reduced sodium soy sauce

- Salsa

- Lemon or lime juice

- Vinegar

- Horseradish

- Fresh ginger

- Sprinkled buttered flavor (not made with real butter)

- Red pepper flakes

- Sprinkle of parmesan cheese (stronger flavor than most cheese)

- Sodium free salt substitute

- Jelly or fruit preserves on toast or bagels

Tips For Healthy Dining Out

Whether or not you're trying to lose weight, you can eat healthfully when dining out or bringing in food, if you know how. The following tips will help you move toward healthier eating as you limit your calories, as well as fat, saturated fat, cholesterol, and sodium when eating out.

You Are The Customer

- Ask for what you want. Most restaurants will honor your requests.

- Ask questions. Don't be intimidated by the menu—your server will be able to tell you how foods are prepared or suggest substitutions on the menu.

- To reduce portion sizes, try ordering appetizers as your main meal or share an entree with a friend or family member.

- General tips: Limiting your calories and fat can be easy as long as you know what to order. Try asking these questions when you call ahead or before you order. Ask the restaurant, whether they would, on request, do the following:
  - Serve fat-free (skim) milk rather than whole milk or cream
  - Reveal the type of cooking oil used
  - Trim visible fat off poultry or meat
  - Leave all butter, gravy, or sauces off a side dish or entree
  - Serve salad dressing on the side
  - Accommodate special requests if made in advance by telephone or in person

Above all, don't get discouraged. There are usually several healthy choices to choose from at most restaurants.

Reading The Menu

- Choose lower calorie, low-fat cooking methods. Look for terms such as, "steamed in its own juice" (au jus), "garden fresh," "broiled," "baked," "roasted," "poached," "tomato juice," "dry boiled" (in wine or lemon juice), or "lightly sautéed."

- Be aware of foods high in calories, fat, and saturated fat. Watch out for terms such as "butter sauce," "fried," "crispy," "creamed," "in cream or cheese sauce," "au gratin," "au fromage," "escalloped," "parmesan," "hollandaise," "bearnaise," "marinated (in oil)," "stewed," "basted," "sautéed," "stir-fried," "casserole," "hash," "prime," "pot pie," and "pastry crust."

Specific Ordering Tips For Healthy Choices

Breakfast

- Fresh fruit or small glass of citrus juice
- Whole grain bread, bagel, or English muffin with jelly or honey
- Whole grain cereal with low-fat (1%) or fat-free milk
- Oatmeal with fat-free milk topped with fruit
- Omelet made with egg whites or egg substitute
- Multigrain pancakes without butter on top
- Fat-free yogurt (try adding cereal or fresh fruit)

Beverages

- Water with lemon
- Flavored sparkling water (noncaloric)
- Juice spritzer (half fruit juice and half sparkling water)
- Iced tea
- Tomato juice (reduced sodium)

Bread

Most bread and bread sticks are low in calories and low in fat. The calories add up when you add butter, margarine, or olive oil to the bread. Also, eating a lot of bread in addition to your meal will fill you up with extra unwanted calories and not leave enough room for fruits and vegetables.

Appetizers

- Steamed seafood

- Shrimp cocktail (limit cocktail sauce—it's high in sodium; also, if you are on a cholesterol-lowering diet, eat shrimp and other shellfish in moderation)

- Melons or fresh fruit

- Bean soups

- Salad with reduced fat dressing (or add lemon juice or vinegar)

Entree

- Poultry, fish, shellfish, and vegetable dishes are healthy choices

- Pasta with red sauce or with vegetables (primavera)

- Look for terms such as "baked," "broiled," "steamed," "poached," "lightly sauteed," or "stir-fried"

- Ask for sauces and dressings on the side

- Limit the amount of butter, margarine, and salt you use at the table

Salads/Salad Bars

- Fresh greens, lettuce, and spinach

- Fresh vegetables—tomato, mushroom, carrots, cucumber, peppers, onion, radishes, and broccoli

- Beans, chickpeas, and kidney beans

- Skip the nonvegetable choices: deli meats, bacon, egg, cheese, croutons

- Choose lower calorie, reduced fat, or fat-free dressing; lemon juice; or vinegar

Side Dish

- Vegetables and starches (rice, potato, noodles) make good additions to meals and can also be combined for a lower calorie alternative to higher calorie entrees

- Ask for side dishes without butter or margarine

- Ask for mustard, salsa, or low-fat yogurt instead of sour cream or butter

Dessert/Coffee

- Fresh fruit

- Fat-free frozen yogurt

- Sherbet or fruit sorbet (these are usually fat-free, but check the calorie content)

- Try sharing a dessert

- Ask for low-fat milk for your coffee (instead of cream or half-and-half)

Tips For Healthy Multicultural Eating Out

If you're dining out or bringing in, it is easy to find healthy foods. Knowing about food terms can help make your dining experience healthy and enjoyable. The following list includes healthy food choices (lower in calories and fat) and terms to look for when making your selection.

Chinese: Choose More Often

- Steamed

- Jum (poached)

- Chu (boiled)

- Kow (roasted)

- Shu (barbecued)

- Hoison sauce with assorted Chinese vegetables: broccoli, mushrooms, onion, cabbage, snow peas, scallions, bamboo shoots, water chestnuts, asparagus

- Oyster sauce (made from seafood)

- Lightly stir-fried in mild sauce

- Cooked in light wine sauce

- Hot and spicy tomato sauce

- Sweet and sour sauce

- Hot mustard sauce

- Reduced sodium soy sauce

- Dishes without MSG added

- Garnished with spinach or broccoli

- Fresh fish filets, shrimp, scallops

- Chicken, without skin

- Lean beef

- Bean curd (tofu)

- Moo shu vegetables, chicken, or shrimp

- Steamed rice

- Lychee fruit

Deli/Sandwich Shop: Choose More Often

- Fresh sliced vegetables in pita bread with low-fat dressing, yogurt, or mustard

- Cup of bean soup (lentil, minestrone)

- Turkey breast sandwich with mustard, lettuce, and tomato

- Fresh fruit

French: Choose More Often

- Dinner salad with vinegar or lemon juice dressing (or other reduced fat dressing)
- Crusty bread without butter
- Fresh fish, shrimp, scallops, steamed mussels (without sauces)
- Chicken breast, without skin
- Rice and noodles without cream or added butter or other fat
- Fresh fruit for dessert

Italian: Choose More Often

- Lightly sautéed with onions
- Shallots
- Peppers and mushrooms
- Artichoke hearts
- Sun-dried tomatoes
- Red sauces—spicy marinara sauce (arrabiata), marinara sauce, or cacciatore
- Light red sauce or light red or white wine sauce
- Light mushroom sauce
- Red clam sauce
- Primavera (no cream sauce)
- Lemon sauce
- Capers
- Herbs and spices—garlic and oregano
- Crushed tomatoes and spices
- Florentine (spinach)
- Grilled (often fish or vegetables)
- Piccata (lemon)
- Manzanne (eggplant)

Middle Eastern: Choose More Often

- Lemon dressing, lemon juice
- Blended or seasoned with Middle Eastern spices
- Herbs and spices
- Mashed chickpeas
- Fava beans
- Smoked eggplant
- With tomatoes, onions, green peppers, and cucumbers
- Spiced ground meat
- Special garlic sauce
- Basted with tomato sauce
- Garlic
- Chopped parsley and/or onion
- Couscous (grain)
- Rice or bulgur (cracked wheat)
- Stuffed with rice and imported spices

- Grilled on a skewer

- Marinated and barbecued

- Baked

- Charbroiled or charcoal broiled

- Fresh fruit

Japanese: Choose More Often

- House salad with fresh ginger and cellophane (clear rice) noodles

- Rice

- Nabemono

- Chicken, fish, or shrimp teriyaki, broiled in sauce

- Soba noodles, often used in soups

- Yakimono (broiled)

- Tofu or bean curd

- Grilled vegetables

Indian: Choose More Often

- Tikka (pan roasted)

- Cooked with, or marinated in yogurt

- Cooked with green vegetables, onions, tomatoes, peppers, and mushrooms

- With spinach (saag)

- Baked leavened bread

- Masala

- Tandoori

- Paneer

- Cooked with curry, marinated in spices

- Lentils, chickpeas (garbanzo beans)

- Garnished with dried fruits

- Chickpeas (garbanzo) and potatoes

- Basmati rice (pullao)

- Matta (peas)

- Chicken or shrimp kebab

Mexican: Choose More Often

- Shredded spicy chicken

- Rice and black beans

- Rice

- Ceviche (fish marinated in lime juice and mixed with spices)

- Served with salsa (hot red tomato sauce)

- Served with salsa verde (green chili sauce)

- Covered with enchilada sauce

- Topped with shredded lettuce, diced tomatoes, and onions

- Served with or wrapped in a corn or wheat flour (soft) tortilla

- Grilled

- Marinated

- Picante sauce

- Simmered with chili vegetarian tomato sauce

Thai: Choose More Often

- Barbecued, sautéed, broiled, boiled, steamed, braised, marinated

- Charbroiled

- Basil sauce, basil, or sweet basil leaves

- Lime sauce or lime juice

- Chili sauce or crushed dried chili flakes

- Thai spices

- Served in hollowed-out pineapple

- Fish sauce

- Hot sauce

- Napa, bamboo shoots, black mushrooms, ginger, garlic

- Bed of mixed vegetables

- Scallions, onions

Steak Houses: Choose More Often

- Lean broiled beef (no more than 6 ounces)—London broil, filet mignon, round and flank steaks

- Baked potato without added butter, margarine, or sour cream. Try low-fat yogurt or mustard.

- Green salad with reduced fat dressing

- Steamed vegetables without added butter or margarine. Try lemon juice and herbs.

- Seafood dishes (usually indicated as "surf" on menus)

Tips For Eating Fast Foods

When you eat in a healthy way, you don't have to give up eating fast foods completely. You can eat right and still eat fast foods if you select carefully. Here are some tips on fast foods to choose:

- Order a small hamburger instead of a larger one. Try the lower fat hamburger. Hold the extra sauce.

- Order roast beef for a leaner choice than most burgers.

- Order a baked potato instead of french fries. Be careful of high fat toppings like sour cream, butter, or cheese.

- Order grilled, broiled, or baked fish and chicken.

- Order skim or 1-percent milk instead of a milkshake. Try the low-fat frozen yogurt or low-fat milkshake.

- Order a salad. Use vinegar and oil or low calorie dressing.

- Create a salad at the salad bar. Choose any raw vegetables, fruits, or beans. Limit high saturated fat toppings of cheese, fried noodles, and bacon bits as well as some salads made with mayonnaise. Also limit salad dressings high in saturated fat and cholesterol.

- For sandwich toppings try lettuce, tomato, onion, mustard, and ketchup instead of toppings high in saturated fat, such as cheese, bacon, special sauces, or butter.

- Order pizza with vegetable toppings such as peppers, mushrooms, or onions instead of extra cheese, pepperoni, or sausage.

Fast Food: Choose More Often

- Grilled chicken breast sandwich without mayonnaise

- Single hamburger without cheese

- Grilled chicken salad with reduced fat dressing

- Garden salad with reduced fat dressing

- Low-fat or fat-free yogurt

- Fat-free muffin

- Cereal with low-fat milk

Moving Forward

Weight management is a long-term challenge influenced by behavioral, emotional, and physical factors. Changing the way you approach weight management can help you be more successful. Most people who are trying to lose weight focus on one thing: weight loss. However, setting goals and focusing on physical activity changes is much more productive.

Set The Right Goals

Setting the right goals is an important first step. Did you know that the amount of weight loss needed to improve health may be much less than you want to lose to look thinner? Ask your healthcare provider what your weight goals should be.

It's important to set diet and/or physical activity goals. People who are successful at managing their weight set only two to three goals at a time.

Effective goals are specific, realistic, and forgiving (less than perfect). For example: "Exercise more" is a fine goal, but it's not specific enough. "Walk five miles every day" is specific and measurable, but is it achievable if you're just starting out? "Walk 30 minutes every day" is more attainable, but what happens if there's a thunderstorm during your walking time? "Walk 30 minutes, five days each week" is specific, achievable, and forgiving. A great goal!

Achieving And Reward Success

Shaping is a technique where you set some short-term goals that get you closer and closer to the ultimate goal. It is based on the concept that "nothing succeeds like success." Shaping uses two important behavioral principles:

- Continuous goals that move you ahead in small steps to reach a distant point
- Continuous rewards to keep you motivated to make changes

Rewards that you control can encourage achievement of your goals, especially ones that have been hard to reach. An effective reward is something that is desirable, timely, and dependent upon meeting your goal. The rewards you choose may be material, (for example, a movie, music CD, or a payment toward buying a larger item) or an act of self-kindness (for example, a massage or personal time). Frequent small rewards earned for meeting smaller goals are more effective than bigger rewards, requiring a long, difficult effort.

Balance Your Food Checkbook

Self-monitoring refers to observing and recording some aspect of your behavior, such as calorie intake, servings of fruits and vegetables eaten, and amount of physical activity, etc., or an outcome of these behaviors, such as weight. Self-monitoring of a behavior can be used at times when you're not sure of how you are doing, and at times when you want the behavior to improve. Self-monitoring of a behavior usually moves you closer to the desired behavior. When you record your behavior, you produce "real time" records for you and your healthcare provider to discuss. For example, keeping a record of your activity can let you and your provider know quickly how you are doing. When your record shows that your activity is increasing, you'll be encouraged to keep it up.

Regular monitoring of your weight is key to controlling it. Remember these four points if you are keeping a weight chart or graph:

- One day's diet and activity routine won't necessarily affect your weight the next day. Your weight will change quite a bit over the course of a few days because of fluctuations in water and body fat.

- Try to weigh yourself at a set time once or twice per week. This can be when you first wake up and before eating and drinking, after exercise, or right before dinner, etc.

- Whatever time you choose, just make sure it is always the same time and use the same scale to help you keep the most accurate records.

- It may also be helpful to create a graph of your weight as a visual reminder of how you're doing, rather than just listing numbers.

Caution: Refeeding Syndrome

If you have been consuming a very low calorie diet for a long time, it's important to discuss a weight gain plan with your doctor before you attempt it. A condition known as refeeding syndrome can be a serious hazard for severe degrees of anorexia nervosa.

When malnutrition is severe, the body becomes depleted of key nutrients and electrolytes, particularly phosphorous. When food becomes available, and cells try to start rebuilding, there can be a rapid and severe drop in blood phosphorous levels. If not properly monitored and treated, this can lead to massive muscle breakdown, seizures, kidney failure, and death. Refeeding syndrome was first described among prisoners kept under starvation conditions during World War II, but it has also affected many people with severe malnutrition due to anorexia nervosa.

If you have a very low body weight, you should be assessed by dietitians and medical specialists with expertise in treating anorexia nervosa. They can assess your risk for refeeding syndrome, and determine whether special precautions need to be taken.

People felt to be at risk for refeeding syndrome are admitted to the hospital for the first few days of resuming a normal diet. Blood levels of phosphorous and other electrolytes are monitored every few hours, and can be supplemented through an IV to prevent dangerous imbalances from developing. After the initial monitoring period, they are discharged home to continue their nutritional recovery.

Source: David A. Cooke, MD, FACP, 2012.

About Weight Loss Programs

If your healthcare provider has said that you need to lose weight, the best way to reach a healthy weight is to follow a sensible eating plan and engage in regular physical activity. If you consider a weight loss program, keep in mind that weight loss programs should encourage healthy behaviors that will help you lose weight and that you can maintain over time. Safe and effective weight loss programs should include these characteristics:

- Healthy eating plans that reduce calories but do not rule out specific foods or food groups

- Regular physical activity and/or exercise instruction

- Tips on healthy behavior changes that also consider your cultural needs

- Slow and steady weight loss of about one to two pounds per week and not more than three pounds per week (Weight loss may be faster at the start of a program.)

- A plan to keep the weight off after you have lost it

If you decide to join any kind of weight loss program, here are some questions to ask before you join.

Is the diet safe? The eating plan should be low in calories but still provide all the nutrients needed to stay healthy, including vitamins and minerals.

Does the program provide counseling to help you change your eating, activity, and personal habits? The program should teach you how to change permanently those eating habits and lifestyle factors, such as lack of physical activity, that have contributed to weight gain.

Is the staff made up of a variety of qualified counselors and health professionals such as nutritionists, registered dietitians, doctors, nurses, psychologists, and exercise physiologists? You need to be evaluated by a physician if you have any health problems, are currently taking any medicine, or plan to lose more than 15–20 pounds. If your weight control plan uses a very low-calorie diet, an exam and followup visits by a doctor are also needed.

Is training available on how to deal with times when you may feel stressed and slip back to old habits? The program should provide long-term strategies to deal with weight problems you may have in the future. These strategies might include things like setting up a support system and establishing a physical activity routine.

Is attention paid to keeping the weight off? How long is this phase? Choose a program that teaches skills and techniques to make permanent changes in eating habits and levels of physical activity to prevent weight gain.

Are food choices flexible and suitable? Are weight goals set by the client and the health professional? The program should consider your food likes and dislikes and your lifestyle when your weight loss goals are planned.

What is healthy weight loss?

It's natural for anyone trying to lose weight to want to lose it very quickly. But evidence shows that people who lose weight gradually and steadily (about one to two pounds per week) are more successful at keeping weight off. Healthy weight loss isn't just about a "diet" or "program." It's about an ongoing lifestyle that includes long-term changes in daily eating and exercise habits.

Once you've achieved a healthy weight, by relying on healthful eating and physical activity most days of the week (about 60—90 minutes, moderate intensity), you are more likely to be successful at keeping the weight off over the long term.

Source: Excerpted from "Losing Weight," Centers for Disease Control and Prevention (www.cdc.gov), August 17, 2011.

Additional Questions

There are other questions you can ask about how well a program works. Because many programs don't gather this information, you may not get answers. But it's still important to ask them the following:

- What percentage of people complete the program?
- What is the average weight loss among people who finish the program?
- What percentage of people maintain their weight loss after one, two, and even five years?
- What percentage of people have problems or side effects? What are they?
- Are there fees or costs for additional items such as dietary supplements?

Remember, quick weight loss methods don't provide lasting results. Weight loss methods that rely on diet aids like drinks, prepackaged foods, or diet pills don't work in the long run. Whether you lose weight on your own or with a group, remember that the most important changes are long term. No matter how much weight you have to lose, modest goals and a slow course will increase your chances of both losing the weight and keeping it off.

Chapter 48

How To Choose A Safe Weight-Loss Program

Choosing a weight-loss program may be a difficult task. You may not know what to look for in a weight-loss program or what questions to ask. This information can help you talk to your health care professional about weight loss and get the best information before choosing a program.

Talk With Your Health Care Professional

If your health care provider tells you that you should lose weight and you want to find a weight-loss program to help you, look for one that is based on regular physical activity and an eating plan that is balanced, healthy, and easy to follow.

You may want to talk with your doctor or other health care professional about controlling your weight before you decide on a weight-loss program. Doctors do not always address issues such as healthy eating, physical activity, and weight management during general office visits. It is important for you to start the discussion in order to get the information you need. Even if you feel uncomfortable talking about your weight with your doctor, remember that he or she is there to help you improve your health. Here are some tips:

- Tell your health care professional that you would like to talk about your weight. Share your concerns about any medical conditions you have or medicines you are taking.

- Write down your questions in advance. Bring pen and paper to take notes.

- Bring a friend or family member along for support if this will make you feel more comfortable.

About This Chapter: "Choosing A Safe And Successful Weight-Loss Program," National Institute of Diabetes and Digestive and Kidney Diseases (www.niddk.nih.gov), April 2010.

- Make sure you understand what your health care provider is saying. Do not be afraid to ask questions if there is something you do not understand.

- Ask for other sources of information like brochures or websites.

- If you want more support, ask for a referral to a registered dietitian, a support group, or a commercial weight-loss program.

- Call your health care professional after your visit if you have more questions or need help.

Ask Questions

Find out as much as you can about your health needs before joining a weight-loss program. Here are some questions you might want to ask your health care professional:

- Do I need to lose weight? Or should I just avoid gaining more? Is my weight affecting my health?

- Could my extra weight be caused by a health problem such as hypothyroidism or by a medicine I am taking? (Hypothyroidism is when your thyroid gland does not produce enough thyroid hormone, a condition that can slow your metabolism—how your body creates and uses energy.)

- What should my weight-loss goal be? How will losing weight help me?

- How should I change my eating habits? What kinds of physical activity can I do? How much physical activity do I need?

- Should I take weight-loss drugs? What about weight-loss surgery? What are the risks of weight-loss drugs or surgery?

What is a nutritionist or dietitian?

A nutritionist or dietitian is a member of an eating disorders treatment team who is trained in nutrition. The dietitian or nutritionist will assess patients' nutritional needs, develop and implement nutrition programs, and evaluate and report the results. They also confer with doctors and other health care professionals to coordinate medical and nutritional needs. Some clinical dietitians specialize in the treatment of clinical eating disorders, though not all dietitians have received such training.

Source: Excerpted from "Eating Disorders Glossary," © 2012 Families Empowered and Supporting Treatment of Eating Disorders (www.feast-ed.org).

A Responsible And Safe Weight-Loss Program

If your health care provider tells you that you should lose weight and you want to find a weight-loss program to help you, look for one that is based on regular physical activity and an eating plan that is balanced, healthy, and easy to follow. Weight-loss programs should encourage healthy behaviors that help you lose weight and that you can stick with every day. Safe and effective weight-loss programs should include:

- Healthy eating plans that reduce calories but do not forbid specific foods or food groups.

- Tips to increase moderate-intensity physical activity.

- Tips on healthy habits that also keep your cultural needs in mind, such as lower-fat versions of your favorite foods.

- Slow and steady weight loss. Depending on your starting weight, experts recommend losing weight at a rate of one-half to two pounds per week. Weight loss may be faster at the start of a program.

- Medical care if you are planning to lose weight by following a special formula diet, such as a very low-calorie diet (a program that requires careful monitoring from a doctor).

- A plan to keep the weight off after you have lost it.

Get Familiar With The Program

Gather as much information as you can before deciding to join a program. Professionals working for weight-loss programs should be able to answer the questions listed below.

What Does The Weight-Loss Program Consist Of?

- Does the program offer one-on-one counseling or group classes?

- Do you have to follow a specific meal plan or keep food records?

- Do you have to purchase special food, drugs, or supplements?

- If the program requires special foods, can you make changes based on your likes and dislikes and food allergies?

- Does the program help you be more physically active, follow a specific physical activity plan, or provide exercise instruction?

- Does the program teach you to make positive and healthy behavior changes?

- Is the program sensitive to your lifestyle and cultural needs?

- Does the program provide ways to keep the weight off? Will the program provide ways to deal with such issues as what to eat at social or holiday gatherings, changes to schedules, lack of motivation, and injury or illness?

What Are The Staff Qualifications?

- Who supervises the program?

- What type of weight management training, experience, education, and certifications do the staff have?

Does The Product Or Program Carry Any Risks?

- Could the program hurt you?

- Could the recommended drugs or supplements harm your health?

- Do participants talk with a doctor?

- Does a doctor run the program?

- Will the program's doctors work with your personal doctor if you have a medical condition such as high blood pressure or are taking prescribed drugs?

- Is there ongoing input and follow-up from a health care professional to ensure your safety while you participate in the program?

How Much Does The Program Cost?

- What is the total cost of the program?

- Are there other costs, such as weekly attendance fees, food and supplement purchases, etc.?

- Are there fees for a follow-up program after you lose weight?

- Are there other fees for medical tests?

What Results Do Participants Typically Have?

- How much weight does an average participant lose and how long does he or she keep the weight off?

- Does the program offer publications or materials that describe what results participants typically have?

Chapter 49

Physical Fitness For Teens

Regular physical activity in children and adolescents promotes health and fitness. Compared to those who are inactive, physically active youth have higher levels of cardiorespiratory fitness and stronger muscles. They also typically have lower body fatness. Their bones are stronger, and they may have reduced symptoms of anxiety and depression.

Youth who are regularly active also have a better chance of a healthy adulthood. Children and adolescents don't usually develop chronic diseases, such as heart disease, hypertension, type 2 diabetes, or osteoporosis. However, risk factors for these diseases can begin to develop early in life. Regular physical activity makes it less likely that these risk factors will develop and more likely that children will remain healthy as adults.

Youth can achieve substantial health benefits by doing moderate- and vigorous-intensity physical activity for periods of time that add up to 60 minutes (one hour) or more each day. This activity should include aerobic activity as well as age-appropriate muscle- and bone–strengthening activities. Although current science is not complete, it appears that, as with adults, the total amount of physical activity is more important for achieving health benefits than is any one component (frequency, intensity, or duration) or specific mix of activities (aerobic, muscle-strengthening, bone strengthening). Even so, bone-strengthening activities remain especially important for children and young adolescents because the greatest gains in bone mass occur during the years just before and during puberty. In addition, the majority of peak bone mass is obtained by the end of adolescence.

About This Chapter: Excerpted from "Chapter 3: Active Children and Adolescents," Physical Activity Guidelines for Americans, U.S. Department of Health and Human Services (www.health.gov), October 16, 2008.

Key Guidelines For Children And Adolescents

Children and adolescents should do 60 minutes (one hour) or more of physical activity daily.

- **Aerobic**: Most of the 60 or more minutes a day should be either moderate- or vigorous-intensity aerobic physical activity, and should include vigorous-intensity physical activity at least three days a week.
- **Muscle-Strengthening:** As part of their 60 or more minutes of daily physical activity, children and adolescents should include muscle-strengthening physical activity on at least three days of the week.
- **Bone-Strengthening:** As part of their 60 or more minutes of daily physical activity, children and adolescents should include bone-strengthening physical activity on at least three days of the week.

It is important to encourage young people to participate in physical activities that are appropriate for their age, that are enjoyable, and that offer variety.

Source: U.S. Department of Health and Human Services, 2008.

Types Of Activity

The guidelines for children and adolescents focus on three types of activity: aerobic, muscle-strengthening, and bone-strengthening. Each type has important health benefits.

Aerobic activities are those in which young people rhythmically move their large muscles. Running, hopping, skipping, jumping rope, swimming, dancing, and bicycling are all examples of aerobic activities. Aerobic activities increase cardiorespiratory fitness. (Children often do activities in short bursts, which may not technically be aerobic activities, but they are considered as aerobic in this chapter.)

Muscle-strengthening activities make muscles do more work than usual during activities of daily life. This is called "overload," and it strengthens the muscles. Muscle-strengthening activities can be unstructured and part of play, such as playing on playground equipment, climbing trees, and playing tug-of-war. Or these activities can be structured, such as lifting weights or working with resistance bands.

Bone-strengthening activities produce a force on the bones that promotes bone growth and strength. This force is commonly produced by impact with the ground. Running, jumping rope, basketball, tennis, and hopscotch are all examples of bone strengthening activities. As these examples illustrate, bone-strengthening activities can also be aerobic and muscle-strengthening.

How Age Influences Physical Activity

Children and adolescents should meet the guidelines by doing activity that is appropriate for their age. Their natural patterns of movement differ from those of adults. For example, children are naturally active in an intermittent way, particularly when they do unstructured active play. During recess and in their free play and games, children use basic aerobic and bone-strengthening activities, such as running, hopping, skipping, and jumping, to develop movement patterns and skills. They alternate brief periods of moderate- and vigorous-intensity physical activity with brief periods of rest. Any episode of moderate- or vigorous–intensity physical activity, however brief, counts toward the guidelines.

Children also commonly increase muscle strength through unstructured activities that involve lifting or moving their body weight or working against resistance. Children don't usually do or need formal muscle-strengthening programs, such as lifting weights.

Regular physical activity in children and adolescents promotes a healthy body weight and body composition.

As children grow into adolescents, their patterns of physical activity change. They are able to play organized games and sports and are able to sustain longer periods of activity. But they still commonly do intermittent activity, and no period of moderate- or vigorous-intensity activity is too short to count toward the guidelines.

Adolescents may meet the guidelines by doing free play, structured programs, or both. Structured exercise programs can include aerobic activities, such as playing a sport, and muscle-strengthening activities, such as lifting weights, working with resistance bands, or using body weight for resistance (such as push-ups, pull-ups, and sit-ups). Muscle-strengthening activities count if they involve a moderate to high level of effort and work the major muscle groups of the body: legs, hips, back, abdomen, chest, shoulders, and arms.

What about stretching?

Stretching improves flexibility, allowing you to move more easily. This will make it easier for you to reach down to tie your shoes or look over your shoulder when you back the car out of your driveway. You should do stretching activities after your muscles are warmed up—for example, after strength training. Stretching your muscles before they are warmed up may cause injury.

Source: Excerpted from "Physical Activity (Exercise) Fact Sheet," Office on Women's Health (www.womenshealth.gov), February 26, 2009.

Levels Of Intensity For Aerobic Activity

Children and adolescents can meet the guidelines by doing a combination of moderate- and vigorous intensity aerobic physical activities or by doing only vigorous-intensity aerobic physical activities.

Youth should not do only moderate-intensity activity. It's important to include vigorous-intensity activities because they cause more improvement in cardiorespiratory fitness.

The intensity of aerobic physical activity can be defined on either an absolute or a relative scale. Either scale can be used to monitor the intensity of aerobic physical activity:

• Absolute intensity is based on the rate of energy expenditure during the activity, without taking into account a person's cardiorespiratory fitness.

• Relative intensity uses a person's level of cardiorespiratory fitness to assess level of effort.

Relative intensity describes a person's level of effort relative to his or her fitness. As a rule of thumb, on a scale of 0 to 10, where sitting is 0 and the highest level of effort possible is 10, moderate-intensity activity is a 5 or 6. Young people doing moderate-intensity activity will notice that their hearts are beating faster than normal and they are breathing harder than normal. Vigorous-intensity activity is at a level of 7 or 8. Youth doing vigorous-intensity activity will feel their heart beating much faster than normal and they will breathe much harder than normal.

What is moderate activity?

During moderate-intensity activities you should notice an increase in your heart rate, but you should still be able to talk comfortably. An example of a moderate-intensity activity is walking on a level surface at a brisk pace (about three to four miles per hour). Other examples include ballroom dancing, leisurely bicycling, moderate housework, and waiting tables.

What is vigorous activity?

If your heart rate increases a lot and you are breathing so hard that it is difficult to carry on a conversation, you are probably doing vigorous-intensity activity. Examples of vigorous-intensity activities include jogging, bicycling fast or uphill, singles tennis, and pushing a hand mower.

Source: Excerpted from "Physical Activity (Exercise) Fact Sheet," Office on Women's Health (www.womenshealth.gov), February 26, 2009.

Examples of Physical Activities For Children And Adolescents

- **Moderate-Intensity Aerobic:** Active recreation, such as hiking, skateboarding, rollerblading; Bicycle riding; Brisk walking

- **Vigorous-Intensity Aerobic:** Active games involving running and chasing, such as tag; Bicycle riding; Jumping rope; Martial arts, such as karate; Running; Sports such as soccer, ice or field hockey, basketball, swimming, tennis; Cross-country skiing

- **Muscle-Strengthening:** Games such as tug-of-war; Modified push-ups (with knees on the floor); Resistance exercises using body weight or resistance bands; Rope or tree climbing; Sit-ups (curl-ups or crunches); Swinging on playground equipment/bars

- **Bone-Strengthening:** Games such as hopscotch; Hopping, skipping, jumping; Jumping rope; Running; Sports such as gymnastics, basketball, volleyball, tennis

Note: Some activities, such as bicycling, can be moderate or vigorous intensity, depending upon level of effort.

Getting And Staying Active: Real-Life Examples

Children and adolescents can meet the physical activity guidelines and become regularly physically active in many ways. Here are just two examples showing how a child and an adolescent can be physically active for at least 60 minutes each day over the course of a week.

These examples illustrate that even though the activity patterns are different, each young person is meeting the guidelines by getting the equivalent of at least 60 minutes or more of aerobic activity each day that is at least moderate intensity. Both are also doing vigorous-intensity, muscle-strengthening, and bone strengthening activities on at least three days a week.

Harold: A 7-Year-Old Child

Harold participates in many types of physical activities in many places. For example, during physical education class, he jumps rope and does gymnastics and sit-ups. During recess, he plays on the playground—often by doing activities that require running and climbing. He also likes to play soccer with his friends and family. When Harold gets home from school, he likes to engage in active play (playing tag) and ride his bicycle with his friends and family.

Harold gets 60 minutes of physical activity each day that is at least moderate intensity. He participates in the following activities each day:

- **Monday:** Walks to and from school (20 minutes), plays actively with family (20 minutes), jumps rope (10 minutes), does gymnastics (10 minutes).

- **Tuesday:** Walks to and from school (20 minutes), plays on playground (25 minutes), climbs on playground equipment (15 minutes).

- **Wednesday:** Walks to and from school (20 minutes), plays actively with friends (25 minutes), jumps rope (10 minutes), runs (5 minutes), does sit-ups (2 minutes).

- **Thursday:** Plays actively with family (30 minutes), plays soccer (30 minutes).

- **Friday:** Walks to and from school (20 minutes), plays actively with friends (25 minutes), bicycles (15 minutes).

- **Saturday:** Plays on playground (30 minutes), climbs on playground equipment (15 minutes), bicycles (15 minutes).

- **Sunday:** Plays on playground (10 minutes), plays soccer (40 minutes), plays tag with family (10 minutes).

Harold meets the guidelines by doing vigorous-intensity aerobic activities, bone-strengthening activities, and muscle-strengthening activities on at least three days of the week:

- Vigorous-intensity aerobic activities six times during the week: jumping rope (Monday and Wednesday), running (Wednesday), soccer (Thursday and Sunday), playing tag (Sunday)

- Bone-strengthening activities six times during the week: jumping rope (Monday and Wednesday), running (Wednesday), soccer (Thursday and Sunday), playing tag (Sunday)

- Muscle-strengthening activities four times during the week: gymnastics (Monday), climbing on playground equipment (Tuesday and Saturday), sit-ups (Wednesday)

Maria: A 16-Year-Old Adolescent

Maria participates in many types of physical activities in many places. For example, during physical education class, she plays tennis and does sit-ups and push-ups. She also likes to play basketball at the YMCA, do yoga, and go dancing with friends. Maria likes to take her dog on walks and hikes.

Maria gets 60 or more minutes of daily physical activity that is at least moderate intensity. She participates in the following activities each day:

- **Monday:** Walks dog (10 minutes), plays basketball at YMCA (50 minutes).

- **Tuesday:** Walks dog (10 minutes), plays tennis (30 minutes), does sit-ups and push-ups (5 minutes), walks briskly with friends (15 minutes).

- **Wednesday:** Walks dog (10 minutes), plays basketball at YMCA (50 minutes).

- **Thursday:** Walks dog (10 minutes), plays tennis (30 minutes), does sit-ups and push-ups (5 minutes), plays with children at the park while babysitting (15 minutes).

- **Friday:** Plays Frisbee in park (45 minutes), mows lawn (30 minutes).

- **Saturday:** Goes dancing with friends (60 minutes), does yoga (30 minutes).

- **Sunday:** Hikes (60 minutes).

Maria meets the guidelines by doing vigorous-intensity aerobic activities, bone-strengthening activities, and muscle-strengthening activities on at least three days of the week:

- Vigorous-intensity aerobic activities four times during the week: basketball (Monday and Wednesday), dancing (Saturday), hiking (Sunday)

- Bone-strengthening activities four times during the week: basketball (Monday and Wednesday), dancing (Saturday), hiking (Sunday)

- Muscle-strengthening activities three times during the week: sit-ups and push-ups (Tuesday and Thursday), yoga (Saturday)

Can I stay active if I have a disability?

A disability may make it harder to stay active, but it shouldn't stop you. In most cases, people with disabilities can improve their flexibility, mobility, and coordination by becoming physically active. Getting regular physical activity can also help you stay independent by preventing illnesses, such as heart disease, that can make caring for yourself more difficult.

Even though you have a disability, you should still aim to meet physical activity goals. Work with a doctor to develop a physical activity plan that works for you.

Source: Excerpted from "Physical Activity (Exercise) Fact Sheet," Office on Women's Health (www.womenshealth.gov), February 26, 2009.

Chapter 50

Fitness Safety Tips

There are many things you need to do to stay safe and injury-free during exercise. Review these items so that you don't get hurt:

Warming Up And Cooling Down

Before you start exercising, you need to warm up your muscles. It is best to warm up your muscles before stretching them. You can warm up by walking at an easy pace before stretching. Then stretch by starting at the top of your body and working your way down. Slowly stretch your calf, quad, groin, and hamstring muscles. Warming up can also include jogging slowly, doing knee lifts, and arm circles.

Make sure to cool down and stretch after exercising, too. A cool-down is a gentle exercise or stretch that helps the body return to its normal state after vigorous exercise. Cool-downs help your pulse (or heart rate) return to normal and can help prevent your muscles from feeling stiff after a workout.

Important Exercise Safety Tips

- See your doctor for a sports physical before you start a sport.

- Don't exercise when it is really hot and humid out. You do not want your body to overheat or get dehydrated. If it's very hot or humid outside, try moving your exercise indoors that day. Also, if you live in an area with high air pollution, exercise early in the day or at night and avoid congested streets and rush hour traffic.

About This Chapter: Excerpted from "Fitness: Keeping Safe and Injury Free," Office on Women's Health (www .girlshealth.gov), October 9, 2009.

- Drink water before, during, and after exercise or sports competitions.

- Make sure you warm up and stretch your muscles for five minutes before and after workouts to make your muscles more flexible. It is easer to get hurt if your muscles are not stretched. It is also important to increase the intensity of your workout gradually. If you exercise intensely right away, you could risk getting hurt.

- If you do get hurt, see a doctor or let your parents/guardian know if: 1) You are in severe pain, 2) you see swelling around where you got hurt, or 3) The pain gets in the way of sleep and activities. Don't jump back to your regular exercise after getting hurt because you could get hurt again. Follow your doctor's orders for how to care for your injury and when you can be active again. This includes following instructions for use of pain medicine.

- Follow the rules of the game. The rules are there, in part, to keep you safe.

Using The Right Equipment

When you exercise or play sports, it is important to use the right safety equipment.

- Helmets are needed for sports such as baseball, softball, biking, snow skiing, and rollerblading. Make sure you wear the right helmet for the sport you are playing and that it fits well. Also make sure that the helmet you wear for biking has a sticker from the Consumer Product Safety Commission (CPSC), which means that it is safe for this activity.

- Mouth guards protect your mouth, teeth, and tongue. You should wear a guard if there's a chance you could get hit in the head while taking part in activities such as volleyball, basketball, or martial arts. You can find mouth guards at sport stores or your dentist. It will also help keep your mouth safe to take out your retainer.

- Special eye protection is needed for sports such as ice hockey, soccer, and basketball. Goggles and face masks should fit snugly and have cushion for a comfortable fit. If you wear glasses, you need to get fitted for guards that fit over your glasses. You could also buy special prescription goggles, which cost about $60 or more. These guards and goggles are made with a special plastic called polycarbonate. This special plastic will not hurt your eyes.

- It is important to wear the right footwear for your sport. Check with your coach or an athletic shoe salesperson about what shoes to wear.

- Wrist, knee, and elbow pads can help prevent broken bones when you are inline skating/rollerblading, skate or snow boarding, or playing sports such as hockey.

Female Athlete Triad

Some girls who play sports or exercise intensely are at risk for a problem called female athlete triad. Female athlete triad is a combination of three conditions: disordered eating, amenorrhea (or missed periods), and osteoporosis. A female athlete can have one, two, or all three parts of the triad.

- **Eating Disorders:** Most female athletes who develop an eating disorder are trying to lose weight so they can be better at their sport. This kind of eating disorder can range from avoiding certain types of food the athlete thinks are "bad" (such as foods containing fat) to serious eating disorders like anorexia nervosa or bulimia nervosa.

- **Menstrual Dysfunction:** A missed period is a concern for girls and women who over-exercise. Your body needs a certain amount of fat to function and to have regular periods. Eating right and exercising is important for having a healthy body, but some girls take it too far. Too much exercising or very strict dieting can use up your body fat and delay your period, or cause it to stop until you gain some weight back. Not having menstrual periods is called amenorrhea—a sign that hormone patterns have changed. Oligomenorrhea is having very few periods, usually with cycles that last longer than 35 days. Women who suffer from anorexia and elite women athletes who train seriously for competition often have amenorrhea or oligomenorrhea.

- **Low Bone Mineral Density:** Osteopenia and osteoporosis is when your bones become weak. If a female athlete doesn't eat a balanced diet that includes plenty of calcium, she can develop osteopenia or osteoporosis. This can ruin a female athlete's career because it may lead to stress fractures and other injuries. Usually, the teen years are a time when girls should be building up their bone mass to their highest levels—called peak bone mass. Not getting enough calcium during the teen years can also have a lasting effect on how strong a girl's bones are later in life.

Osteoporosis

Osteoporosis is when your bones become weak and break easily. If a female athlete doesn't eat a balanced diet that includes plenty of calcium, she can develop osteoporosis. This can ruin a female athlete's career because it may lead to stress fractures and other injuries.

The teen years are the most important time for girls to build up their bone mass to their highest levels—called peak bone mass. Not getting enough calcium, vitamin D, and physical activity during the teen years can have a lasting effect on how strong a girl's bones are later in life.

Over-Exercising Can Actually Be Harmful

Sometimes you really can have too much of a good thing. If you over-exercise your emotional health can suffer. It is linked to depression and eating disorders.

Sometimes, teens over-exercise along with having an eating disorder such as anorexia. People with anorexia take extreme steps to lose weight, including not eating at all. This combination puts your health in danger.

If you think that you may be over-exercising or have an eating disorder, talk about it with someone you can trust. Talk to a school counselor or nurse. The longer you wait, the harder it will be to bring it up. If you think that your friend may have one of these problems, help them find someone to talk to. Be supportive and let them know you care about them.

Chapter 51

Mental Fitness

Meaning Of Mental Health

Definitions of mental health are changing. It used to be that a person was considered to have good mental health simply if they showed no signs or symptoms of a mental illness. But in recent years, there has been a shift towards a more holistic approach to mental health.

Today, we recognize that good mental health is not just the absence of mental illness. Nor is it absolute—some people are more mentally healthy than others, whether you are mentally ill or not. These realizations are prompting a new kind of focus on mental health that identifies components of mental wellness and mental fitness and explores ways to encourage them.

Positive Approach To Psychology

A group of psychologists, led by Martin E.P. Seligman, a psychology professor at the University of Pennsylvania and past-president of the American Psychological Association, wants to shift the emphasis in their discipline from a disease model to a health model, called "positive psychology."

Instead of looking at how society's negative aspects affect us, their aim is to investigate the positive qualities that help people flourish. These include courage, optimism, hope, honesty, interpersonal skills, work ethic and perseverance.

Consider these key characteristics when assessing your own mental health:

- **Ability To Enjoy Life:** Can you live in the moment and appreciate the "now"? Are you able to learn from the past and plan for the future without dwelling on things you can't change or predict?

- **Resilience:** Are you able to bounce back from hard times? Can you manage the stress of a serious life event without losing your optimism and a sense of perspective?

- **Balance:** Are you able to juggle the many aspects of your life? Can you recognize when you might be devoting too much time to one aspect, at the expense of others? Are you able to make changes to restore balance when necessary?

- **Self-Actualization:** Do you recognize and develop your strengths so that you can reach your full potential?

- **Flexibility:** Do you feel, and express, a range of emotions? When problems arise, can you change your expectations—of life, others, yourself—to solve the problem and feel better?

You can gauge your mental health by thinking about how you coped with a recent difficulty. Did you feel there was no way out of the problem and that life would never be normal again? Were you unable to carry on with work or school? With time, were you able to enjoy your life, family and friendships? Were you able to regain your balance and look forward to the future?

Taking the pulse of mental health brings different results for everyone; it's unique to the individual. By reflecting on these characteristics, you can recognize your strengths, and identify areas where your level of mental fitness could be improved.

Benefits Of Good Mental Health

Just as physical fitness helps our bodies to stay strong, mental fitness helps us to achieve and sustain a state of good mental health. When we are mentally healthy, we enjoy our life and environment, and the people in it. We can be creative, learn, try new things, and take risks. We are better able to cope with difficult times in our personal and professional lives. We feel the sadness and anger that can come with the death of a loved one, a job loss or relationship problems and other difficult events, but in time, we are able to get on with and enjoy our lives once again.

Nurturing our mental health can also help us combat or prevent the mental health problems that are sometimes associated with a chronic physical illness. In some cases, it can prevent the onset or relapse of a physical or mental illness. Managing stress well, for instance, can have a positive impact on heart disease.

Chances are, you are already taking steps to sustain your mental health, as well as your physical health—you just might not realize it.

Three important ways to improve your mental fitness are to get physical, eat right, and take control of stress.

Get Physical

We've known for a long time about the benefits of exercise as a proactive way to enhance our physical condition and combat disease; now, exercise is recognized as an essential element in building and maintaining mental fitness.

So, if you already do exercise of some kind, give yourself two pats on the back—you're improving your physical and mental fitness.

Exercise has many psychological benefits. For example:

- Physical activity is increasingly becoming part of the prescription for the treatment of depression and anxiety. Exercise alone is not a cure, but it does have a positive impact.

- Research has found that regular physical activity appears as effective as psychotherapy for treating mild to moderate depression. Therapists also report that patients who exercise regularly simply feel better and are less likely to overeat or abuse alcohol and drugs.

- Exercise can reduce anxiety. Many studies have come to this conclusion. People who exercise report feeling less stressed or nervous. Even five minutes of aerobic exercise (exercise which requires oxygen, such as a step class, swimming, walking) can stimulate anti-anxiety effects.

- Physical exercise helps to counteract the withdrawal, inactivity, and feelings of hopelessness that characterize depression. Studies show that both aerobic and anaerobic exercise (exercise which does not require oxygen, such as weightlifting) have anti-depressive effects.

- Moods such as tension, fatigue, anger, and vigor are all positively affected by exercise.

- Exercising can improve the way you perceive your physical condition, athletic abilities and body image. Enhanced self-esteem is another benefit.

- Last, but not least, exercise brings you into contact with other people in a non-clinical, positive environment. For the length of your walk or workout or aqua-fit class, you engage with people who share your interest in that activity.

Feel The Rush

We may not realize what caused it, but most of us have felt it. Whether we're engaged in a leisurely swim or an adrenaline-charged rock climb, there is that moment when suddenly pain or discomfort drops away and we are filled with a sense of euphoria.

We have endorphins to thank for these moments of bliss. Endorphins are chemicals produced in the brain, which bind to neuro-receptors to give relief from pain.

Discovered in 1975, the role of endorphins is still being studied. They are believed to: relieve pain; enhance the immune system; reduce stress; and delay the aging process. Exercise stimulates the release of endorphins, sending these depression-fighting, contentment-building chemicals throughout the body. No wonder we feel good after a workout or brisk walk.

Endorphin release varies from person to person; some people will feel an endorphin rush, or second wind, after jogging for 10 minutes. Others will jog for half an hour before their second wind kicks in.

You don't have to exercise vigorously to stimulate endorphin release: meditation, acupuncture, massage therapy, even eating spicy food or breathing deeply—these all cause your body to produce endorphins naturally.

So enjoy some moderate exercise and feel the endorphin rush.

Eat Right

Here's some food for thought: Making the right nutritional choices can affect more than the fit of our clothes; it can have an impact on our mental health.

A new study by the UK's Mental Health Foundation suggests that poor diet has played a role in the significant increase in mental health problems over the past 50 years.

The trend away from eating less fresh produce and consuming more saturated fats and sugars, including substances like pesticides, additives, and trans fats, can prevent the brain from functioning properly, says the Feeding Minds study. It makes a persuasive link between changing food fads and increases in attention deficit hyperactivity disorder, Alzheimer disease and schizophrenia.

The message is not a new one, but it is perhaps the most forceful argument yet for paying more attention to the nutrition-mental health connection. What we put on our plates becomes the raw material for our brains to manufacture hormones and neurotransmitters—chemical substances that control our sleep, mood and behavior. If we shortchange the brain, we also shortchange our intellectual and emotional potential.

Our diet also supplies the vitamins which our bodies cannot create, and which we need to help speed up the chemical processes that we need for survival and brain function. Vitamin deficiencies sometimes manifest themselves as depression and can cause mood swings, anxiety, and agitation, as well as a host of physical problems.

Mental health professionals point out that good eating habits are vital for people wanting to optimize the effectiveness of and cope with possible side effects of medications used to treat mental illnesses.

Clearly, selecting which foods to eat has consequences beyond immediate taste bud satisfaction. To optimize our brain function, we need to eat a balanced diet of:

- Fresh fruits and vegetables
- Foods high in omega-3 fatty acids, such as fish, nuts, seeds and eggs
- Protein
- Whole grains

Take Control Of Stress

Stress is a fact of life. No matter how much we might long for a stress-free existence, the fact is, stress is actually necessary. It's how we respond to stress that can negatively affect our lives.

Stress is defined as any change that we have to adapt to. This includes difficult life events (bereavement, illness) and positive ones. Getting a new job or going on vacation are certainly perceived to be happy occurrences, but they, too, are changes, also known as stress, that require some adaptation.

Learning to effectively cope with stress can ease our bodies and our minds. Meditation and other relaxation methods, exercise, visualization are all helpful techniques for reducing the negative impact of stress.

Stress can be beneficial—in moderation. That's because short episodes of stress trigger chemicals that improve memory, increase energy levels, and enhance alertness and productivity. But chronic stress has debilitating effects on our overall health. Physically, it can contribute to migraines, ulcers, muscle tension, and fatigue. Canadian researchers found that chronic stress more than doubled the risk of heart attacks.

Persistent stress also affects us emotionally and intellectually, and can cause:

- Decreased concentration and memory
- Confusion

- Loss of sense of humor

- Anxiety

- Anger

- Irritability

- Fear

The link between stress and mental illness has yet to be fully understood, but it is known that stress can negatively affect an episode of mental illness.

Managing Stress

First, it's important to recognize the source(s) of your stress. Events such as the death of a loved one, starting a new job or moving house are certainly stressful.

However, much of our stress comes from within us. How we interpret things—a conversation, a performance review, even a look—determines whether something becomes a stressor. Negative self-talk, where we focus on self-criticism and pessimistic over-analysis, can turn an innocent remark into a major source of stress.

Understanding where your stress originates can help you decide on a course of action. External stressors, like bereavement or career changes, can be managed over time and with the support of family and friends. Internal stressors, caused by our own negative interpretation, require changes in attitude and behavior.

The goal of managing stress is to cue the "relaxation response." This is the physiological and psychological calming process our body goes through when we perceive that the danger, or stressful event, has passed.

Here are some tips for triggering the relaxation response:

- **Learn Relaxation Techniques:** Practicing meditation or breathing awareness every day can relieve chronic stress and realign your outlook in a more positive way. Good breathing habits alone can improve both your psychological and physical well-being.

- **Set Realistic Goals:** Learning to say no is essential for some people. Assess your schedule and identify tasks or activities that you can or should let go. Don't automatically volunteer to do something until you've considered whether it is feasible and healthy for you to do so.

- **Exercise:** You don't have to train for a marathon, but regular, moderate exercise helps ease tension, improves sleep and self-esteem. Making exercise a habit is key.

- **Enjoy Yourself:** Taking the time for a favorite hobby is a great way of connecting with and nurturing your creative self.

- **Visualization:** Athletes achieve results by picturing themselves crossing the finish line first. Use the same technique to practice "seeing" yourself succeed in whatever situation is uppermost in your mind.

- **Maintain A Healthy Lifestyle:** A good diet is often the first thing to go when we're feeling stressed. Making a meal instead of buying one ready-made may seem like a challenge, but it will be probably cheaper and certainly better for you and the simple action of doing something good for yourself can soothe stressful feelings.

- **Talk About It:** Sharing your troubles with a friend may help you to put things in perspective and to feel that you're not alone. You may also learn some other ways to manage stress effectively.

Mental Fitness Tips

Think about your emotional well-being. Assess your emotional health regularly. Consider the particular demands or stresses you are facing and how they are affecting you. Give yourself permission to take a break from your worries and concerns. Recognize that dedicating even a short time every day to your mental fitness will reap significant benefits in terms of feeling rejuvenated and more confident.

Here are some simple ways to practice mental fitness:

- **Daydream:** Close your eyes and imagine yourself in a dream location. Breathe slowly and deeply. Whether it's a beach, a mountaintop, a hushed forest or a favorite room from your past, let the comforting environment wrap you in a sensation of peace and tranquility.

- **"Collect" Positive Emotional Moments:** Make it a point to recall times when you have experienced pleasure, comfort, tenderness, confidence, or other positive emotions.

- **Learn Ways To Cope With Negative Thoughts:** Negative thoughts can be insistent and loud. Learn to interrupt them. Don't try to block them (that never works), but don't let them take over. Try distracting yourself or comforting yourself, if you can't solve the problem right away.

- **Do One Thing At A Time:** For example, when you are out for a walk or spending time with friends, turn off your cell phone and stop making that mental "to do" list. Take in all the sights, sounds and smells you encounter.

- **Exercise:** Regular physical activity improves psychological well-being and can reduce depression and anxiety. Joining an exercise group or a gym can also reduce loneliness, since it connects you with a new set of people sharing a common goal.

- **Enjoy Hobbies:** Taking up a hobby brings balance to your life by allowing you to do something you enjoy because you want to do it, free of the pressure of everyday tasks. It also keeps your brain active.

- **Set Personal Goals:** Goals don't have to be ambitious. You might decide to finish that book you started three years ago; to take a walk around the block every day; to learn to knit or play bridge; to call your friends instead of waiting for the phone to ring. Whatever goal you set, reaching it will build confidence and a sense of satisfaction.

- **Keep A Journal (Or Even Talk To The Wall!):** Expressing yourself after a stressful day can help you gain perspective, release tension and even boost your body's resistance to illness.

- **Share Humor:** Life often gets too serious, so when you hear or see something that makes you smile or laugh, share it with someone you know. A little humor can go a long way to keeping us mentally fit!

- **Volunteer:** Volunteering is called the "win-win" activity because helping others makes us feel good about ourselves. At the same time, it widens our social network, provides us with new learning experiences and can bring balance to our lives.

- **Treat Yourself Well:** Cook yourself a good meal. Have a bubble bath. See a movie. Call a friend or relative you haven't talked to in ages. Sit on a park bench and breathe in the fragrance of flowers and grass. Whatever it is, do it just for you.

Chapter 52

Developing Resilience

Introduction

How do people deal with difficult events that change their lives? The death of a loved one, loss of a job, serious illness, terrorist attacks, and other traumatic events: these are all examples of very challenging life experiences. Many people react to such circumstances with a flood of strong emotions and a sense of uncertainty.

Yet people generally adapt well over time to life-changing situations and stressful conditions. What enables them to do so? It involves resilience, an ongoing process that requires time and effort and engages people in taking a number of steps.

This chapter is intended to help readers with taking their own road to resilience. The information within describes resilience and some factors that affect how people deal with hardship. Much of the chapter focuses on developing and using a personal strategy for enhancing resilience.

What Is Resilience?

Resilience is the process of adapting well in the face of adversity, trauma, tragedy, threats, or even significant sources of stress—such as family and relationship problems, serious health problems, or workplace and financial stressors. It means "bouncing back" from difficult experiences.

Research has shown that resilience is ordinary, not extraordinary. People commonly demonstrate resilience. One example is the response of many Americans to the September 11, 2001 terrorist attacks and individuals' efforts to rebuild their lives.

Being resilient does not mean that a person doesn't experience difficulty or distress. Emotional pain and sadness are common in people who have suffered major adversity or trauma in their lives. In fact, the road to resilience is likely to involve considerable emotional distress.

Resilience is not a trait that people either have or do not have. It involves behaviors, thoughts, and actions that can be learned and developed in anyone.

Resilience Factors And Strategies

Factors In Resilience

A combination of factors contributes to resilience. Many studies show that the primary factor in resilience is having caring and supportive relationships within and outside the family. Relationships that create love and trust, provide role models, and offer encouragement and reassurance help bolster a person's resilience.

Several additional factors are associated with resilience, including:

- The capacity to make realistic plans and take steps to carry them out
- A positive view of yourself and confidence in your strengths and abilities
- Skills in communication and problem solving
- The capacity to manage strong feelings and impulses

All of these are factors that people can develop in themselves.

Strategies For Building Resilience

Developing resilience is a personal journey. People do not all react the same to traumatic and stressful life events. An approach to building resilience that works for one person might not work for another. People use varying strategies.

Some variation may reflect cultural differences. A person's culture might have an impact on how he or she communicates feelings and deals with adversity—for example, whether and how a person connects with significant others, including extended family members and community resources. With growing cultural diversity, the public has greater access to a number of different approaches to building resilience.

Some or many of the ways to build resilience in the following pages may be appropriate to consider in developing your personal strategy.

10 Ways To Build Resilience

- **Make Connections:** Good relationships with close family members, friends, or others are important. Accepting help and support from those who care about you and will listen to you strengthens resilience. Some people find that being active in civic groups, faith-based organizations, or other local groups provides social support and can help with reclaiming hope. Assisting others in their time of need also can benefit the helper.

- **Avoid Seeing Crises As Insurmountable Problems:** You can't change the fact that highly stressful events happen, but you can change how you interpret and respond to these events. Try looking beyond the present to how future circumstances may be a little better. Note any subtle ways in which you might already feel somewhat better as you deal with difficult situations.

- **Accept That Change Is A Part Of Living:** Certain goals may no longer be attainable as a result of adverse situations. Accepting circumstances that cannot be changed can help you focus on circumstances that you can alter.

- **Move Toward Your Goals:** Develop some realistic goals. Do something regularly—even if it seems like a small accomplishment—that enables you to move toward your goals. Instead of focusing on tasks that seem unachievable, ask yourself, "What's one thing I know I can accomplish today that helps me move in the direction I want to go?"

- **Take Decisive Actions:** Act on adverse situations as much as you can. Take decisive actions, rather than detaching completely from problems and stresses and wishing they would just go away.

- **Look For Opportunities For Self-Discovery:** People often learn something about themselves and may find that they have grown in some respect as a result of their struggle with loss. Many people who have experienced tragedies and hardship have reported better relationships, greater sense of strength even while feeling vulnerable, increased sense of self-worth, a more developed spirituality, and heightened appreciation for life.

- **Nurture A Positive View Of Yourself:** Developing confidence in your ability to solve problems and trusting your instincts helps build resilience.

- **Keep Things In Perspective:** Even when facing very painful events, try to consider the stressful situation in a broader context and keep a long-term perspective. Avoid blowing the event out of proportion.

- **Maintain A Hopeful Outlook.** An optimistic outlook enables you to expect that good things will happen in your life. Try visualizing what you want, rather than worrying about what you fear.

- **Take Care Of Yourself:** Pay attention to your own needs and feelings. Engage in activities that you enjoy and find relaxing. Exercise regularly. Taking care of yourself helps to keep your mind and body primed to deal with situations that require resilience.

Additional Ways Of Strengthening Resilience May Be Helpful: For example, some people write about their deepest thoughts and feelings related to trauma or other stressful events in their life. Meditation and spiritual practices help some people build connections and restore hope.

The key is to identify ways that are likely to work well for you as part of your own personal strategy for fostering resilience.

Learning From Your Past

Some Questions To Ask Yourself

Focusing on past experiences and sources of personal strength can help you learn about what strategies for building resilience might work for you. By exploring answers to the following questions about yourself and your reactions to challenging life events, you may discover how you can respond effectively to difficult situations in your life.

What are coping skills and mechanisms?

A coping skill or coping mechanism is a behavior or thought process utilized to decrease anxiety, discomfort or the experience of stress. Coping is done in a deliberate manner and, to some degree, is considered conscious behavior. A central goal of psychotherapy treatment for eating disorders is enabling patients to develop effective means of coping with negative thoughts, feelings, and/or impulses.

Source: Excerpted from "Eating Disorders Glossary," © 2012 Families Empowered and Supporting Treatment of Eating Disorders (www.feast-ed.org).

Consider the following:

- What kinds of events have been most stressful for me?

- How have those events typically affected me?

- Have I found it helpful to think of important people in my life when I am distressed?

- To whom have I reached out for support in working through a traumatic or stressful experience?

- What have I learned about myself and my interactions with others during difficult times?

- Has it been helpful for me to assist someone else going through a similar experience?

- Have I been able to overcome obstacles, and if so, how?

- What has helped make me feel more hopeful about the future?

Staying Flexible

Resilience involves maintaining flexibility and balance in your life as you deal with stressful circumstances and traumatic events. This happens in several ways, including:

- Letting yourself experience strong emotions, and also realizing when you may need to avoid experiencing them at times in order to continue functioning

- Stepping forward and taking action to deal with your problems and meet the demands of daily living, and also stepping back to rest and reenergize yourself

- Spending time with loved ones to gain support and encouragement, and also nurturing yourself

- Relying on others, and also relying on yourself

Places To Look For Help

Getting help when you need it is crucial in building your resilience. Beyond caring family members and friends, people often find it helpful to turn to:

- **Self-Help And Support Groups:** Such community groups can aid people struggling with hardships such as the death of a loved one. By sharing information, ideas, and emotions, group participants can assist one another and find comfort in knowing that they are not alone in experiencing difficulty.

- **Books And Other Publications** by people who have successfully managed adverse situations such as surviving cancer. These stories can motivate readers to find a strategy that might work for them personally.

- **Online Resources:** Information on the web can be a helpful source of ideas, though the quality of information varies among sources.

For many people, using their own resources and the kinds of help listed above may be sufficient for building resilience. At times, however, an individual might get stuck or have difficulty making progress on the road to resilience.

A licensed mental health professional such as a psychologist can assist people in developing an appropriate strategy for moving forward. It is important to get professional help if you feel like you are unable to function or perform basic activities of daily living as a result of a traumatic or other stressful life experience.

Different people tend to be comfortable with somewhat different styles of interaction. A person should feel at ease and have good rapport in working with a mental health professional or participating in a support group.

Continuing On Your Journey

To help summarize several of the main points in this chapter, think of resilience as similar to taking a raft trip down a river.

On a river, you may encounter rapids, turns, slow water, and shallows. As in life, the changes you experience affect you differently along the way.

In traveling the river, it helps to have knowledge about it and past experience in dealing with it. Your journey should be guided by a plan, a strategy that you consider likely to work well for you.

Perseverance and trust in your ability to work your way around boulders and other obstacles are important. You can gain courage and insight by successfully navigating your way through white water. Trusted companions who accompany you on the journey can be especially helpful for dealing with rapids, upstream currents, and other difficult stretches of the river.

You can climb out to rest alongside the river. But to get to the end of your journey, you need to get back in the raft and continue.

Part Six
If You Need More Information

Chapter 53

For More Information About Eating Disorders

Academy for Eating Disorders

111 Deer Lake Road, Suite 100
Deerfield, IL 60015
Phone: 847-498-4274
Fax: 847-480-9282
Website: http://www.aedweb.org
E-mail: info@aedweb.org

Alliance for Eating Disorders Awareness

P.O. Box 2562
West Palm Beach, FL 33402
Toll-Free: 866-662-1235
Phone: 561-841-0900
Fax: 561-653-0043
Website: www.eatingdisorderinfo.org
E-mail: info@eatingdisorderinfo.org

Binge Eating Disorder Association (BEDA)

637 Emerson Place
Severna Park, MD 21146
Phone: 855-855-BEDA (855-855-2332)
Fax: 410-741-3037
Website: http://www.bedaonline.com
E-mail: info@bedaonline.com

Bulimia Nervosa Resource Guide

ECRI Institute
Attn: Bulimia Guide Webmaster
5200 Butler Pike
Plymouth Meeting, PA 19462
Website: http://www.bulimiaguide.org

Caring Online

Website: http://www.caringonline.com

About This Chapter: The resources listed in this chapter were compiled from many sources deemed accurate. Inclusion does not constitute endorsement and there is no implication associated with omission. All contact information was verified in July 2012.

Casa Palmera

14750 El Camino Real
Del Mar, CA 92014
Phone: 866-768-6719
Website:
http://www.casapalmera.com

Children's Hospital Colorado Eating Disorder Program

Anschutz Medical Campus
13123 East 16th Avenue
Aurora, CO 80045
Phone: 720-777-6452
Website:
http://www.childrenscolorado.org/
conditions/psych/eatingdisorders/
index.aspx

Eating Disorder Expert

Daresbury Point
Green Wood Drive
Manor Park
Cheshire, WA7 1UP
UK
Website: http://www.eating
disorderexpert.co.uk

Eating Disorder Foundation

1901 East 20th Avenue
Denver, CO 80205
Phone: 303-322-3373
Website:
http://www.eatingdisorderfoundation.org

Eating Disorder Referral and Information Center

2923 Sandy Pointe, Suite 6
Del Mar, CA 92014-2052
Phone: 858-792-7463
Fax: 858-220-7417
Website: http://www.edreferral.com
E-mail: edreferral@aol.com

Eating Disorders Coalition (EDC)

720 7th Street NW, Suite 300
Washington, DC 20001
Phone: 202-543-9570
Website:
http://www.eatingdisorderscoalition.org
E-mail:
manager@eatingdisorderscoalition.org

Eating Disorders Foundation of Victoria

1513 High Street
Glen Iris, VIC 3146
Australia
Website:
http://www.eatingdisorders.org.au
E-mail: help@eatingdisorders.org.au

Eating Disorders Recovery Center

232 Vance Road, Suite 206
St. Louis, MO 63088
Phone: 636-225-3700
Website: http://www.addictions.net

F.E.A.S.T. (Families Empowered And Supporting Treatment of Eating Disorders)

P.O. Box 331
Warrenton, VA 20188
Phone: 540-227-8518
Website: http://feast-ed.org
E-mail: info@feast-ed.org

Female Athlete Triad Coalition

Website:
http://www.femaleathletetriad.org

Harris Center for Education and Advocacy in Eating Disorders

2 Longfellow Place, Suite 200
Boston, MA 02114
Phone: 617-726-8470
Website:
http://www2.massgeneral.org/
harriscenter/index.asp

Mirror, Mirror

Website:
http://www.mirror-mirror.org

Multi-Service Eating Disorders Association

92 Pearl Street
Newton, MA 02458
Toll-Free: 866-343-MEDA
(866-343-6332)
Phone: 617-558-1881
Website: http://www.medainc.org
E-mail: info@medainc.org

National Association of Anorexia Nervosa and Associated Disorders (ANAD)

800 E Diehl Road #160
Naperville, IL 60563
Phone: 630-577-1330
Website: http://www.anad.org
E-mail: anadhelp@anad.org

National Center for Overcoming Overeating

Website:
http://www.overcomingovereating.com

National Eating Disorder Information Centre (DEDIC)

ES 7-421, 200 Elizabeth Street
Toronto, Ontario M5G 2C4
Canada
Toll-free: 866-NEDIC-20
(866-633-4220)
Phone: 416-340-4156
Fax: 416-340-4736
Website:
http://www.nedic.ca/index.shtml
E-mail: nedic@uhn.on.ca

National Eating Disorders Association (NEDA)

165 West 46th Street
New York, NY 10036
Toll-Free: 800-931-2237
Phone: 212-575-6200
Fax: 212-575-1650
Website:
http://www.nationaleatingdisorders.org
E-mail: info@nationaleatingdisorders.org

Overeaters Anonymous

P.O. Box 44020
Rio Rancho, NM 87174-4020
Phone: 505-891-2664
Fax: 505-891-4320
Website: http://www.oa.org

Rader Programs

Toll-Free: 800-841-1515
Website: http://www.raderprograms.com

Remuda Ranch

Toll-Free: 855-219-5266 (Information)
Toll-Free: 888-484-2926 (Hotline)
Website: http://www.remudaranch.com

River Centre Clinic

5465 Main Street
Sylvania, OH 43560
Toll-Free: 877-212-5457
Phone: 419-885-8800
Fax: 419-885-8600
Website: http://www.river-centre.org

Sheena's Place

87 Spadina Road
Toronto, Ontario
Canada M5R 2T1
Phone: 416-927-8900
Fax: 416-927-8844
Website: http://www.sheenasplace.org
E-mail: info@sheenasplace.org

Something Fishy

Website:
http://www.something-fishy.org

Chapter 54

For More Information About Nutrition And Weight Management

Academy of Nutrition and Dietetics

120 South Riverside Plaza, Suite 2000
Chicago, IL 60606-6995
Toll-Free: 800-877-1600
Phone: 312-899-0040
Website: http://www.eatright.org

American Diabetes Association

1701 North Beauregard Street
Alexandria, VA 22311
Toll-Free: 800-DIABETES
(800-342-2383)
Website: http://www.diabetes.org
E-mail: AskADA@diabetes.org

American Heart Association

7272 Greenville Avenue
Dallas, TX 75231-4596
Toll-Free: 800-AHA-USA1
(800-242-8721)
Website: http://www.americanheart.org

Ask the Dietitian®

Website:
http://www.dietitian.com/
Healthy Body Calculator:
http://www.dietitian.com/calcbody.php

Center for Science in the Public Interest

1220 L Street NW, Suite 300
Washington, DC 20009
Phone: 202-332-9110
Fax: 202-265-4954
Website: http://www.cspinet.org
E-mail: cspi@cspinet.org

The resources listed in this chapter were compiled from many sources deemed accurate. Inclusion does not constitute endorsement and there is no implication associated with omission. All contact information was verified in July 2012.

Centers for Disease Control and Prevention (CDC)

Division of Nutrition, Physical Activity, and Obesity (DNPAO)
1600 Clifton Road
Atlanta, GA 30333
Toll-Free: 800-CDC-INFO
(800-232-4636)
Toll-Free TTY: 888-232-6348
Nutrition Website: http://www.cdc.gov/nutrition/index.html
E-mail: cdcinfo@cdc.gov

ChooseMyPlate.gov

Center for Nutrition Policy and Promotion
3101 Park Center Drive, 10th Floor
Alexandria, VA 22302-1594
Website: http://www.choosemyplate.gov
E-mail: support@cnpp.usda.gov

Food and Nutrition Information Center

National Agricultural Library
10301 Baltimore Avenue, Room 108
Beltsville, MD 20705-2351
Phone: 301-504-5414
Fax: 301-504-6409
Website: http://www.nal.usda.gov/fnic
E-mail: fnic@nal.usda.gov

GirlsHealth.gov

Department of Health and Human Services
200 Independence Avenue SW
Room 712E
Washington, DC 20201
Website: http://www.girlshealth.gov

International Food Information Council Foundation

1100 Connecticut Avenue NW
Suite 430
Washington, DC 20036
Phone: 202-296-6540
Website: http://www.foodinsight.org
E-mail: foodinfo@ific.org

Kidshealth.org

Nemours Foundation
10140 Centurion Parkway
Jacksonville, FL 32256
Phone: 904-697-4100
Fax: 904-697-4220
Website: http://www.kidshealth.org

Milk Matters Calcium Education Campaign

National Institute of Child Health and Human Development (NICHD)
31 Center Drive, Room 2A32
Bethesda, MD 20892-2425
Toll-Free: 800-370-2943
Toll-Free TTY: 888-320-6942
Toll-Free Fax: 866-760-5947
Website: http://www.nichd.nih.gov/milk
E-mail: NICHDMilkMatters@nail.nih.gov

National Agricultural Library

Food and Nutrition Information Center
Nutrition.gov Staff
10301 Baltimore Avenue
Beltsville, MD 20705-2351
Website: http://www.nutrition.gov

National Center for Complementary and Alternative Medicine

NCCAM Clearinghouse

P.O. Box 7923

Gaithersburg, MD 20898

Toll-Free: 888-644-6226

Toll-Free TTY: 866-464-3615

Toll-Free Fax: 866-464-3616

Website: http://nccam.nih.gov

National Heart, Lung, and Blood Institute

NHLBI Health Information Center

P.O. Box 30105

Bethesda, MD 20824-0105

Phone: 301-592-8573

TTY: 240-629-3255

Fax: 240-629-3246

Website: http://www.nhlbi.nih.gov

E-mail: nhlbiinfo@ nhlbi.nih.gov

National Institute of Child Health and Human Development

P.O. Box 3006

Rockville, MD 20847

Toll-Free: 800-370-2943

Toll-Free TTY: 888-320-6942

Toll-Free Fax: 866-760-5947

Website: http://www.nichd.nih.gov

E-mail:

NICHDInformationResourceCenter

@mail.nih.gov

National Women's Health Information Center

Office on Women's Health

Department of Health and Human

Services

200 Independence Avenue, SW

Room 712E

Washington, DC 20201

Toll-free: 800-994-9662

Toll-Free TDD: 888-220-5446

Phone: 202-690-7650

Fax: 202-205-2631

Website: http://www.womenshealth.gov

Obesity Society

8757 Georgia Avenue, Suite 1320

Silver Spring, MD 20910

Phone: 301-563-6526

Fax: 301-563-6595

Website: http://www.obesity.org

E-mail: fdea@obesity.org

Office of Dietary Supplements

National Institutes of Health

6100 Executive Boulevard

Room 3B01, MSC 7517

Bethesda, MD 20892-7517

Phone: 301-435-2920

Fax: 301-480-1845

Website: http://ods.od.nih.gov

E-mail: ods@nih.gov

U.S. Department of Agriculture

1400 Independence Avenue SW
Washington, DC 20250
Phone: 202-720-2791
TDD: 202-720-2600 (Voice–TDD,
TARGET Center)
Fax: 202-720-2681
Website: http://www.usda.gov
MyPlate: http://www.choosemyplate.gov
E-mail: agsec@usda.gov

U.S. Food and Drug Administration (FDA)

Consumer Inquiries
10903 New Hampshire Avenue
Silver Spring, MD 20993
Toll-Free: 888-INFO-FDA
(888-463-6332)
Fax: 301-847-8622
Website: http://www.fda.gov
E-mail: ConsumerInfo@fda.hhs.gov

Vegetarian Resource Group

P.O. Box 1463
Baltimore, MD 21203
Phone: 410-366-8343
Website: http://www.vrg.org
E-mail: vrg@vrg.org

Weight-Control Information Network

National Institute of Diabetes and
Digestive and Kidney Diseases
1 WIN Way
Bethesda, MD 20892-3665
Toll-Free: 877-946-4627
Fax: 202-828-1028
Website: http://win.niddk.nih.gov
E-mail: win@info.niddk.nih.gov

Chapter 55

For More Information About Physical And Mental Fitness

Physical Fitness And Exercise

Action for Healthy Kids
600 West Van Buren Street, Suite 720
Chicago, IL 60607
Toll-Free: 800-416-5136
Fax: 312-212-0098
Website:
http://www.actionforhealthykids.org

Aerobics and Fitness Association of America
15250 Ventura Boulevard, Suite 200
Sherman Oaks, CA 91403
Toll-Free: 877-YOUR-BODY
(877-968-7263)
Website: http://www.afaa.com

American Alliance for Health, Physical Education, Recreation, and Dance
1900 Association Drive
Reston, VA 20191-1598
Toll-Free: 800-213-7193
Phone: 703-476-3400
Fax: 703-476-9527
Website: http://www.aahperd.org

American Council on Exercise (ACE)
4851 Paramount Drive
San Diego, CA 92123
Toll-Free: 888-825-3636
Phone: 858-279-8227
Fax: 858-576-6564
Website: http://www.acefitness.org
E-mail: support@acefitness.org

About This Chapter: The resources listed in this chapter were compiled from many sources deemed accurate. Inclusion does not constitute endorsement and there is no implication associated with omission. All contact information was verified in July 2012.

American Health and Fitness Alliance

P.O. Box 20750
New York, NY 10021
Phone: 212-808-0765
Fax: 212-988-3130
Website: www.health-fitness.org

American Running Association (ARA)

4405 East-West Highway, Suite 405
Bethesda, MD 20814
Phone: 800-776-2732 (ext. 13 or ext. 12)
Fax: 301-913-9520
Website:
http://www.americanrunning.org

Aquatic Exercise Association

P.O. Box 1609
Nokomis, FL 34274-1609
Toll-Free: 888-232-9283
Website: http://www.aeawave.com

Centers for Disease Control and Prevention (CDC)

Division of Nutrition, Physical Activity,
and Obesity (DNPAO)
1600 Clifton Road
Atlanta, GA 30333
Toll-Free: 800-CDC-INFO
(800-232-4636)
Toll-Free TTY: 888-232-6348
Website: http://www.cdc.gov/nccdphp/
dnpao/index.html
E-mail: cdcinfo@cdc.gov

Fitness Institute Australia

Level 3, 815 -825 George Street
Sydney NSW 2000 Australia
Website: http://www.fia.com.au
E-mail: admin@fia.com.au

Girls Health

Department of Health
and Human Services
200 Independence Ave. SW, Rm. 712E
Washington, DC 20201
Website: http://www.girlshealth.gov

HealthyWomen

157 Broad Street, Suite 106
Red Bank, NJ 07701
Toll-Free: 877-986-9472
Fax: 732-530-3347
Website: http://www.healthywomen.org
E-mail: info@healthywomen.org

IDEA Health & Fitness Association

10455 Pacific Center Court
San Diego, CA 92121
Toll-Free: 800-999-4332, ext. 7
Phone: 858-535-8979, ext. 7
Fax: 858-535-8234
Website: http://www.ideafit.com
E-mail: contact@ideafit.com

International Fitness Association

12472 Lake Underhill Road, #341
Orlando, FL 32828-7144
Toll-Free: 800-227-1976
Phone: 407-579-8610
Website: http://www.ifafitness.com

International Health, Racquet and Sportsclub Association (IHRSA)

70 Fargo Street
Boston, MA 02210
Toll-Free: 800-228-4772
Phone: 617-951-0055
Fax: 617-951-0056
Website: http://www.ihrsa.org
E-mail: info@ihrsa.org

Kidshealth.org

Nemours Foundation
10140 Centurion Parkway
Jacksonville, FL 32256
Phone: 904-697-4100
Fax: 904-697-4220
Website: http://www.kidshealth.org

LiveStrong

Website: http://www.livestrong.com

National Alliance for Youth Sports

National Headquarters
2050 Vista Parkway
West Palm Beach, FL 33411
Toll-Free: 800-688-KIDS
(800-729-2057)
Phone: 561-684-1141
Fax: 561-684-2546
Website: http://www.nays.org
E-mail: nays@nays.org

National Coalition for Promoting Physical Activity

1100 H Street NW, Suite 510
Washington, DC 20005
Phone: 202-454-7521
Fax: 202-454-7598
Website: http://www.ncppa.org
E-mail: info@ncppa.org

National Institute for Fitness and Sport

250 University Boulevard
Indianapolis, IN 46202
Phone: 317-274-3432
Fax: 317-274-7408
Website: http://www.nifs.org

National Recreation and Park Association

22377 Belmont Ridge Road
Ashburn, VA 20148-4501
Toll-Free: 800-626-NRPA
(800-626-6772)
Website: http://www.nrpa.org
E-mail: customerservice@nrpa.org

National Strength and Conditioning Association

1885 Bob Johnson Drive
Colorado Springs, CO 80906
Toll-Free: 800-815-6826
Phone: 719-632-6722
Fax: 719-632-6367
Website: http://www.nsca-lift.org
E-mail: nsca@nsca-lift.org

PE Central

P.O. Box 10262
1995 South Main Street, Suite 902
Blacksburg, VA 24062
Phone: 540-953-1043
Fax: 540-301-0112
Website: http://www.pecentral.org
E-mail: pec@pecentral.org

President's Challenge

501 North Morton Street
Suite 203
Bloomington, IN 47404
Toll-Free: 800-258-8146
Fax: 812-855-8999
Website:
http://www.presidentschallenge.org
E-mail: preschal@indiana.edu

President's Council on Fitness, Sports, and Nutrition

Tower Building, Suite 560
1101 Wootton Parkway
Rockville, MD 20852
Phone: 240-276-9567
Fax: 240-276-9860
Website: http://www.fitness.gov
E-mail: fitness@hhs.gov

Spark Teens

Website:
http://www.sparkteens.com

SportsMD

Toll-Free: 800-679-1765
Website: http://www.sportsmd.com
E-mail: contactus@sportsmd.com

Women's Sports Foundation

Eisenhower Park
1899 Hempstead Turnpike
Suite 400
East Meadow, NY 11554
Toll-Free: 800-227-3988
Phone: 516-542-4700
Fax: 516-542-4716
Website:
http://www.womenssportsfoundation.org
E-mail:
Info@WomensSportsFoundation.org

Mental Wellness

American Academy of Child and Adolescent Psychiatry

3615 Wisconsin Avenue, NW
Washington, DC 20016-3007
Phone: 202-966-7300
Fax: 202-966-2891
Website: www.aacap.org

American Counseling Association

5999 Stevenson Avenue
Alexandria, VA 22304
Toll-Free: 800-347-6647
TDD: 703-823-6862
Toll-Free Fax: 800-473-2329
Fax: 703-823-0252
Website: www.counseling.org
E-mail: webmaster@counseling.org

American Psychiatric Association

1000 Wilson Boulevard, Suite 1825
Arlington, VA 22209-3901
Toll-Free: 888-35-PSYCH
(888-357-7924)
Phone: 703-907-7300
Website: www.psych.org
E-mail: apa@psych.org

American Psychological Association

750 First Street NE
Washington, DC 20002-4242
Toll-Free: 800-374-2721
Phone: 202-336-5500
TDD/TTY: 202-336-6123
Website: http://www.apa.org
E-mail: public.affairs@apa.org

Association for Behavioral and Cognitive Therapies

305 7th Avenue, 16th Floor
New York, NY 10001
Phone: 212-647-1890
Fax: 212-647-1865
Website: www.abct.org

Canadian Mental Health Association

Phenix Professional Building
595 Montreal Road, Suite 303
Ottawa ON K1K 4L2
Fax: 613-745-5522
Website: http://www.cmha.ca

Canadian Psychological Association

141 Laurier Avenue West, Suite 702
Ottawa, ON K1P 5J3
Toll-Free: 888-472-0657
Phone: 613-237-2144
Fax: 613-237-1674
Website: www.cpa.ca
E-mail: cpa@cpa.ca

Center for Mental Health Services

5600 Fishers Lane, Room 17C-20
Rockville, MD 20857
Phone: 240-276-1310
Website: mentalhealth.samhsa.gov
E-mail: info@mentalhealth.org

Centre for Clinical Interventions

223 James Street,
Northbridge, Western Australia 6003
Phone: + 011 61 (08) 9227 4399
Fax: + 011 61 (08) 9328 5911
Website: http://www.cci.health.wa.gov.au
E-mail: info.cci@health.wa.gov.au

Mental Health America

(formerly National Mental Health Assn.)
2000 North Beauregard Street, 6th Floor
Alexandria, VA 22311
Toll-Free: 800-969-6642
Crisis Line: 800-273-TALK (800-273-8255)
Phone: 703-684-7722
Fax: 703-684-5968
Website: www.nmha.org
E-mail: webmaster@mentalhealthamerica.net

Mind

15-19 Broadway
Stratford, London, UK E15 4BQ
Phone: +44 208-519-2122
Fax: +44 208-522-1725
Website: www.mind.org.uk
E-mail: contact@mind.org.uk

National Alliance on Mental Illness (NAMI)

3803 North Fairfax Drive
Suite 100
Arlington, VA 22203
Toll-Free: 888-999-NAMI
(888-999-6264)
Toll-Free: 800-950-NAMI
(800-950-6264 Helpline)
Phone: 703-524-7600
Fax: 703-524-9094
Website: www.nami.org
E-mail: info@nami.org

National Institute of Mental Health (NIMH)

6001 Executive Boulevard
Room 8184 MSC 9663
Bethesda, MD 20892-9663
Toll-Free: 866-615-NIMH
(866-615-6464)
Toll-Free TTY: 866-415-8051
Phone: 301-443-4513
TTY: 301-443-8431
Fax: 301-443-4279
Website: http://www.nimh.nih.gov
E-mail: nimhinfo@nih.gov

Psych Central

55 Pleasant Street, Suite 207
Newburyport, MA 01950
Phone: 978-992-0008
Website: www.psychcentral.com
E-mail: talkback@psychcentral.com

Royal College of Psychiatrists

17 Belgrave Square
London SW1X 8PG
Phone: 020 7235 2351
Fax: 020 7245 1231
Website: mentalhealthuk.org

Substance Abuse and Mental Health Services Administration (SAMHSA)

1 Choke Cherry Road
Rockville, MD 20857
Toll-Free: 877-SAMHSA-7
(877-726-4727)
Fax: 240-221-4295
Website: mentalhealth.samhsa.gov
Mental Health Services Locator:
mentalhealth.samhsa.gov/databases

Index

Index

Page numbers that appear in *Italics* refer to tables or illustrations. Page numbers that have a small 'n' after the page number refer to information shown as Notes at the beginning of each chapter. Page numbers that appear in **Bold** refer to information contained in boxes on that page (except Notes information at the beginning of each chapter).

A

"About Body Image"
   (Office on Women's Health) 37n
Academy for Eating Disorders
   contact information 349
   publications
      eating disorders diagnosis 209n
      eating disorders treatment 213n
Academy of Nutrition and Dietetics,
   contact information 353
Action for Healthy Kids, contact information 357
A.D.A.M., Inc., publications
   eating disorders 17n
   eating disorders complications 127n
ADHD *see* attention deficit hyperactivity disorder
advertising *see* media
aerobic activities
   described 322
   intensity levels 324–25
Aerobics and Fitness Association of America,
   contact information 357
age factor
   binge eating disorder 78
   calorie needs *276*

age factor, continued
   eating disorders 20
   eating disorders risk factor 32
   physical activity 323
"Aim for a Healthy Weight" (NHLBI) 295n
alcohol abuse
   bulimia nervosa 128
   eating disorders **106**
Alliance for Eating Disorders Awareness
   abused substances publication 105n
   contact information 349
Ambien (zolpidem) 91
amenorrhea, female athlete triad 114, 331
American Academy of Child and Adolescent
   Psychiatry, contact information 360
American Alliance for Health, Physical Eduction,
   Recreation, and Dance, contact information 357
American Council on Exercise,
   contact information 357
American Counseling Association,
   contact information 360
American Diabetes Association,
   contact information 353

American Health and Fitness Alliance,
contact information 358
American Heart Association,
contact information 353
American Pregnancy Association,
eating disorders publication 159n
American Psychiatric Association,
contact information 361
American Psychological Association
contact information 361
resilience publication 341n
American Running Association,
contact information 358
aminoketone, eating disorders 221
amitriptyline 220
amphetamines, eating disorders **106**
amygdala, eating disorders 18
ana *see* pro-ana
anabolic steroids, muscles **26**
ANAD *see* National Association of Anorexia
Nervosa and Associated Disorders
Anafranil (clomipramine) 220
anemia, anorexia nervosa 132
animal assisted therapy, defined 225
anorexia nervosa
antidepressant medications **69**
behavioral signs **194**
bodily damage, depicted *68*
described 4
diabetes 24
diagnosis 209
medical consequences 128–33
oral health 152
osteoporosis 155–58
overview 65–70
symptoms 25
"Anorexia Nervosa Fact Sheet"
(Office on Women's Health) 65n
anticonvulsant medications, eating disorders 221
antidepressant medications
anorexia nervosa **69**
binge eating disorder **5**
black box warning label **69**, 75, **175**
defined 224

antiemetics, eating disorders 221
anxiety disorders
eating disorders 21–22, 163–64
media influence 51
overview 176–82
purging 38
"Anxiety Disorders" (NIMH) 171n
Aquatic Exercise Association,
contact information 358
Ask the Dietitian, website address 353
Association for Behavioral and Cognitive
Therapies, contact information 361
athletes
compulsive exercise 110
eating disorders statistics 61
see also female athlete triad; sports activities
attention deficit hyperactivity disorder (ADHD),
eating disorder risk **23**
avoidant personality disorder, described 20–21

B

BDD *see* body dysmorphic disorder
Beals, Katherine 30–34
Becker, Anne 51
behavior therapy
defined 224
obesity 148–49
Benazide (isocarboxazid) 220
"Benefits of Good Mental Health"
(Canadian Mental Health Association) 333n
bigorexia, defined **122**
binge eating, diabetes 24
binge eating disorder (BED)
defined **5, 78**
diagnosis 210–11
overview 77–81
"Binge Eating Disorder"
(Binge Eating Disorder Association) 77n
Binge Eating Disorder Association
contact information 349
publications
binge eating disorder 77n
EDNOS 9n, 97n

binge eating disorder episodes, defined **78**
biological changes, eating disorders **18–19**
biologic factors, eating disorders 17–20, 33
biology
    anorexia nervosa 66
    bulimia nervosa 73
black box warning label,
    antidepressant medications **69**, 75, **175**
blood problems, anorexia nervosa 132
body dysmorphic disorder (BDD)
    defined **121**
    described 22, 165
    overview 119–24
"Body Dysmorphic Disorder"
    (Nemours Foundation) 119n
body image
    bulimia nervosa 74
    compulsive exercise 111–12
    defined **38**
    media influence 52–54
    overview 37–40
    self-esteem 229–32
    sports activities 33–34
"Body Image and Self-Esteem"
    (Nemours Foundation) 229n
body image distortion, defined **38**
"Body Image: Eating Disorders"
    (Office on Women's Health) 37n
body mass index (BMI)
    chart *297*
        boys **141**
        girls **142**
    described 140–43
    EAT-26 **201**
    emotional eating 85
    media influence 49, 53
    online calculator 9
    weight management 295–96
    weight range 248–49
Bolvidon (mianserin) 221
Bonci, Tina 25–28
bone density
    anorexia nervosa 132
    female athlete triad 331

bone mineral density test,
    osteoporosis 158
bone-strengthening activities,
    described 322m325
borderline personality disorder (BPD),
    described 21
boys
    body mass index chart **141**
    excessive exercise 24
    see also gender factor; men
BPD *see* borderline personality disorder
brain and neurobiology of eating disorders,
    defined **43**
Bratman Steven 93, 95
brofaromine 220
Brownell, Kelly 48
"Build a Healthy Meal: 10 Tips for
    Healthy Meals" (USDA) 253n
bulimia nervosa
    behavioral signs **194**
    bodily damage, depicted *75*
    brain activity study **72–73**
    described 4
    diabetes 24
    diagnosis 210
    medical consequences 127–28
    oral health 151–52
    overview 71–76
    symptoms 25
"Bulimia Nervosa Fact Sheet"
    (Office on Women's Health) 71n
Bulimia Nervosa Resource Guide,
    contact information 349
bupropion, FDA warning 221

C

caffeine, eating disorders **106**
calcium
    food sources **256**
    nutritional requirements 11
    osteoporosis 157
    sports activities 293
    sports nutrition **294**

calories
    age factor *276*
    athletes 288
    food labels 14
    healthy eating 254
    obesity 144
    overview 265–77
    sports nutrition **288**
"Calories: How Many Can I Have?" (USDA) 265n
Canadian Mental Health Association
    contact information 361
    mental fitness publication 333n
Canadian Psychological Association,
  contact information 361
carbohydrate loading, described 290
carbohydrates
    food sources **280**
    nutrition myths 15–16
    sports activities 289–90
    sports nutrition **291**
Carbolith (lithium carbonate) 221
Caring Online, website address 349
Casa Palmera, contact information 350
Celexa (citalopram) 220
Center for Mental Health Services,
  contact information 361
Center for Science in the Public Interest,
  contact information 353
Centers for Disease Control and Prevention
  (CDC), contact information 354, 358
Centre for Clinical Interventions,
  contact information 361
"Chapter 3: Active Children and
  Adolescents" (DHHS) 321n
Children's Hospital Colorado
    contact information 350
    eating disorders publication 3n
cholesterol levels, nutrition myths 14–15
ChooseMyPlate.gov, contact information 354
"Choosing A Safe And Successful Weight-Loss
  Program" (NIDDK) 317n
Cibalith-S (lithium carbonate) 221
citalopram 220
clinical trials, antidepressant medications **175**

clomipramine 220
coaches
    female athletes 31, 32
    female athlete triad 24, 117
    weight loss influence 34
cocaine, eating disorders **106**
cognitive analytic therapy, defined 224
cognitive behavioral therapy (CBT)
    binge eating disorder **5**, 80–81
    body dysmorphic disorder **121**, 123
    bulimia nervosa 74
    defined 224
    eating disorders 188–89
    EDNOS 99
    self-guided 228
cognitive orientation therapy, defined 224
cognitive remediation therapy, defined 224
cognitive therapy, defined 224
Colorado Department of Public Health and
  Environment, oral health publications 151n
comfort foods, described 84
comorbidity, described 163
compensatory behaviors, defined **79**
compulsive actions, body dysmorphic disorder 120
compulsive exercise
    described 39–40, 332
    overview 109–12
"Compulsive Exercise" (Nemours Foundation) 109n
comradery **55**
Consonar (brofaromine) 220
Cooke, David A. 89n, 93n, 151n, 197n, 205n, 295n
coping skills, described **344**
coping skills training, eating disorders 189
cortisol, anorexia nervosa 156
creatine, muscles **26**
cultural pressures
    anorexia nervosa 66
    body dysmorphic disorder 122
    bulimia 72
    eating disorders 20
    media influence 51–52
    pica 103
cutting 165, **185**
Cymbalta (duloxetine) 221

D

"Dairy: Health Benefits and Nutrients"
(USDA) 253n
dance therapy, defined 227
"Dealing with and Eating Disorder Relapse"
(Remuda Ranch) 241n
deliberate self-harm **185**
dental complications, purging **153**
Department of Health and Human
Services *see* US Department of Health
and Human Services
depression
bulimia nervosa 74–75
eating disorders 22, 164–65
overview 171–76
"Depression" (NIMH) 171n
desipramine 220
Desyrel (trazodone) 221
DHHS *see* US Department of
Health and Human Services
diabetes mellitus
anorexia nervosa 133
defined **168**
eating disorders 24, 167–70
obesity 139–40
diabetic ketoacidosis, diabulimia **169**
diabulimia
defined **169**
described 169
"Diagnosis of Eating Disorders"
(Academy for Eating Disorders) 209n
Diagnostic and Statistical Manual IV (DSM-IV)
binge eating disorder 78
eating disorders not otherwise specified 97, 211
dialectical behavior therapy
defined **225**
eating disorders 189
diet, defined **16**
diet and nutrition
athletes 287–94
body image **39**
everyday foods **255**
mental health 336–37
orthorexia 94–95

diet and nutrition, *continued*
osteoporosis 157
power foods **256–57**
vegetarians **284–85**
see also nutritional requirements
dietitians, described **318**
"Diet Pills" (Alliance for Eating
Disorders Awareness) 105n
diet pills, eating disorders 105
diets
described **262**
media influence 49–50
disabilities, physical activity **327**
disordered eating
female athlete triad 114
men 27
"Diuretics" (Alliance for Eating
Disorders Awareness) 105n
diuretics, eating disorders 106–7
dopamine, reward seeking behavior 19–20
DOVE campaign 32
Doyle, Angela 25–28
dual diagnosis, described 163
duloxetine 221
Duralith (lithium carbonate) 221
dysmorphia *see* body dysmorphic disorder

E

early puberty, eating disorders 24
"Eat Fewer Empty Calories" (USDA) 265n
Eating Attitudes Test (EAT-26) 197–204
"Eating Attitudes Test (EAT-26)"
(Garner, et al.) 197n
"Eating Attitudes Test (EAT-26):
Scoring and Interpretation" (Garner) 197n
Eating Disorder Coalition,
contact information 350
Eating Disorder Expert, contact information 350
Eating Disorder Foundation,
contact information 350
Eating Disorder Referral and
Information Center, contact information 350
"Eating Disorder Relapse Prevention:
Support Is Key" (Remuda Ranch) 241n

eating disorders
    defined **6**
    diagnosis overview 209–11
    overview 3–7
    recovery statistics **211**
    re-establishing normal eating 237–39
    relapse 241–44
    symptoms overview 193–96
    treatment overview 213–17
    treatment study **214–15**
"Eating Disorders" (NIMH) 171n
"Eating Disorders and Oral Health"
    (Colorado Department of Public
    Health and Environment) 151n
"Eating Disorders during Pregnancy"
    (American Pregnancy Association) 159n
Eating Disorders Foundation of Victoria,
    contact information 350
"Eating Disorders: In-Depth Report"
    (A.D.A.M., Inc.) 17n, 127n
eating disorders not otherwise specified (EDNOS)
    described 211
    overview 97–100
"Eating Disorders Not Otherwise
    Specified (EDNOS)" (Binge Eating
    Disorder Association) 9n, 97n
Eating Disorders Recovery Center,
    contact information 350
"Eating Disorders Signs and Symptoms"
    (ANAD) 193n
"Eating Disorder Statistics" (ANAD) 59n
eating patterns
    overview 9–16
    vegetarians **284–85**
eating plans
    described **299**
    overview 253–63
    vegetarians 283–86
    weight management 144–46, 296–300
    see also diet and nutrition;
                healthy eating guidelines
"Eat the Right Amount of
    Calories for You" (USDA) 265n
EDNOS *see* eating disorders
    not otherwise specified

Effexor (venlafaxine) 221
Elavil (amitriptyline) 220
electrolytes, described 288–89
EMDR *see* eye movement
    desensitization and reprocessing
emotional concerns
    eating disorders 6, 10
    obesity 138
"Emotional Eating"
    (Nemours Foundation) 83n
emotional eating, overview 83–87
emotional resilience *see* resilience
empty calories, foods, listed *276*
endorphins
    described 109
    mental health 336
energy balance
    described **266**
    obesity 136
environment
    genes 43–44
    obesity 137
equine assisted therapy, defined 225
ERP *see* exposure with response prevention
escitalopram 220
Eskalith (lithium carbonate) 221
esteem *see* self-esteem
ethnic factors, eating disorders 20
exercise
    body image **39**
    daily guidelines **322**
    eating disorders 190
    emotional eating 87
    moderate activity described **324**
    osteoporosis 157
    safety considerations 329–32
    stretching **323**
    vigorous activity described **324**
    see also compulsive exercise;
                physical activity
exercise-induced anorexia, described 33
exercise therapy, defined 225
exposure with response prevention (ERP),
    defined 225
expressive therapy, defined 225

eye movement desensitization and
  reprocessing (EMDR)
    defined 225
    trauma treatment 188

F

"Facts about Eating Disorders, including Anorexia
  and Bulimia" (Children's Hospital Colorado) 3n
Families Empowered and Supporting
  Treatment of Eating Disorders (F.E.A.S.T.)
    contact information 351
    other conditions publication 163n
family issues
    anorexia nervosa 66
    bulimia 72
family therapy, defined 225
fats
    eating plans 300
    food sources **280**
    nutrition myths 14–15
FDA *see* US Food and Drug Administration
Female Athlete Coalition, website address 351
female athlete triad
    described 24
    overview 113–17
    safety considerations 331
    see also girls
Female Athlete Triad" (Nemours Foundation) 113n
fertility, eating disorders 159–61
fiber
    food sources **257**
    nutritional requirements 12
fitness, overview 321–27
Fitness Institute Australia, contact information 358
"Fitness: Keeping Safe and Injury Free"
  (Office on Women's Health) 329n
fluoxetine 220
    binge eating disorder **5**
    bulimia nervosa 75, 219–20
fluvoxamine 220
"Focus on Foods You Need" (USDA) 265n
folate (folic acid), food sources **256**
Food and Drug Administration
  see US Food and Drug Administration

Food and Nutrition Information Center,
  contact information 354
food groups
    eating plans 298–300
    overview 255–62
    see also diet and nutrition
"Food Label Helps Consumers Make
  Healthier Choices" (FDA) 279n
food labels
    described 12–14
    overview 279–82
    see also Nutrition Facts labels
friends
    anorexia nervosa 69–70
    bulimia nervosa 76
    eating disorders 7, 205–8
    female athlete triad 117
    quick tips **206, 208**
    self-harm **177, 185**

G

Garner, David M. 197n
gastrointestinal problems, anorexia nervosa 133
gender factor
    eating disorders 20
    EDNOS 98
    nutritional requirements 11–12
generalized anxiety disorder (GAD),
  described 181
genes
    anorexia nervosa 66
    binge eating disorder 80
    bulimia nervosa 73
    defined **43**
    obesity 137–38
    overview 41–45
genetic predisposition, defined **43**
gestational diabetes, defined **168**
girls
    ADHD, eating disorders **23**
    body mass index chart **142**
    excessive exercise 24
    see also female athlete triad;
      gender factor; women

Girls Health, contact information 358
GirlsHealth.gov, contact information 354
group therapy, binge eating disorder 80
gum disease, purging **153**

H

Halcion (triazolam) 91
Harris Center for Education
  and Advocacy in Eating Disorders,
  contact information 351
health care teams
    anorexia nervosa 67
    eating disorders treatment 215–16
    weight control 143
    weight loss programs 317–18
healthy eating guidelines
    orthorexia 95
    overview 10–16
    weight management 295–316
    see also eating plans
HealthyWomen, contact information 358
heart disease, anorexia nervosa 129–30
heredity
    body shape 250–51
    eating disorders 4, 17
    see also genes
HHS *see* US Department of
  Health and Human Services
hormonal changes,
  anorexia nervosa 128–29, 156
"How Can I Improve My Self-Esteem?"
  (Nemours Foundation) 229n
"How to Eat for Health"
  (Office on Women's Health) 253n
"How to Help a Friend with
  Eating and Body Image Issues"
  (National Eating Disorders
  Association) 205n
HPA system, described 17–19
hypnobehavioral therapy, defined 225
hypnosedative induced complex behaviors,
    described 91–92
hypothalamus, eating disorders 17

I

IDEA Health and Fitness Association,
  contact information 358
imipramine 220
"The Impact of Other Conditions
  on Eating Disorder Symptoms and
  Treatment - Also Called 'Co-Morbidity'"
  (Families Empowered and Supporting
  Treatment of Eating Disorders) 163n
impulsive behavior, bulimia nervosa 128
inner voice, described **234**
International Fitness Association,
  contact information 358
International Food Information
  Council Foundation,
  contact information 354
International Health, Racquet and Sportsclub
  Association (IHRSA),
  contact information 359
interpersonal therapy (IPT), defined 226
ipecac syrup
    abuse results 196
    defined **107**
IPT *see* interpersonal therapy
iron
    food sources **257**
    healthy eating 259
    nutritional requirements 11
    sports activities 292
    sports nutrition **293**
isocarboxazid 220
"Is Unresolved Trauma Preventing a
  Full Eating Disorder Recovery?"
  (Ross) 187n

J

Jade, Deanne 47n
Janimine (imipramine) 220
Jasper, Karin 41n

K

Kidshealth.org *see* Nemours Foundation

L

"Laxatives" (Alliance for Eating
   Disorders Awareness) 105n
laxatives, eating disorders 107
"Let's Eat for the Health of It!" (USDA) 253n
Lexapro 220
LifeMedia, Inc., diabetes publication 167n
lifestyles
   anorexia nervosa 66
   bulimia nervosa 73
   mental health 339
   obesity 136–37
   oral health 153–54
   osteoporosis 157
   weight control 143–44
light therapy, defined 226
Lithane (lithium carbonate) 221
lithium carbonate 221
Lithizine (lithium carbonate) 221
Lithobid (lithium carbonate) 221
Lithonate (lithium carbonate) 221
Lithotabs (lithium carbonate) 221
LiveStrong, website address 359
Lock, James 183
Luvox (fluvoxamine) 220

M

magnesium, food sources **257**
"Male Eating Disorders May
   Be More Common than We Think"
   (Weisensee) 25n
malnourishment, body image distortion **38**
malnutrition, pica 102
Manerix (moclobemide) 220
massage therapy, defined 226
Maudsley method, defined 226
mealtime support therapy, defined 226
"Meaning of Mental Health"
   (Canadian Mental Health Association) 333n
media
   eating disorders statistics 60
   overview 47–58
"The Media and Eating Disorders" (Jade) 47n

medical consequences
   anorexia nervosa 128–33
   binge eating disorder 79
   bulimia nervosa 127–28
   eating disorders **129**
   EDNOS 99
   obesity **144**
   substance abuse 107–8
medications
   anorexia nervosa 67–68
   body dysmorphic disorder **121**
   bulimia nervosa 75
   eating disorders 216, 219–21
   hypnosedative induced complex
          behaviors 91–92
   night eating syndrome 90
   obesity 138
   osteoporosis 158
men
   body image **26**
   eating disorders 25–28
   eating disorders statistics 60
   see also boys; gender factor
"Mental Fitness Tips"
   (Canadian Mental Health Association) 333n
mental health, overview 333–40
Mental Health America, contact information 361
Merikangas, Kathleen **214–15**
MET *see* motivational enhancement therapy
mianserin 221
Milk Matters Calcium Education
   Campaign, contact information 354
Mind, contact information 362
mind-body therapies, eating disorders 190
minerals
   food sources **280**
   sports activities 291
   sports nutrition **292**
Minnesota Experiment, described **130–31**
Mirror, Mirror, website address 351
mirtazapine 221
moclobemide 220
moderate activity, described **324**
modified cyclic antidepressant, eating disorders 221
monoamine oxidase inhibitors, eating disorders 220

monounsaturated fats (MUFA), described 14
mortality rates, eating disorders statistics 61
motivational enhancement therapy (MET),
    defined 226
movement therapy, defined 227
multiorgan failure, anorexia nervosa 133
Multi-Service Eating Disorders Association,
    contact information 351
muscle building damage **26**
muscle dysmorphia
    defined **122**
    described 22–23
muscle-strengthening activities,
    described 322, 325

N

Nalorex (naltrexone) 221
naltrexone 221
narcissistic personality disorder,
    described 21
Nardil (phenelzine) 220
National Agricultural Library,
    contact information 354
National Alliance for Youth Sports,
    contact information 359
National Alliance on Mental Illness (NAMI),
    contact information 362
National Association of Anorexia Nervosa
    and Associated Disorders (ANAD)
        contact information 351
        publications
            eating disorders statistics 59n
            eating disorders symptoms 193n
National Center for Complementary and
    Alternative Medicine, contact information 355
National Center for Overcoming Overeating,
    website address 351
National Centre for Eating Disorders,
    media influence publication 47n
National Coalition for Promoting
    Physical Activity, contact information 359
National Eating Disorder Information Centre
    contact information 351
    genetic influences publication 41n

National Eating Disorders Association
    contact information 351
    publications
        friends, eating disorders 205n
        orthorexia nervosa 93n
        treatment options 219n
National Heart, Lung,
    and Blood Institute (NHLBI)
        contact information 355
        publications
            obesity 135n
            weight management 295n
National Institute for Fitness and Sport,
    contact information 359
National Institute of Arthritis
    and Musculoskeletal and Skin Diseases (NIAMS),
    anorexia nervosa, osteoporosis publication 155n
National Institute of Child Health and Human
    Development (NICHD), contact information 355
National Institute of Diabetes and
    Digestive and Kidney Diseases (NIDDK),
    weight-loss programs publication 317n
National Institute of Mental Health (NIMH)
    contact information 362
    publications
        anxiety 171n
        depression 171n
National Mental Health Association
    see Mental Health America
National Recreation and Park Association,
    contact information 359
National Strength and Conditioning Association,
    contact information 359
National Women's Health Information Center
    (NWHIC), contact information 355
Nemours Foundation
    contact information 354, 359
    publications
        body dysmorphic disorder 119n
        compulsive exercise 109n
        emotional eating 83n
        female athlete triad 113n
        pica 101n
        self-esteem 229n
        weight/height ratio 247n

neurological problems, anorexia nervosa 132
neurotransmitters
    appetite regulation 19–20
    defined **43**
    women 33
NHLBI *see* National Heart,
  Lung, and Blood Institute
NIAMS *see* National Institute of Arthritis
  and Musculoskeletal and Skin Diseases
nicotine abuse, eating disorders **106**
night eating syndrome, described 89–90
"Night Eating Syndrome and
  Sleep-Related Eating Disorder" (Cooke) 89n
NIMH *see* National Institute of Mental Health
nocturnal eating syndrome 89–90
non-suicidal self-injury **185**
norepinephrine, described 19
"Normal Eating" (Thompson) 237n
Norpramin (desipramine) 220
Northwestern University,
  male eating disorders publication 25n
nutraceuticals, eating disorders 190
nutritional requirements
    athletes 287–94
    described 11–12
    eating disorders treatment 216, 223
    see also diet and nutrition
nutritional therapy, defined 227
Nutrition Facts labels
    content information 280–81, **282**
    depicted *281*
    described 12–14, 263
nutritionists
    described **318**
    emotional eating 87
Nutrition Labeling and Education Act (1990) 13
nuts, nutrition myths 16

O

obesity
    binge eating disorder 211
    media influence 56–57
    night eating syndrome 89
    overview 135–49

Obesity Society, contact information 355
obsessive-compulsive disorder (OCD)
    described 21–22, 178–79
    medications 220
    pica 103
OCD *see* obsessive-compulsive
  disorder
Office of Dietary Supplements,
  contact information 355
Office on Women's Health,
  publications
    anorexia nervosa 65n
    body image 37n
    bulimia nervosa 71n
    diet and nutrition 253n
    fitness safety 329n
    oral health 151n
omega 3 fatty acids
    healthy eating 260
    nutritional requirements 11–12
ondansetron 221
opioid antagonist, eating disorders 221
opioid antagonists, defined 227
"Oral Health"
  (Office on Women's Health) 151n
oral health, eating disorders 151–54
orthorexia, overview 93–96
"Orthorexia Nervosa"
  (National Eating
  Disorders Association) 93n
osteopenia, anorexia nervosa 132, 156
osteoporosis
    anorexia nervosa 132, 155–58
    described **33**
    eating disorders 6
    female athlete triad 114
Overeaters Anonymous,
  contact information 352
over eating *see* binge eating disorder
over-exercising *see* compulsive exercise
overweight
    binge eating disorder 80
    body mass index **248**
    eating disorders 22
    overview 135–49

P

panic disorder
    described 177–78
    eating disorders 22
Parnate (tranylcypromine) 220
paroxetine 220
Paxil (paroxetine) 220
peak bone mass, described **33**
PE Central, contact information 360
Peebles, Rebecka 183–84
perfectionists, described **234**
perimylolysis, described **153**
personality traits
    anorexia nervosa 66
    bulimia nervosa 73
    eating disorders 20–21, 165–66
    eating disorders risk factor 31
Pertofrane (desipramine) 220
pharmacotherapy, defined 227
phenelzine 220
phobias
    described 180–81
    eating disorders 22
phototherapy, defined 226
physical activity
    daily guidelines **322**
    disabilities **327**
    mental health 335–36
    obesity 146–48
    overview 321–27
    see also exercise
"Physicians missing self-injury behavior in
  youths with eating disorders, study finds"
  (Stanford School of Medicine) 183n
"Pica" (Nemours Foundation) 101n
pica, overview 101–4
pituitary gland, eating disorders 18
Popcorn, Faith 48
posttraumatic stress disorder (PTSD)
    described 179–80
    eating disorders 22
potassium
    eating disorders 6
    food sources **257**

power foods, described **256–57**
pregnancy
    anorexia nervosa 131
    eating disorders 159–61
    gestational diabetes **168**
    nutrition myths 16
    obesity 139
    pica 103
President's Challenge, contact information 360
President's Council on Fitness, Sports, and Nutrition
    contact information 360
    sports nutrition publication 287n
"Prevent Eating Disorders in Female Athletes"
  (Zeigler) 29n
pro-ana, defined **55**
progressive muscle relaxation, defined 227
protein
    food sources **280**
    healthy eating 259
    muscle mass 291–92
    nutritional requirements 12
    sports nutrition **293**
Prozac (fluoxetine) 75, 220
Psych Central
    contact information 362
    unresolved trauma publication 187n
psychoanalysis, defined 227
psychodrama, defined 227
psychodynamic group therapy, defined 227
psychodynamic therapy, defined 227
psychoeducational therapy, defined 228
psychosocial consequences, eating disorders **129**
psychosocial factors, female athletes 30–31
psychotherapy
    anorexia nervosa 68
    binge eating disorder **5**, 80
    bulimia nervosa 74
    coping skills **344**
    defined 227
    eating disorders 216, 222–23
    night eating syndrome 90
PTSD *see* posttraumatic stress disorder
puberty
    eating disorders **18–19**
    weight range 247–48

purging
  compensatory behaviors **79,** 97
  dehydration 25
  electrolyte loss 6
  heart failure 99
  oral health 151–52, **153**
  psychological therapies 75, 222, 225–26
  statistics 59
  see also binge eating disorder;
    bulimia nervosa; laxatives

Q

quality of life, eating disorders **129**
"Questions Most Frequently
  Asked about Sports Nutrition"
  (President's Council
  on Fitness, Sports, and Nutrition) 287n

R

racial factor, eating disorders 20
Rader Programs, contact information 352
ramelteon 91
refeeding syndrome
  defined **239**
  described **314**
"Reflections on Genes and
  Eating Disorders" (Jasper) 41n
relapse, defined **243**
relapse prevention, overview 241–44
Remeron (mirtazapine) 221
Remuda Ranch
  contact information 352
  relapse publication 241n
renutrition, defined **239**
residential programs,
  eating disorders treatment 217
resilience
  described **231**
  mental health 334
  overview 341–46
Restoril (temazepam) 91
reverse anorexia, defined **122**
reverse thinspiration, described **55**

risk factors
  anorexia nervosa 65–66
  bulimia 71–73
  eating disorder 54
  eating disorders 20–21, 39
  eating disorders, female athletes 29–35
  eating disorders, men 27–28
rituals, obsessive-compulsive disorder 21
River Centre Clinic, contact information 352
"The Road to Resilience" (American
  Psychological Association) 341n
Ross, Carolyn Coker 187n
Royal College of Psychiatrists,
  contact information 362
Rozerem (ramelteon) 91

S

safety considerations
  fitness activities 329–32
  weight loss programs 317–20
sample menus
  described **267, 268**
  healthy choices 306–12
  overview 267–73
"Sample Menus for a 2000
  Calorie Food Pattern" (USDA) 265n
Sarafem (fluoxetine) 220
Schneeman, Barbara 279–82
selective serotonin reuptake inhibitors (SSRI)
  body dysmorphic disorder **121**
  eating disorders 220
  night eating syndrome 90
self-esteem
  female athletes 32
  media influence 51
  orthorexia 96
  overview 229–35
self-guided cognitive behavior therapy,
  defined 228
self-help, eating disorders 189
self-injury
  Cornell research program **185**
  described 165
  overview 183–85

self psychology, defined 228
Seligman, Martin E.P. 333
serotonin
    body dysmorphic disorder 121–22
    described 19
    women 33
serotonin and norepinephrine reuptake inhibitors
    (SNRI), eating disorders 221
sertraline 220
serving size, food labels 14
Sheena's Place, contact information 352
"Signs of Eating Disorders"
    (LifeMedia, Inc.) 167n
Sindy dolls 50
sleep disorders, obesity 139
sleep related eating disorder, described 90–91
social phobia, described 180
sociocultural environment
    body image 44–45
    female athletes 30
Something Fishy, website address 352
Sonata (zaleplon) 91
Spark Teens, website address 360
specific phobias, described 180–81
sports activities
    diet and nutrition 287–94
    excessive exercise 23–24
    female athletes 29–35, **116**
    female athlete triad 114–15
SportsMD
    contact information 360
    female eating disorders publication 29n
stages of change, motivational
    enhancement therapy 226
Stanford School of Medicine,
    self-injury publication 183n
starvation syndrome, described **130–31**
State of Missouri Department of Health
    and Senior Services,
    diabetes publication 167n
statistics
    binge eating disorder 78
    eating disorders 59–61
    night eating syndrome 90
    television watching 47

stress management
    body image **39**
    coping mechanisms 31
    eating disorders 166
    female athletes 34–35
    mental health 337–39
    purging 38
stretching, exercise **323**
substance abuse
    anorexia nervosa 128
    bulimia nervosa 128
    eating disorders 105–8, **106**
Substance Abuse and Mental
    Health Services Administration
    (SAMHSA), contact information 362
suicide attempts
    antidepressant medications **69, 175**
    body dysmorphic disorder 22
    self-injury 184
support groups
    binge eating disorder 80–81
    eating disorders 189
supportive therapy, defined 228
surgical procedures, body
    dysmorphic disorder 22, 123
susceptibility genes, described 42–43

T

teeth
    perimylolysis **153**
    protection tips **152**
telephone therapy, defined 228
temazepam 91
tests
    eating attitudes 197–204
    osteoporosis 158
tetracyclics, eating disorders 221
thinspiration, defined **55**
Thompson, Colleen 237n
"Tips for Vegetarians" (USDA) 283n
tobacco use
    bulimia nervosa 128
    obesity 138–39
    osteoporosis 157

Tofranil (imipramine) 220
Topamax (topiramate) 221
topiramate 90, 221
tranylcypromine 220
trauma
    female athletes 34–35
    overview 187–90
trazodone 221
"Treatment" (Academy for
   Eating Disorders) 213n
"Treatments Available for Eating Disorders"
   (National Eating Disorders Association) 219n
triazolam 91
tricyclic antidepressants, eating disorders 220
twins studies, eating disorders 17

U

Uniquely ME! 32
US Department of Agriculture (USDA)
    contact information 356
    publications
        diet and nutrition 253n
        vegetarians 283n
US Department of Health and Human Services
   (DHHS; HHS), physical fitness publication 321n
US Food and Drug Administration (FDA)
    contact information 356
    food labels publication 279n

V

Vegetarian Resource Group, contact information 356
vegetarians, healthy eating 283–86
venlafaxine 221
vigorous activity, described **324**
vitamin A, food sources **256**
vitamin C, food sources **256**
vitamin D, osteoporosis 157
vitamin E, food sources **256**
vitamins
    food sources **280**
    healthy eating 259
    sports activities 291
    sports nutrition **292**

W

Weight-Control Information Network
   (WIN), contact information 356
weight-cutting, wrestlers 24
weight gain
    benefits **300**
    binge eating disorder 79
weight loss
    compulsive exercise 110
    eating disorders 4
    lifestyle changes **316**
    sports activities 33–34
    wrestlers 24
weight loss programs
    described 315–16
    safety considerations 317–20
weight management
    healthy eating guidelines 295–316
    men, eating disorders 28
    overview 247–51
Weisensee, Kimberly 25n
Wellbutrin (bupropion), FDA warning 220, 221
"What Are Empty Calories?" (USDA) 265n
"What Are Overweight And Obesity"
   (NHLBI) 135n
"What People with Anorexia Nervosa Need to
   Know about Osteoporosis" (NIAMS) 155n
"What Should I Say?" (National Eating
   Disorders Association) 205n
"What's the Right Weight for My Height?"
   (Nemours Foundation) 247n
"Why Is It Important to Eat Fruit?" (USDA) 253n
"Why Is It Important to Eat Grains,
   Especially Whole Grains?" (USDA) 253n
"Why Is It Important to Eat Vegetables?"
   (USDA) 253n
"Why Is It Important to Make Lean or Low-Fat
   Choices from the Protein Foods Group?"
   (USDA) 253n
Wilson, Jenny 184
women, eating disorder statistics 60–61
    see also gender factor; girls
Women's Sports Foundation,
   contact information 360

Z

zaleplon 91
Zeigler, Terry 29n
Zofran (ondansetron) 221

Zoloft (sertraline) 220
zolpidem 91
Zyban (bupropion) FDA warning 221